lateral curvature spine

E. W. Hodgkins.

Flexion = Process of Bending

Abduction = From median line

Adduction = Toward   "   "

Eversion = Turning out.

Adductor = Effecting adduction
as a muscle.

Coxa - Farm - distortion neck of
P. 68.   the femur -

ORTHOPEDIC SURGERY

BY

EDWARD H. BRADFORD, M.D.

Surgeon to the Boston Children's Hospital; Consulting Surgeon to the Boston City
Hospital; Professor of Orthopedic Surgery, Harvard Medical School

AND

ROBERT W. LOVETT, M.D.

Associate Surgeon to the Boston Children's Hospital; Surgeon to the Infants'
Hospital, the Peabody House for Crippled Children and the Massa-
chusetts Hospital School for Cripples; Assistant Professor
of Orthopedic Surgery, Harvard Medical School

———

NEW YORK
WILLIAM WOOD AND COMPANY
MDCCCCXIII

Printed by
The Maple Press
York, Pa.

THIS BOOK IS DEDICATED TO
OUR COLLEAGUES
THE MEMBERS OF THE

American Orthopedic Association

AS A SLIGHT TOKEN
OF
OBLIGATION AND FRIENDSHIP

PREFACE.

THE increasing interest in the surgical treatment of the class of cases which are grouped under the term of Orthopedic Surgery has given rise to a demand for a condensed handbook for the use of students and practitioners embodying a brief statement of the generally accepted opinions as to the nature and treatment of the affections under consideration.

For the sake of brevity the writers have been obliged to omit the presentation and critical discussion of differing views. For these the writers would refer to their previous writings, as well as to the admirable publications of their colleagues. In the present book emphasis is necessarily laid upon such measures of treatment as have been demonstrated to be of value in the clinical work at the Boston Children's Hospital in the past 30 years.

This is not done in any spirit of ignorance or disparagement of the work of others, but in the need of condensed statement. References and bibliographical notes have also been largely omitted for the same reason.

The writers wish, however, to express their indebtedness to the teaching and investigations of others, by which they have been largely influenced in the views which they venture to present.

E. H. BRADFORD.
R. W. LOVETT.

CONTENTS.

CONTENTS

ORTHOPEDIC SURGERY.

CHAPTER I.

TUBERCULOUS DISEASE OF THE BONES AND JOINTS.

ORTHOPEDIC surgery deals with the prevention and correction of deformity, and demands not only a study of the deformities of the human body, but also some knowledge of the affections which produce them. Of these the most important are the tuberculous diseases of the joints.

PATHOLOGY.

Articular tuberculosis begins usually as an affection of the spongy tissue of the epiphysis, or in the juxta-epiphyseal and adjacent region of growing bone.

The common form of tuberculous infection of the epiphysis is the one spoken of as focal, when the first change is the formation of single or multiple foci of tuberculous degeneration. On section of the diseased epiphysis the first noticeable change consists of a local hyperæmia of some part of the spongy tissue.

From the stage of tuberculous infiltration the process may follow any one of three courses: the diseased focus may be absorbed and so cured; it may extend to the periphery of the bone and break through the periosteum and empty itself there; or, lastly and probably most commonly, it may extend to the joint, which becomes involved.

1. The absorption of the diseased focus is theoretically possible up to a late stage in the process, so long as the disease remains strictly local.

2. The next most favorable termination to the disease is when the focus does not infect the joint, but breaks through the periosteum and discharges into the periarticular structure.

3. Usually after extensive involvement of the epiphysis an arthritis results, with attendant injury to the joint.

Repair is brought about by the formation of fibrous tissue, probably arising from the layer of non-tuberculous granulation tissue which grows into and replaces the tuberculous material. Caseous material is largely absorbed, and the inspissated remainder is replaced by fibrous tissue or is calcified and encapsulated. Fibrous, cartilaginous, or bony ankylosis may result from the process of repair.

It is most important to note that the process of repair may be incomplete, and that small areas of tuberculous material encapsulated by fibrous tissue may persist for a long time and under certain conditions (i.e., trauma, or imperfect hygiene) may become active and

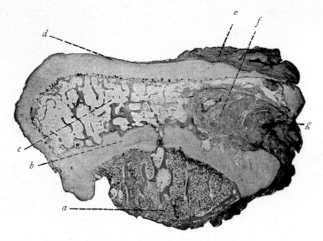

FIG. 1.—Tuberculous Epiphysis. Vertical section through the head of the radius. *a,* Shaft of radius; *b,* epiphyseal cartilage; *c,* epiphysis; *d,* joint surface; cartilage; *e,* tuberculous primary focus; *f,* perforation of joint cartilage and infection of joint; *g,* tuberculous "pannus" extending over joint cartilage. (Nichols.)

cause a recurrence of the disease. Or the repair may be complete and the previously inflamed tissue be converted into cicatricial bone—usually more firm than the original structure.

While synovial tuberculosis undoubtedly exists as a primary affection, in a large majority of cases of tuberculous arthritis the affection arises in the bone.

Cold Abscesses.—If the tuberculous process in the bone reaches the surrounding tissues by perforation of the cortex and periosteum or by rupture of the joint capsule, an abscess is likely to occur. The area of tuberculous softening in the periarticular tissues is formed by the coalescence and caseation of tubercles. Surrounding the softened area is a layer of tuberculous tissue, about which is another layer of œdematous and vascular granulation tissue. This process may extend until a large cavity has been formed.

The contents of these abscesses are composed of caseous material from the degeneration of the tubercles and exuded serum with necrotic pieces of bone. In the fluid are polymorphonuclear leucocytes, often taking up little or no stain on cover slips. Pyogenic organisms are absent unless present by secondary infection. The fluid may be like true pus; it may be so thick that it will hardly flow; it may be thin and watery and contain coagula, or it may be red or brownish from hemorrhage. Microscopically tubercle bacilli may be found in the abscess, but they are to be identified, even after prolonged search, in only about one-third of the cases. In such cases inoculation experiments must be relied upon to establish their presence.

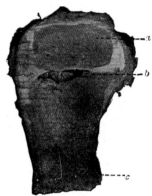

Fig. 2.—Tumor Albus. Small focus in upper epiphyseal line of tibia. Synovitis of joint, but no tuberculous process apart from focus as noted. Death from miliary tuberculosis. *a*, Epiphysis; *b*, primary focus; *c*, shaft. (Nichols.)

The wall of these abscess cavities is composed of an inner layer of tuberculous tissue, outside of which is a layer of secondary inflammatory tissue. The inner layer may be granular or necrotic and ulcerated. The abscess extends by peripheral enlargement in the line of least resistance. The walls of tuberculous sinuses consist of an inner layer of tuberculous tissue, outside of which is a zone of œdematous granulation tissue.

Instead of forming a " bone abscess " the process may result in the formation of a sequestrum composed of necrotic trabeculæ retaining their shape and lying in a cavity in the bone. About the sequestrum is a layer of granulation tissue. The sequestrum may take the shape of a wedge having its base toward the joint, in which case it is known as a " bone infarct."

ETIOLOGY.

Heredity.—That heredity is a factor in causing tuberculous joint disease has long been claimed. Whether the tuberculous virus can be directly transmitted as such from father or mother to the offspring must still be held open to question, but that the surroundings of certain families weaken the resistance and favor tuberculous invasion appears not improbable.

Traumatism.—Experimentally it has been shown that trauma to the joint of a tuberculous animal may cause tuberculous joint disease, but that it does not do so in the healthy animal. It has been established that contusions and wrenches cause the effusion of blood in the spongy tissue of the bone. It would therefore seem rational to assume that trauma may cause tuberculous joint disease in children with a tuberculous tendency.

The fact that there is a preponderance of joint tuberculosis in the lower extremity when contrasted with the joints of the upper points to the influence of slight traumatism and weight-bearing as factors in the development of the affection.

It is probable that whatever continuously diminishes the power of resistance and of repair in growing children increases what may be termed the vulnerability of the epiphyses, and furnishes the soil for the development of tubercle bacilli and the consequent results.

Age.—Tuberculous joint disease is pre-eminently a disease of childhood. It is not congenital, and under one year it is not common. The majority of cases occur between three and ten years of age, but the liability of the aged to tuberculous joint disease must not be overlooked.

The reasons why tuberculous joint disease affects children to so great an extent are as follows:

In the active period of growth more change is going on and therefore more instability exists and consequently greater liability to disease. Children are more liable to falls and injuries, which are such a fertile source of joint and bone lesions. It is not till after puberty that the process of natural selection has eliminated the weaklings from the stock. Children are kept quiet less easily than adults, and a slight injury may develop into a formidable disease. Tuberculosis in general is common in childhood.

Sex is not a factor of any prominence, but there is a slightly larger proportion of tuberculous joint disease among boys than among girls.

Distribution of Chronic Tuberculous Joint Disease.—The relative frequency with which tuberculosis attacks the various joints in children may be estimated from the following figures:

At the Children's Hospital, from 1869 to 1903 inclusive, 5,950 cases of tuberculosis of the joints were distributed as follows: spine, 2,867; hip, 2,281; knee, 375; ankle, 394; elbow, 33. These practically all occurred in children under the age of twelve.

In 211 cases of joint tuberculosis among the out-patients occurring in children under two years, there were 120 cases of Pott's disease, 61 of hip disease, and 29 of tuberculosis of the knee-joint.

In joint disease, when one or more articulations are involved, any combination may be found; but the most common are hip disease and Pott's disease, knee disease and Pott's disease, and double hip disease. Disease of the knee- and hip-joint at the same time is not common, and double tumor albus is unusual.

DIAGNOSIS.

The recognition of tuberculous joint disease is to be based upon certain general phenomena modified by the anatomical conditions of the joint affected. These diagnostic signs are considered in connection with the individual joints.

The use of *tuberculin* as a means of diagnosis is open to the criticism that its results are attended with so much uncertainty that its value in the individual case is always open to question and cannot be assumed to be a reliable demonstration that tuberculosis is either present or absent in that case. It has been demonstrated that in a certain per cent of well-marked cases of pulmonary or other tuberculosis, tuberculin gives a negative result, while in other cases, presumably non-tuberculous, a certain percentage of positive results is obtained. The great frequency of tuberculous invasion has been shown by the autopsies of Babes, for example, who found lesions of the bronchial glands in more than one-half of his autopsies on children; and those of Naegeli, who found, in 508 consecutive autopsies, that 97 to 98 per cent showed evidences of tuberculosis. Under these circumstances tuberculin must necessarily be unreliable in demonstrating joint tuberculosis.

The *inoculation* of material from suspected joints into guinea-pigs forms a reliable means in the diagnosis of tuberculosis of the joints.

The *x-ray* is an aid in the diagnosis of joint tuberculosis where the process is sufficiently advanced to have caused the absorption of lime salts in the affected area or to have destroyed any part of the bony structure. In early cases the radiograph may be normal when disease is present.

PROGNOSIS.

The destructive process which is so prominent a feature of joint tuberculosis is almost from the first accompanied by a reparative process tending to limit the destruction, protect the surrounding tissues, and prevent generalization. The prognosis depends in the individual case upon which of these two processes prevails over the other. The former is favored by inefficient local treatment, bad inheritance, poor general condition, unfavorable surroundings, and, in general, what may be termed poor resistance to the tuberculous process. The reparative process is favored by the reverse of these conditions. In the majority of all cases of joint tuberculosis, properly treated at a fairly early stage, the outlook is favorable. The prognosis is more favorable in children than in adults.

TREATMENT.

Since bone tuberculosis has been shown to be one manifestation of tuberculous infection and not the result of an unknown evil, the principles of treatment are more clear.

Resistance to the infection by the tubercle bacillus is furnished when the individual is in a normal state. The antidotes to be relied upon to check its advance after it has found lodgment are not only good air and food, but such general activity as will promote normal metabolism. Tuberculosis is prevalent and fatal among caged animals —a fact which is to be borne in mind in the treatment of bone tuberculosis.

The treatment is both general and local. The general treatment consists in giving the patient the best possible environment and in furnishing such conditions that normal activity will cause the least possible injury to the part locally affected. Treatment by immunization through the repeated injection of tuberculin is as yet of unproved value.

In tuberculosis of the lung the patient is in constant danger of self-infection or increase of the process from the inhalation of infected material; but in bone tuberculosis no such danger exists. Strong, well ossified bone does not offer suitable soil for the bacillus, for bone tissues when invaded resist the advance of tuberculous infection by surrounding the diseased area with a thick enveloping mass of tissue and by subsequently repairing the invaded region by the development of strong bone. Traumatism, which injures this bone construction and furnishes undeveloped cells instead of firm bony structure, favors the spread of the tuberculous process. The treatment of bone tuberculosis, therefore, consists in promoting such general conditions as will favor repair (general treatment) and the protection of the parts from injury during the disease (local treatment).

General Treatment.—The patient should be placed in the most favorable environment available in the matter of food, home surroundings, air, sunlight, proper clothing, exercise, avoidance of fatigue, and similar requirements.

OUTDOOR TREATMENT.—Of these requirements outdoor air is of the utmost importance, and the open-air treatment of surgical tuberculosis is nowhere more beneficial than in joint disease. The outdoor method recognized as of such value in the treatment of pulmonary tuberculosis is advisable.

The importance of the treatment by fresh air and sunlight has been recognized in Europe in the establishment of seaside sanatoriums for children with tuberculous joint disease. It is being recognized in America that a convalescent home in the country is an almost necessary part of a surgical hospital for children.

Local Treatment.—*Fixation, distraction,* and *protection,* along with *operative treatment,* are considered in speaking of the individual joints.

CHAPTER II.

TUBERCULOUS DISEASE OF THE SPINE.

Definition.—Pott's disease is the name applied to a destructive pathological process which attacks the bodies of the vertebræ. It is also called caries of the spine and angular curvature.

PATHOLOGY.

Pott's disease represents the result of a destructive ostitis affecting the spongy tissue of one or more of the vertebral bodies. This ostitis is tuberculous in type and follows the same course as tuberculous ostitis occurring at the epiphyses of the long bones, as in hip disease, tumor albus, etc.

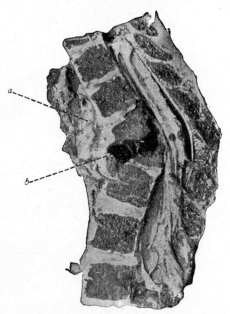

The focus of tuberculous material may either be absorbed or calcified, or as happens much more commonly, the ostitis may increase until it has destroyed a large part or the whole of a vertebral body. In its course of enlargement it may include portions of bone, the nutrition of which is cut off by the adjacent inflammatory destruction; which portions necessarily become necrosed, and with caseous matter, granulation tissue,

FIG. 3.—Lower Dorsal Region. Opposite half of specimen rested on knuckle while hardening, so that gravity extended the spine. Marked separation of diseased vertebræ. *a*, Tuberculous disease beneath prevertebral ligaments; *b*, cavity between diseased vertebræ. (Nichols.)

and the products of inflammation constitute an area of altered and degenerated structure in the vertebral body. If this diseased area has become large enough, the vertebral body gradually becomes incapable of sustaining as much pressure as before. From the peculiar weight-

8

bearing function of the vertebral column, the pressure upon each vertebral body is always considerable when the vertebral column is in the erect position. If one vertebral body is becoming excavated, a point will be reached where it can no longer sustain the weight, but must give way slowly or suddenly. A forward tilt of the whole vertebral column above the seat of disease is then inevitable, with a cer-

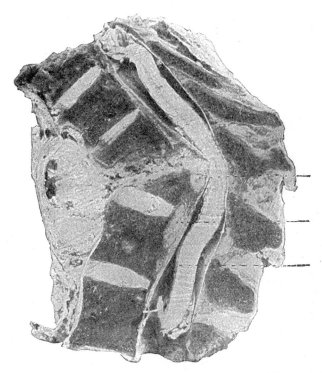

Fig. 4.—Sagittal Section of the Spine from the 9th Dorsal to the 2nd Lumbar. Compression of cord and abscess. (Schulthess.)

tain amount of backward angular deformity at the diseased vertebra. This is the mechanism of the production of the knuckle in the back.

This process is limited, as a rule, to the vertebral bodies; the transverse, articular, or spinous processes are rarely affected secondarily or primarily, their structure of hard bone apparently protecting them from tuberculous invasion. The intervertebral cartilage between the diseased vertebræ becomes disintegrated and disappears.

There may be two or more foci in one vertebra, or the whole body may be equally affected; the disease may be limited to one spot, forming a localized abscess of the bone, or it may extend so as to involve the adjacent vertebræ. If the disease remains limited to the centre of the vertebra, but little deformity may result.

In certain cases the formation of tuberculous detritus is a characteristic of the disease from the first, and in these cases abscesses are apt to be a conspicuous feature. The tuberculous pus finds its way, during or after the destruction of the body of the vertebra, into the surrounding tissues and gravitates downward. It appears usually in the course of the sheath of the psoas muscle when the disease is situated in the lower half of the spine, but the site of the abscess necessarily depends upon the place of the original disease, and may be in the mouth—as in retropharyngeal abscess— in the neck, in the axilla, or in the back, lungs, abdomen, or groin. The contents of such abscess as a rule contain no pyogenic bacteria.

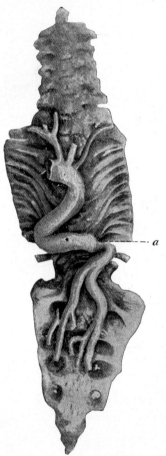

Fig. 5.—Distortion of Aorta. From a case of spinal caries in an adult. At one point marked constriction of the aorta. Angular deformity very marked. a, Constriction of aorta. (Dwight.)

Paralysis.—In certain cases meningitis and myelitis are present in the cord opposite the seat of disease, accompanied sometimes by what is virtually the destruction of the cord at that point. The paralysis is very rarely caused by direct pressure of bone, as it is uncommon for even very marked deformities of the spine to narrow the spinal canal to any great extent. Many cases with extreme deformity are never paralyzed at all.

In proportion to the extent of the disease and the number of vertebræ involved, an angular deformity of the spine may be present to any extent. In severe cases this angular deformity leads to many secondary pathological changes. The shape and capacity of the chest are necessarily very much altered, and the ribs sometimes sink into the pelvis. As a result of these changes in chest capacity, hypertrophy of the heart, often accompanied by valvular disease, is common. The aorta may be distorted as a result of the deformity. Dwight reports a case in which its course " might be compared to an S lying on its side, with the ends bent strongly back to fit around the prominence of the spine." Lannelongue found a very marked narrowing of the calibre of the aorta in many cases. Sometimes it was reduced even to a mere slit.

OCCURRENCE AND ETIOLOGY.

Sex.—Sex does not appear to be an important factor in causing Pott's disease, though statistics vary somewhat.

Age.—The disease is more common in childhood.

Localization.—Any of the vertebræ may be attacked, but in varying frequency.

Although the locations of relative frequency given by different observers do not agree, it would appear that certain portions of the

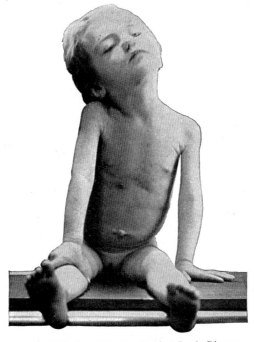

Fig. 6.—Attitude of Head in Cervical Pott's Disease.

spine are more liable to attack than certain others, and that the regions most liable to the disease were those which were the most exposed to jars or increased pressure; and that the disease would be more frequent where the hinges of motion at the spinal column came, varying to a degree according to age and occupation, or where there was the greatest exposure to the effects of violent jars.

Causation.—It may be assumed that the localizing cause of Pott's disease is jar or superincumbent pressure; the influential cause being that physical state which is incapable of resisting slight trauma, exposing the tissue probably to the invasion of the tubercle bacillus.

SYMPTOMS.

Typical cases of Pott's disease are so characteristic in their symptoms that the diagnosis is evident almost at a glance. The guarded character of all the movements is perhaps the most striking feature. In walking, in stooping, or in lying down, the spine is most carefully

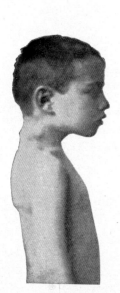
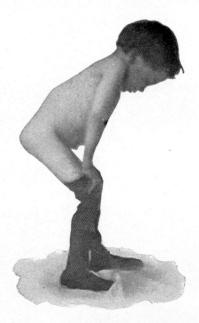

FIG. 7.—Attitude in Cervical Caries of only Moderate Severity.

FIG. 8.—Attitude Assumed by Children with Acute Pott's Disease, and in Other Cases Necessitated by Psoas Contraction.

guarded against jar and against motion, attitudes are assumed which relieve the vertebral column of some of the weight of the body, and a glance at the naked child shows unnatural modes of standing and walking.

A prominence of the vertebræ is ordinarily present as early as at this stage, and oftener than not pain is acute and aggravated by motion.

Peculiarity of attitude and gait, muscular stiffness, and referred pain are the most prominent of the earlier symptoms, and they may be present before a projection has been noticed. The importance of recognizing these early symptoms can hardly be overstated, as it is on an early recognition of the affection that the hope of a ready cure is to be based.

Attitude.—These attitudes necessarily vary according to the point of the spine attacked. In disease of the upper cervical region, the most common attitude is that of wryneck.

When the disease is in the *lower cervical* or *upper dorsal* region, the chin is held somewhat raised, suggesting the position of a seal's head when out of water. The spinal column below the point of disease is abnormally straight, and in some instances curved slightly forward, while in the lower dorsal region an exaggerated backward projection of the spinous processes may be seen; this projection, due to a compensating curve, is sometimes so marked as to suggest that the disease has attacked another part of the spine.

In the *middle dorsal* region the attitude to be noticed most frequently is an elevation of the shoulders. Temporarily a slight lateral deviation of the spine is to be seen.

In the *lumbar* region, the patients in the early stage frequently will be noticed to lean backward, like pregnant women or adults with large abdomens. A peculiar position and characteristic

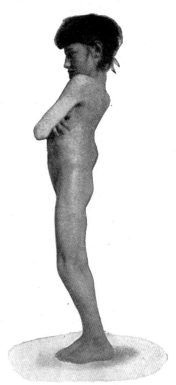

Fig. 9.—Lordosis in Lumbar Pott's Disease.

sidling gait, which is sometimes seen at a comparatively early stage of the disease in the lower dorsal or lumbar region, is due to a slight contraction of the psoas and iliacus muscles. In a late stage, when psoas contraction is present, a limitation to the arc of extension of the thigh on the trunk develops.

In general, in addition to the square position of the shoulders, the peculiar position of the head, and the erect attitude of the upper part of the spine, which prevents the superincumbent weight of the trunk and upper extremities (above the diseased portion of the spine) from falling forward upon the diseased vertebral body, the gait is peculiar; the patient walks more on the toes than on the heels, and with the

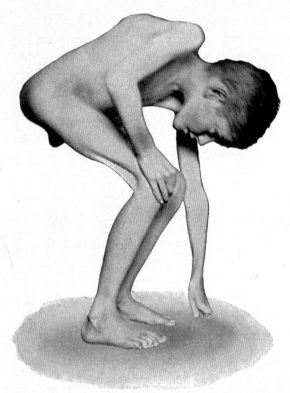

FIG. 10.—Attitude Assumed in Dorsal Pott's Disease when Rising from Floor.

knees slightly bent—in such a way that all possible springs may be brought into play to diminish the jarring of the spine.

A certain amount of muscular rigidity of the muscles of the back will be felt on palpation in affections of the middle dorsal and lumbar regions; stooping which involves arching of the back forward is diffi-cult or impossible in disease of the lower spine, and in attempting to stoop in order to pick up any article from the floor the patient will keep the spine erect and reach the floor, lowering himself with an erect trunk, by bending the knees.

It will often be noticed that children become tired more easily than usual, and after playing about for a time will desire to lie down, to rest their arms upon a chair or seat, or to support the head with their hands, or the trunk by holding on to the thighs, according to the part of the spine affected.

The amount of muscular stiffness, rigidity, and difficulty in maintaining the spine erect is in a measure an index of the degree of activity of the disease.

Lateral deviation of the spine is an attitude sometimes to be found in Pott's disease and is discussed in its relation to lateral curvature under the head of diagnosis.

Pain.—In certain cases of Pott's disease pain is absent altogether, but it is often present to a distressing degree. The pain is rarely complained of in the back, but is referred to the peripheral ends of the nerves, and is thus described as being felt in the abdomen, chest, or limbs. Abdominal pain passes for " stomach-ache," and pains in the limbs for " growing pains " or rheumatism. In general, it may be said here that persistent localized pain in

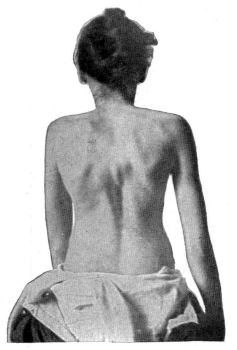

Fig. 11.—Deformity in Dorsal Pott's Disease Showing Spasm of Muscles.

the case of a child is a symptom demanding very great attention.

The pain is usually subacute, and may be only occasional. At times the attack may be very severe, accompanied by intense hyperæsthesia, so that the pressure of the bedclothes cannot be tolerated, and patients in this condition have been supposed to have intense peritonitis or pleurisy. The subacute form is more common, and this, together with muscular stiffness, often gives rise to a diagnosis of rheumatism, sciatica, or neuralgia. Analogous to these attacks of pain are disturbances of the functions of other nerves—manifested in cough, peculiar grunting respiration, dyspnœa with cyanosis, gastric disorders, obstinate and recurring vomiting, and troubles of the bladder, with or without pain at the end of the penis. Patients suffering in this way have been treated for bronchitis, pneumonia, gastritis, or cystitis.

Deformity.—The most characteristic feature of Pott's disease is the deformity—that is, the projection backward of one or more

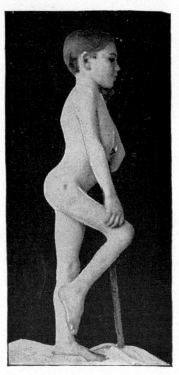

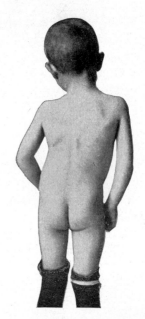

FIG. 12.—Severe Grade of Psoas Contraction.

FIG. 13.—Lateral Deviation of Spine in Dorsal Pott's Disease. Back view.

spinous processes. This is occasioned by the destruction of the vertebral bodies. The projection is primarily of the vertebræ first affected, but following this other vertebræ are more or less involved, and the curve increases, with the establishment of secondary curves. The sharper the projection, as a rule, the more acute is the process; but this rule, however true in the upper dorsal region, has occasional exceptions in the lower dorsal and upper lumbar regions.

It is most important to keep a record of the deformity in each case under observation. This record is most easily taken by a simple method.

A strip of sheet lead half an inch wide, of the quality known to the dealers as " four pounds to the foot," is made straight by pressing out the curves, and is laid along the spinous processes of the child, who lies on his face on a flat table without a pillow, with his hands at his sides and his head turned to one side. With the fingers the lead is pressed against the spinous processes, and when it is removed it is stiff enough to keep its shape. The curve is then drawn upon a piece of cardboard by means of this lead strip, placed on its side and used as a ruler. The cardboard curve is cut out with scissors and the concavity is then applied to the child's back to see if it fits accurately. If not, it should be trimmed with the scissors until it does. The slightest change in the outline of the back can then be detected at any subsequent visit, because any increase or diminution of the deformity will cause the cardboard cutting to fit the outline of the back imperfectly.

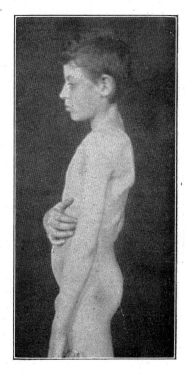

FIG. 14.—Result in Severe Case of Dorsal Pott's Disease.

If the deformity is left to itself, its tendency is to increase until a spontaneous cure results or death ensues. In many cases in dorsal Pott's disease this result is reached only after an extensive deformity has occurred. In cervical and lumbar Pott's disease spontaneous cure is more likely to occur, and, when it occurs, is accompanied by much less deformity than in the dorsal region.

When this spontaneous cure occurs, the change takes place gradually and does not cause narrowing of the spinal canal. The secondary curvatures are: in cervical Pott's disease, a dorsal incurvation below the disease, with a slight lumbar excurvation; in dorsal disease, an increased hollowing in above and below the gibbosity of the disease; in lumbar disease, a long curvature with convexity inward above the disease. The neck becomes shortened and thickened in cervical Pott's disease; the trunk is shortened in disease of other parts of the spine;

occasionally there is also in cases of long duration a diminution in the growth of the whole body, so that adults recovered from Pott's disease of ordinary severity are of less than average height.   An alteration in the shape of the lower part of the face takes place in marked dorsal disease, with a facial expression which is characteristic. Cases in which the deformity is rapidly increasing are, as a rule, characterized by much pain.

Deformity of the chest is a constant accompaniment of dorsal Pott's disease.   The vertebral column cannot give way and form an

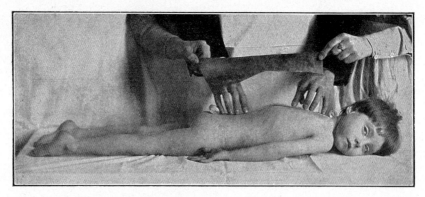

FIG. 15.—Method of Measurement of Deformity in Pott's Disease. Shows lead strip and cardboard tracing.   (Children's Hospital Report.)

angular deformity without altering the position of the sternum and ribs.   The deformity is usually a thrusting downward and forward of the sternum with a lateral flattening of the chest.   In short, it results in the formation of a pigeon-breast.   There may, however, be a prominence of the ribs on both sides of the sternum, where a depression of the sternum is seen.   Sometimes the pigeon-breast is the first symptom to attract the attention of the parents, and for that alone the children are brought to the surgeon.

High Temperature.—Cases with Pott's disease not infrequently have an elevation of the temperature in the afternoon.   This temperature is diminished or often reduced to normal in cases under bed treatment.   The rise of temperature is from one to three degrees in average cases and occurs independently of abscesses.

COMPLICATIONS.

Paralysis.—Partial or complete paralysis of the legs is a frequent complication of Pott's disease.   It may occur in early or late, in mild or severe cases, and frequently no apparent exciting cause can be assigned for its appearance. The motor paralysis varies from mere muscular weakness to complete loss of power. It begins as a sense of fatigue, a dragging of the feet; then there is inability to hold one's self erect. Unless the disease is in the lumbar region, the reflexes are exaggerated, and muscular spasms may start from the least irritation; they frequently appear spontaneously. In severe cases the muscles are flaccid and the legs may be powerless. With the secondary degenerations in the cord, rigidity sets in. The bladder and rectum are paralyzed toward the end of all severe cases of paralysis, and whenever the lumbar enlargement is involved; in milder cases they escape. The arms are paralyzed in exceptional instances of dorsal Pott's disease. Of the sensory paralysis below the lesion there is less to be said; it is apt to begin as paræsthesia; anæs-

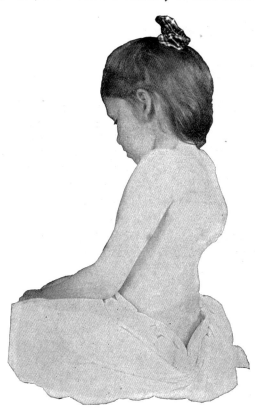

Fig. 16.—Rounded Deformity from Old Disease in the Dorsal Region.

thesia afterward may come on to a greater or less extent. Trophic disturbances are not to be seen unless in exceptional cases.

The wasting of the muscles and diminution of electric contractility are usually only such as disuse would cause.

In a few instances affections of the joints, supposed to be secondary to lesions of the cord, have been noted, and instances are mentioned in which herpes zoster, apparently due to the same cause, was present.

Paralysis is rarely an early symptom in Pott's disease, though it has been observed before the stage of deformity. The frequency of paralysis is indicated by the figures collected in 700 cases observed by Dollinger. Forty-one cases of paralysis were noted (5.8 per cent). In 26 of the 41 cases the disease involved the region from the third to the seventh dorsal vertebræ inclusive.

Paralysis is usually bilateral; it may, however, be unilateral, and in some unusual instances it occurs above the point of deformity. Taylor and Lovett [1] found, in an examination of 59 cases of paralysis (out of 445 cases of Pott's disease), that the location of the disease was as follows: 1 cervical, 7 cervico-dorsal, 37 dorsal, 7 dorso-lumbar, 4 lumbar, 3 unclassified. The deformity was large in 20, medium in 10, small in 17 (in 12 unclassified). The paralyzed cases presented no worse deformity than that seen in average cases. In 26 the outline of the deformity was rounded and gradual; in 16 it was distinctly sharp. The paralysis occurred on the average about two years after the beginning of the disease. It came on immediately after a fall in 4 cases. The duration of the paralysis was never, in the cases reported, over three years, except in one case, when it persisted with but little improvement for six years; in 2 cases it lasted three years; in 5 cases it lasted two years. A recurrence of the paralysis was noted in 6 cases, 4 having two attacks and 2 having three.

Paralysis is not a common occurrence in Pott's disease under efficient protective treatment. Its prognosis is extremely favorable in mild cases, or in severe ones if they can be treated early. Recovery, when it occurs, is generally complete, leaving no trace of the disability of the limbs.

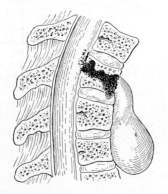

FIG. 17.—Diagram of Abscess from Pott's Disease.

Abscess.—In most cases of Pott's disease, especially in those under efficient treatment, the whole course is run without any evidence of suppuration, but in others abscesses form a distressing complication.

The earlier treatment is begun and the more efficiently it is carried out, the less liable are abscesses to form; but it must not be assumed that the occurrence of abscesses is evidence of incomplete treatment. In certain cases of severe disease an abscess cannot be avoided.

[1] Med. Rec., 1886, xxix., 699.

The causes of development of an abscess are the same in Pott's disease as in bone tuberculosis elsewhere. And the most common form is psoas abscess, so-called from its localization in the region of the insertion of the psoas muscle.

Abscesses may accumulate in the inguinal region above Poupart's ligament, simulating hernia. Before passing down the sheath of

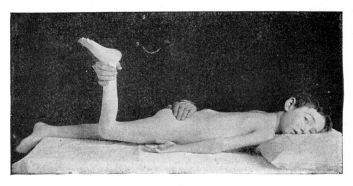

FIG. 18.—Examination for Psoas Contraction.   (Children's Hospital Report.)

the psoas muscle, they may enlarge in the abdominal cavity beneath the peritoneum, constituting a layer of subperitoneal abscesses. In time these abscesses descend down the thigh, but they may remain for a long time large, threatening, abdominal tumors.

A *lumbar abscess* appears as a swelling in the loin on one side or the other just outside the quadratus lumborum.

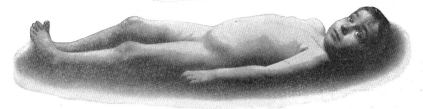

FIG. 19.—Psoas Abscess.

Abscess in *dorsal* disease may pass between the ribs and appear as a tumor on one side of the spine, or the accumulation of pus may remain in the posterior mediastinum, giving rise to cough and dyspnœa, and may be detected as an area on one side of the spine, dull to percussion.

Cervical abscess appears as a tumor at the side of the neck, simulating the ordinary deep cervical abscess, or it may appear as a bunch at the back of the pharynx, causing difficulty in breathing and swallowing. The latter is known as a *retropharyngeal* abscess.

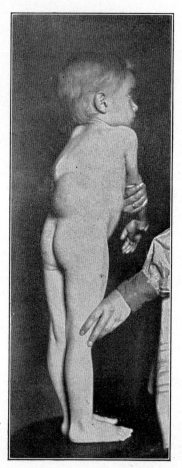

FIG. 20.—Lumbar Abscess.

Abscesses may exceptionally burst into the mouth, trachea, bronchi, mediastinum, œsophagus, or pleura. They may rupture into the intestines, bladder, vagina, rectum, or the abdominal cavity; and one case is reported in which spinal abscess simulated a fistula in ano. Abscesses may also burst into the spinal canal or the hip-joint. Occasionally they burst in the alimentary canal, not so rarely in the lungs, and exceptionally in the peritoneum or larger vessels.

Abscesses in the lung give rise to less disturbance than would be supposed; in reality they present the rational and physical signs of a low form of localized pneumonia, of a chronic or subacute type.

An abscess may remain stationary in size and quiescent for a long time—a condition which may be compatible with fair general health. Instances are not uncommon in which adults have been able to attend to active work and children to play about, although suffering from large cold abscesses.

When absorption takes place the fluid contents disappear, and the caseous and purulent detritus, if present, in all probability becomes encapsulated. This sometimes happens even in large psoas abscesses.

DIAGNOSIS.

The diagnosis is based on physical signs:

These are:

1. Stiffness of the spine in walking and in passive manipulation.

2. Peculiarity of gait and attitudes assumed, according to the location of the disease.

3. Lateral deviation of the spine.

For all examinations children should be stripped.

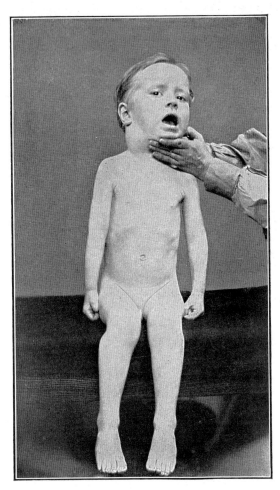

FIG. 21.—Cervical Abscess.

1. **Muscular Stiffness.**—On examining for muscular stiffness of the spine, the child is most conveniently laid face downward on a table or bed, and lifted by the feet. In a normal back the lumbar and lower dorsal spine can be markedly bent, and a general mobility of the whole column is seen. In patients in whom Pott's disease is

present the region affected is held rigidly by muscular contraction when manipulation is attempted. Lifting the patient by the feet in this way will show the existence of lumbar or lower dorsal rigidity,

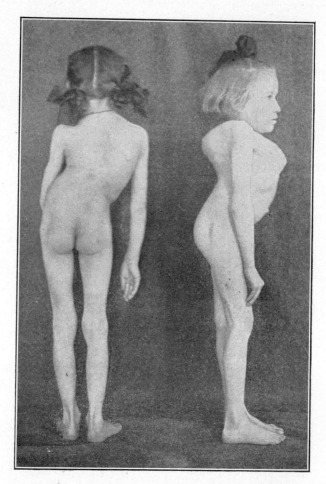

FIG. 22.—On Left Scoliosis.   On Right Old Dorsal Pott's Disease.

but it does not detect high dorsal Pott's disease. In lumbar Pott's disease lateral mobility of the spine, as well as antero-posterior flexibility, is lost.

   2. **Peculiar Gait and Attitudes.**—In general the walk is careful, and steps are taken with such care that jars to the spine are avoided.

   CERVICAL POTT'S DISEASE.—The most common symptom of the

disease in this region is the occurrence of wry-neck with stiffness of the muscles of the back and neck.

In disease of the upper cervical vertebræ the head, however, may be held sharply flexed and sunk upon the chest. It may be hyperextended with the occiput resting on the upper part of the spine, or it may be held laterally bent.

UPPER DORSAL POTT'S DISEASE.—In this region detection of the disease is less difficult, because bony destruction at once results in

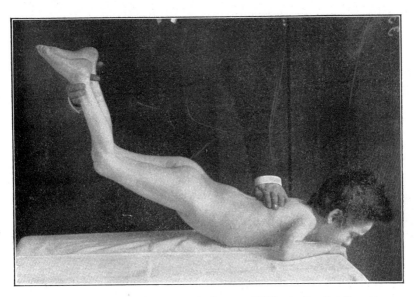

FIG. 23.—Rigidity of Spine in Pott's Disease. (Children's Hospital Report.)

angular deformity, on account of the posterior curve of the spine in this part.

The shoulders are, however, held high and squarely, the gait is careful. In Pott's disease, paralysis may exceptionally be the first perceptible symptom.

From *round shoulders,* Pott's disease is generally to be distinguished by the fact that in the former the spine is flexible and the deformity rounded and not angular. The distinction is generally easily made.

LUMBAR POTT'S DISEASE.—Vertebral disease in this region of the spine is sometimes difficult of detection at an early stage, as a knuckle is not developed in as early a stage as in other parts of the spinal column, but stiffness in gait and peculiarity of attitude are characteristic. The attitude is that of lordosis, which in some cases becomes very marked; the gait is military and careful, and lateral deviation is generally present, sometimes to a very marked degree. It is in this region of the spine that it is most conspicuous.

Lumbar Pott's disease is occasionally mistaken for single or double hip disease, or is regarded as a rhachitic curvature.

When the hip symptoms are due to Pott's disease and are caused by psoas irritability, the restriction of motion in the hip is simply in

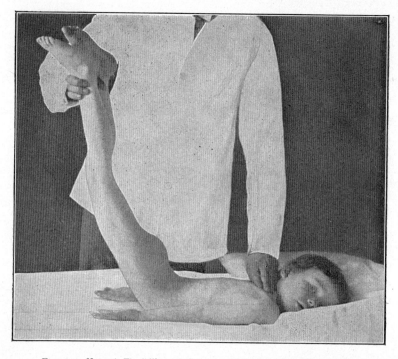

Fig. 24.—Normal Flexibility of Spine.   (Children's Hospital Report.)

the loss of hyperextension, while abduction and internal rotation are free and not affected. This limitation of motion in only one direction is generally sufficient, in connection with the other symptoms, to establish the presence of Pott's disease. On the other hand, in some cases the limitation of the hip's motion is in all directions, and simulates very closely the limitation of true hip disease.

Rhachitic deformity of the spine is a posterior curvature, is usually, though not always, rounded and not angular. It is less sharp and there is less muscular stiffness than in Pott's disease. It occurs at the junction of the dorsal and the lumbar regions. This junction is also a frequent site of Pott's disease.

Hyperæsthetic spine is characterized by tenderness in certain portions of the back, sometimes accompanied by pain or ache. This condition is more common in neurotic persons, but may be seen in others who have been suffering from nervous exhaustion from any cause. As a rule, no real stiffness in the back is present, but in severe cases, or in cases which may have remained in bed for some time, muscular stiffness may be present.

Malignant disease of the spine presents, when a projection is found, a more rounded and less sharp projection than is seen in the beginning of caries. Carcinoma of the spine is usually secondary. The symptoms, however—pseudo-neuralgias, paresis, paralysis, and muscular stiffness—are the same in both, and sometimes only a conjectural diagnosis can be made. Sarcoma of the spine is a rare affection in childhood.

In curvatures of the spine caused by *aneurism,* the diagnosis is usually made by auscultation or by the rational symptoms before the spine is noticeably affected.

Tumors pressing on the spinal cord may cause stiffness of the back and pain referred to the peripheral ends of the nerves. Angular deformity, however, is absent, and the symptoms of nervous disturbance predominate over the ordinary ones of Pott's disease.

Acute Osteomyelitis of the spine may be secondary or primary. The transverse and articular processes as well as the vertebral bodies may be affected, and tenderness is present at the seat of disease. Suppuration elsewhere occurs in sixty per cent of all cases. There is much constitutional disturbance, fever is high, and the course rapid. Œdema of the affected parts appears early; abscesses of a very acute and extensive character as well as paralysis are other early features. The formation of a kyphus of any extent is unusual.

A subacute or chronic form of vertebral osteomyelitis is met with more often secondary to a germ infection. This has been termed " typhoid " spine and may resemble Pott's disease. The affection is more rapid than the tuberculous process. It is less common in children.

Spondylitis deformans of the spine is an affection most frequent in adult life, characterized on superficial examination by stiffness and some arching of the spine; in some instances the ribs are ankylosed to the spine, so that no expansion of the chest is possible. Stiffness of the back is present, but the whole spine is rigid and other joints may be involved. These cases may occur in connection with gonor-rhœa.

Spondylolisthesis, or dislocation forward of one of the lumbar vertebræ, may cause pain, lordosis, and peculiarity of gait and posture.

With regard to the symptoms of *sacro-iliac* disease, *perinephritis,* and *appendicitis,* it may be said that a mistake in diagnosis may happen, but that ordinarily there is no obscurity. It should, however, be borne in mind that in appendicitis and in perinephritis, when an abscess is present, a contraction of the thigh may occur, resembling that seen in psoas abscess. The absence of a projection or irregularity of the back, and the power of muscular movement of the back in these cases, will help to establish the fact that they are not due to disease of the spine.

Skiagrams in early cases of Pott's disease sometimes aid in the diagnosis, but are often negative.

PROGNOSIS.

Pott's disease will always be regarded as one of the most formidable of diseases; its long course, the deformity entailed, the severity of the complications, and the occasional termination in death give both to the surgeon and to the non-professional public a natural dread of the affection. These inferences are, however, drawn from the severer cases, and facts show that the disease has a tendency to recovery, that the deformity can be prevented, and that in few affections does the work of the surgeon give greater benefit than in Pott's disease.

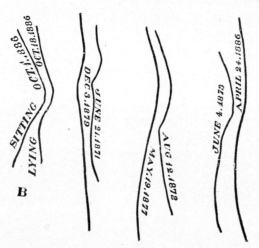

FIG. 25.—Tracings from Cases of Pott's Disease Showing the Recession of the Deformity under Mechanical Treatment.

Mortality.—No statistics of value exist as to the percentage of mortality and recovery.

The tendency of the deformity is to increase, during the years of growth, and this is specially marked in the upper dorsal region.

Instances of arrest without great deformity are not rare in upper cervical disease and in lumbar disease, but in the upper and middle dorsal regions the tendency is for an increase of the deformity proportionate to the extent of the disease.

The disease varies greatly as to its self-limitation in individuals, and according to the situation and extent of the disease. Necessarily there will be a difference in individual cases in the result of treatment.

It may be said that, as the bodies in the cervical region are smaller than those in the lumbar, the time required for self-limitation here is shorter than in the lumbar region. In the latter region, also, the superincumbent weight is a more important factor than in the upper part of the spine.

The occurrence of bony formation firm enough to support the column in its weight-bearing function must be a process requiring a long time for its completion, to judge from it as observed elsewhere; and nowhere is protection more urgently demanded during convalescence than in the vertebral column. This is especially true in growing children. Cases of supposed cure of Pott's disease have redeveloped symptoms at the period of rapid growth at the approach of puberty. It should especially be borne in mind that protection to the spine may be needed at this period.

TREATMENT.

This varies according to the stage and condition of the pathological process.

Treatment, therefore, is different in the acute, the subacute, and the convalescent stages. In the acute stage recumbency is the most efficient method. In the subacute and convalescent stage ambulatory treatment with more or less efficient spinal protection is advisable.

Treatment by Recumbency.

If the patient lies upon his back or upon his face on a hard surface, there is no superincumbent weight pressing upon any portion of the spine. If the patient lies upon his back upon a spring-bed, and the bed sags, the spine is of course bent, and pressure upon the vertebræ, proportional in amount to the extent of the curve, results.

If treatment by recumbency is to be adopted, it is not sufficient simply to place the child in bed. Sagging of the mattress, moving of the patient from side to side, twisting and turning are all injurious,

in that they cause motion between the vertebræ and change interarticular pressure, both of which are undesirable.

It is necessary that the child should be fixed in a suitable position
in bed. This can be done by securing the child in such a manner that
the vertebral column at the seat of the disease is arched forward,

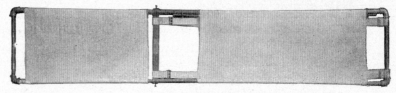

FIG. 26.—Gas-Pipe Frame.

diminishing the interarticular pressure. The simplest way of doing
this is by means of a frame.

The rectangular bed frame consists of a stretcher of heavy cloth
attached to a rectangular gas-pipe frame. The child lying upon this
frame can be secured by means of straps across the shoulders and
pelvis and knees, and can be carried about without jar. When the
frame is placed upon the bed, the cloth covering is no more uncom-
fortable than the surface of the bed.

But simple recumbency alone is not sufficient to promote cicatricial
ostitis. The removal of intervertebral pressure is also necessary.
This is to be accomplished by arching the spinal column forward at

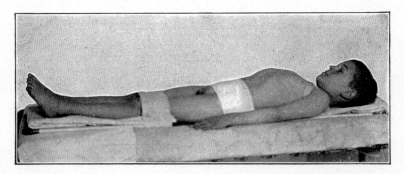

FIG. 27.—Method of Securing Child to Bed Frame for Recumbent Treatment of Dorsal Pott's
Disease.

the point of the kyphotic curve, by placing under the curve of the
child lying upon the back a firm pad, pressing upon each side of the
spinous process, and sufficiently high to press this part upward while
the rest of the spinal column drops back by its own weight. The

pads can be furnished by properly folded sheets or towels, by a bag of fine sawdust, by felt padding, or by a plaster-of-Paris back moulded to a corrected position of the spine, or by arching the frame, as has been suggested by Silva, Hunkin, and Whitman. If the frame is made narrow the child's outer clothing can be placed around the frame and child, which is an advantage in carrying the child about. This holds the spine hyperextended throughout its length.

In cervical caries head traction in a recumbent position will be found of use in cases of torticollis; and in severe neuralgia from cervi-

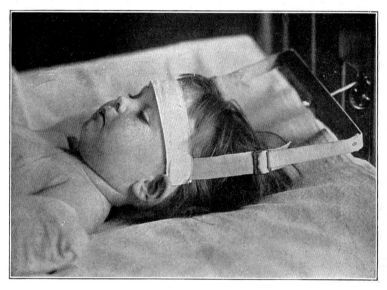

Fig. 28.—Traction in Cervical Caries. (Children's Hospital Report.)

cal caries the relief afforded is often very marked. Traction can be furnished by means of a head sling passing over the forehead and occiput, which is attached to a weight and pulley running over the head of the bed or to the head of the frame. The counter pull may be furnished by the weight of the body in case the head of the bed is raised, by a downward pull upon the trunk through a waist band, or by means of traction applied to the limbs.

Treatment by recumbency, if used, should be thorough. Half measures have the evils of the imprisonment without the benefit of fixation. The objections to treatment by recumbency are evident. Pott's disease is a tuberculous affection and close confinement is injurious to patients with a tuberculous taint. Patients of this sort need all possible help from fresh air and exercise, and the method of treatment by recumbency for years, formerly the only thorough method possible, is not now regarded as necessary in all cases.

AMBULATORY TREATMENT.

Treatment by Plaster Jackets.—The purpose of the treatment by plaster jackets is to fix the spine so firmly that there will be no injury to the affected vertebræ from the jar incident to locomotion.

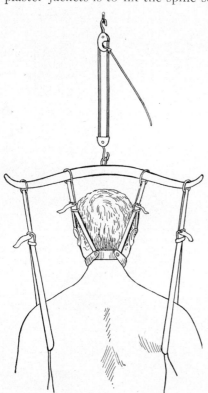

Plaster jackets are made by applying successive layers of properly prepared bandages to the patient's trunk, which has been placed in a suitable position.

The patient during the application of a plaster jacket is either upright or recumbent (on back or face), with or without a suspension or a traction pull.

APPLICATION OF JACKET WITH THE PATIENT SUSPENDED. —Suspending a healthy person by the head diminishes the physiological curves (cervical and lumbar lordosis, dorsal kyphosis), and the spine becomes straight so far as its formation will allow.

The patient's clothes are removed and a thin, tightly fitting undershirt is applied, put on so as to present no wrinkles. The patient is thickly padded by felt or sheet-wadding pads over the pelvis and two thick felt pads are

FIG. 29.—Sayre Headpiece for Suspension in Pott's Disease.

placed longitudinally at the sides of the kyphus. The patient is then suspended; the head is secured in a sling, which is attached to a strong cord playing in a pulley, or series of pulleys, fastened to a point above the patient's head. An assistant pulling on the cord raises the patient so that the heels are free from the floor. It is desirable to diminish the strain upon the neck, and padded loops connected with the bar, which is raised by the cord and pulley, can be passed under each axilla, or handles may be held in each hand, connected with cords which play over pulleys.

The bandages are then wound smoothly around the patient. If the plaster is fresh and of the best quality, it should harden in five minutes. After the plaster is hard or nearly hard, the patient is to be placed on a soft flat surface, care being taken not to crack the plaster in so doing. The edges of the jacket are smoothed down and cut off if they press uncomfortably on the thighs or axillæ.

It is important that the jacket should be strong in front as well as behind, and should be wound as high as possible in front, in order to prevent the spinal column from falling forward. If the jacket becomes broken or softened, it should be removed and another applied.

If the disease is in the cervical, or upper dorsal region, the plaster bandages should be carried up around the back of the head and neck and under the chin, leaving the face and upper part of the head exposed, and so fixation and support may be obtained in that part of the vertebral column.

CALOT'S METHOD.—The modified method of Calot consists in the application of a highly efficient plaster jacket, followed by recumbency in a corrective jacket for a period of two years. The jacket is applied in strong suspension by means of sheets of crinoline impregnated with plaster cream, which are secured in place by ordinary plaster bandages wound outside. In all cases the shoulders are included in the jacket, which terminates above in a "military collar." In the upper dorsal region a plaster headpiece is used. A square window is cut over the kyphus and layers of absorbent wool are placed between the square of plaster removed and the back. This square of plaster is then fastened in place by bandages making compression on the kyphus. The number of layers is subsequently increased to keep up an increasing corrective pressure at the same time a larger window, triangular in shape with the apex upward, is removed from the front of the jacket to allow the spine to be pushed forward at the level of the kyphus. The details of the method are given in the reference.[1]

APPLICATION DURING RECUMBENCY ON THE FACE.—The patient is laid face downward with the arms above the head on a hammock, which consists of a stout cloth a little wider than the child, stretched over the ends of a rectangular gas-pipe frame. One end of this cloth is attached to the upper end of the frame and does not move. The

[1] F. Calot: "L' Orthopédie Indispensable," Paris, 1909, p. 7.

other end is attached to a movable bar connected with the other end of the frame by a rope. By a ratchet this bar can be pulled upon and the tension of the cloth regulated. The hammock may be made very tight or allowed to sag to any extent. In this way hyperextension of the spine may be produced as desired.

The hammock cloth is cut along the sides of the child's body longitudinally and the parts not under the child's body are drawn aside

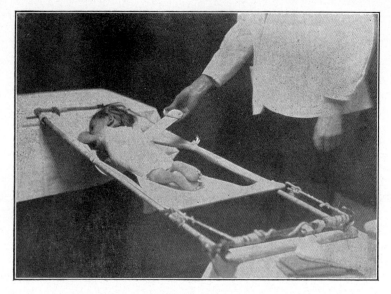

FIG. 30.—Method of Applying a Plaster Jacket in Recumbency, on the Hammock Frame.

and fastened or cut away. The plaster rollers are then applied, including both child and hammock.

Instead of the stretched hammock cloth, the patient may be placed on two pieces of stout webbing stretched along the length of a rectangular frame. These should be placed sufficiently near together to support the trunk without pressure upon the chest. Cross straps of webbing are necessary at the hips and shoulders when the jacket is applied. The webbing straps are untied and patient released, after which they are pulled out.

APPLICATION OF A JACKET WITH THE PATIENT PLACED UPON THE BACK.—In applying a jacket with the patient lying upon the face some compression of the chest and flattening of the abdomen take place. To avoid this, a jacket can be applied with the patient placed upon his back. If this were done with the patient lying upon a stretched sheet, the sagging of the material would prevent the necessary hyperextension of the spine.

An upright steel rod is arranged with a forked top on which can be placed two attachable pad plates. The rod fits in a stand and can be raised or lowered by means of a screw. If the patient is made to lie in such a way that, while the head, shoulders, and pelvis are supported the kyphus rests upon the pad plates, a hyperextending force is exerted on the kyphus. As the rod bearing the pad plates is raised

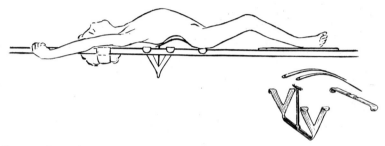

Fig. 31.—Frame for Applying Jacket with Patient Recumbent upon the Back. (Metzger-Goldthwait.)

or lowered, the pressure on the kyphus is increased or diminished. Any desired amount of hyperextension of the spine can be furnished.

Exaggerated lordosis can be prevented by flexing the thighs.

JACKETS APPLIED WITH THE PATIENT SITTING.—The patient may be seated during the application of the jacket if it is desired to prevent lordosis in the lumbar region.

In disease of the lumbar region, since lordosis is desirable to separate the lumbar vertebræ, suspension is not necessary. The jacket can be applied with the patient steadied and the back arched forward to secure exaggerated lordosis.

It is desirable that the surgeon should familiarize himself with the application of plaster jackets by the different methods mentioned, as it will be found that they are of assistance in different cases.

The most acceptable form of permanent jacket is one applied over a seamless woven shirt. These shirts are made very long and reach the knees; one of them is put on the patient and the jacket applied over it. The lower part of the shirt is then turned up over the outside of the jacket and reaches to the top of it. It is there stitched to the upper part of the shirt along the upper edge of the jacket.

REMOVABLE JACKETS.—After a jacket has been applied by any one of these methods, it may be converted into a removable jacket by splitting it and furnishing it with lacings or buckles and straps. Removable jackets are not, however, such efficient supports as fixed jackets during the acute stage of the disease. They are, as a rule, to be used in convalescent cases, in exceptional cases in the acute stage when the skin is very sensitive and requires bathing, when sloughs or excoriations are present, and in similar conditions.

As a substitute for plaster jackets, corsets are made of leather,

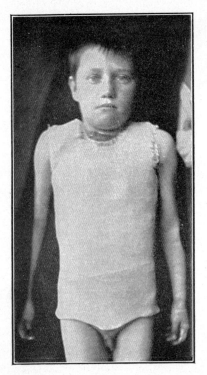
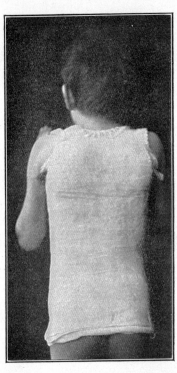

FIG. 32.—Plaster Jacket. Front view.   FIG. 33.—Plaster Jacket. Back view.

wood, aluminum, celluloid gauze dipped in celluloid paste, papier-mâché, and other materials.

There are certain practical details with regard to the application of plaster jackets and removable jackets that are important.

PLASTER-OF-PARIS BANDAGES.—Plaster-of-Paris jackets depend for their durability, lightness, and efficiency largely upon the material from which they are made and the skill with which they are applied. The most durable bandages are those made from slow-setting plaster. The quicker-setting plaster offers distinct advantages, but jackets made of it are more friable and less durable. The material which the writers use as a foundation for the plaster is a crinoline, which is sized with starch, and not with glue, which is especially prepared. This crinoline should be torn into strips, four yards long and four or five inches wide. After the crinoline is torn, the loose threads

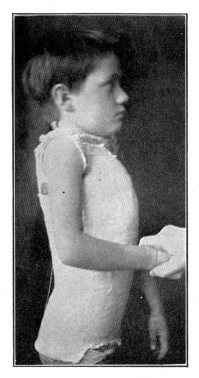

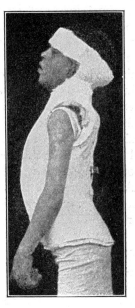

FIG. 34.—Plaster Jacket. Side view.

FIG. 35.—Plaster Jacket and Head-piece. (Wullstein.)

should be removed from the edges, and the strips folded ready for the rubbing-in of the plaster.

PLASTER.—If a quick-setting jacket is desired dental plaster should be used, and if a slow-setting bandage, a high-grade of commercial plaster-of-Paris. The durability and the tensile strength of the jacket are increased if to either kind of plaster is added five per cent of Portland cement, thoroughly mixed with the plaster.

The plaster is incorporated in the bandage by laying the crinoline strip flat on a table, on which is placed a heap of the plaster. A handful of this plaster is then placed on the strip and swept along with the hand or with a flat piece of splint wood, the excess being brushed aside, and the bandage thus impregnated with plaster is rolled loosely, as, if it is tightly rolled, the water does not reach the inner layers. If it is desired to secure bandages of the highest efficiency each bandage, after being rolled, should be wrapped in three paper napkins, applied one at a time and folded over the ends of the bandage. After the third napkin is put on, a rubber elastic strap is placed around the end of the bandage, and the bandage is ready for use. In this way the plaster is all kept in the bandage and does not escape into the water.

When the plaster jacket is to be applied the bandages should be immersed in a pail containing at least eight inches of warm water. If it is desired to hasten the setting of the bandage a teaspoonful of salt may be added to the water, but this increased speed of setting is obtained at the expense of durability. If it is desired to delay the setting a teaspoonful of alum or a small amount of glue should be added to the water. When the bandage is taken from the water the hands of the assistant should be placed over each end of it and it should be squeezed until it no longer drips. If the paper napkins are used the covered bandage should be immersed in the water, allowed to soak, squeezed, and the wet paper then removed before use.

APPLICATION OF BANDAGES.—Bandages should be applied with a smooth even pressure and uniform tension throughout each turn. There should never be reverse turns, and each layer should be rubbed into the next layer by the hand. From eight to ten layers of a properly prepared and applied bandage are in general enough to make a strong jacket. Extra resistance may be secured, and in many cases a lighter jacket constructed, by reinforcing it by means of a plaster rope. A bandage is taken from the water and strips two or three feet long are unrolled. After four or five strips have been loosened they are held by one end, and by the other hand sliding down are incorporated into a plaster rope about an inch in diameter, which is then laid over the light part which it is desired to strengthen, and secured in place by circular turns.

When a jacket is to be removed it is perfectly safe, if a sufficient layer of sheet-wadding has been placed under it in the line of intended removal, to cut the jacket with a sharp knife, making the strokes of the knife parallel to the skin. The form of knife most available for this is a shoe knife with a blunt point and a concave curved edge. There are various forms of plaster shears in use for the same purpose.

REMOVABLE JACKETS.—Although plaster makes a light and, when

properly constructed, a fairly durable jacket, it is injured by constant springing open and the inner surface is apt to be rather rough, consequently various substitutes are used when it is likely that a removable jacket will have to be worn for some time. Celluloid forms one of the most acceptable of these. For the manufacture of this form of jacket the plaster-of-Paris jacket is removed, and filled with a thick mixture of plaster-of-Paris and water. The mould is then removed and the cast smoothed, dried, and shellacked.

CELLULOID.—An undervest is then placed over the cast, and strips of crinoline, cheesecloth, or stockinet laid over the undervest. These strips are then painted with a mixture consisting of celluloid chips dissolved in acetone. This paste is allowed to dry, and other coats are applied so long as the cloth material takes up more celluloid. When it ceases to be absorbed more cloth is laid on in the same way, and the process is repeated. The number of layers necessary will depend upon the thickness of the material. The jacket is left on the cast until it is thoroughly dry inside and out. When it is thoroughly dry it is cut and removed, the inside is painted with celluloid, the edges trimmed and bound with leather, the splint is perforated with holes throughout, and straps, studs, or lacings are put along the edges.

LEATHER SPLINTS AND JACKETS.—Moulded leather jackets are made from oak-tanned English leather, which should not be " filled " or " stuffed." The leather is cut of the desired pattern and softened by soaking in water. When it is thoroughly flexible it is stretched over a plaster cast of the limb or trunk and made to conform to all the curves of it. After being shaped, it is allowed to dry on the cast and removed, as it will retain the shape which it assumed when wet if it is thoroughly dry. If it is wished to stiffen the leather in order to secure a firmer support, especially in the case of jackets, the moulded leather splint is painted with hot bayberry wax until it ceases to absorb it, and it is then allowed to dry. The jacket is now painted with a solution of shellac inside and outside and allowed to dry thoroughly. If desired such jackets or splints can be reinforced with strips of steel fastened on the outside and riveted to the jacket. Jackets should be provided with leather lacings or straps and buckles.

LEATHER AND CELLULOID JACKETS.—A fairly durable and light jacket may be made by a combination of these two processes. A leather jacket, too light to be of much support, is made as described and thoroughly dried out. The inner surface of the jacket is then painted with the celluloid mixture described, over strips of crinoline

or cheesecloth. The jacket is kept on the cast in the interval between
the painting in order that no warping may occur, and as many layers
of cloth are painted on as may seem necessary to secure the desired

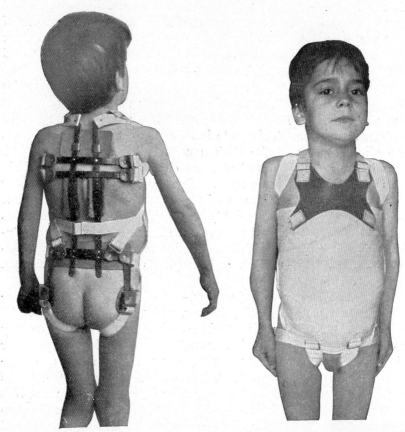

FIG. 36.—Antero-Posterior Brace for Dorsal Pott's
Disease Applied.

FIG. 37.—Antero-Posterior Brace for
Pott's Disease; showing Apron
and Leather Gorget.

firmness. When the last layer has been applied, enough celluloid is
painted on to give a smooth surface to the inside of the jacket.

TREATMENT BY STEEL APPLIANCES.

The basis of ambulatory treatment of Pott's disease in the subacute or convalescent stage is fixation, as complete as possible, of
the spine in as advantageous a position as obtainable. This may be
done by means of a properly made appliance.

As the chief motion of the spine to be guarded against is the forward motion, the principle of the appliance being that of an antero-posterior support. The construction and application of a brace should be superintended directly by the surgeon, and not relegated to an instrument-maker. For the construction of a splint a cardboard tracing of the back should be made at one side of the spinous processes.

The simplest antero-posterior apparatus consists of two uprights of annealed steel. The uprights are joined together below by an inverted U-shaped piece of steel which runs as far down on the buttock as possible without reaching the chair or bench when the patient sits down. At the top the uprights end in shoulder pieces running over the shoulders.

The brace, after being put together but before being finished, should be tried on the patient, who should be lying on his face. Any alteration necessary in the curves of the steel, in order to have the appliance fit closely to the back along its whole length, can be made with wrenches. The brace can be faced with hard rubber or covered smoothly with leather. An accurate fit is essential; the covering is merely a matter of detail.

Accurately fitting pad plates covered with felt and leather or hard rubber are needed, but in some instances, the bars of the brace, if well padded at the points of greatest pressure, answer every purpose. Buckles are needed at various levels.

If properly designed, the appliance will press firmly at the deformity, i.e., the pad plates and pressure should be uniform at this point and closely fitted to the contour of the deformity in all places. The appliance will also touch necessarily at the top and bottom, but the chief pressure should be at the kyphus. It should be borne in mind that, besides accuracy of fit and proper design, it is of importance that the apparatus be stiff enough not to yield as the weight of the trunk falls upon it, inasmuch as yielding involves intervertebral pressure.

It is, of course, essential that the trunk be properly secured to the brace. This can be done in part by means of an apron, of cloth or leather, which covers the front of the trunk, the abdomen, and the chest, reaching from the clavicles nearly to the symphysis pubis. The apron is provided with webbing (non-elastic) straps, which are fastened into buckles attached to the brace. Padded straps, passing from the top of the brace around the arms, under the axillæ, and attached to buckles in the middle of the brace, help to secure it; but the scapulæ, being movable, cannot be relied upon alone to fix the trunk, and the apron must be furnished with straps at the top, which pass over the shoulders to buckles in the top of the brace.

In adults it is often convenient to have the apron split down the front and provided with webbing straps and buckles, so that the patient can adjust it himself by tightening the straps in front.

To secure a proper hold upon the upper segment of the body in dorsal disease some unyielding and rigid chest-piece is necessary.

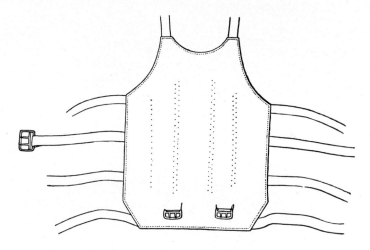

FIG. 38.—Apron for Use with Antero-Posterior Spinal Support.

The brace should be worn day and night, and removed daily that the back may be bathed. While the brace is off, the patient should lie on the face or the back. On no account should he sit erect. The back, after being washed, should be rubbed with alcohol and then powdered with face powder, corn starch, or fuller's earth. The brace should then be applied and buckled tightly into place.

In applying the brace the patient should lie upon his face, and the apron be spread under him. The brace should then be placed in position upon the bare back, or upon a thin, smooth cloth without wrinkles, and the apron strapped to it as tightly as is possible. The more tightly the two are strapped together, the more thorough is the fixation. The position of the straps and their number will vary in cases according to the situation of the disease, etc. The brace must, of course, if it is to exert pressure, always be straighter than the spine.

Head Supports.—In the upper region, as elsewhere, it is desirable to prevent the weight of the head from falling upon the diseased bodies of the vertebræ.

An efficient arrangement is one devised by Dr. Taylor, of New York; an ovoid steel ring passes around the neck, made so that it can open, and be secured when closed, and arranged so that it can serve as a rest for the chin, and so that pressure can also be exerted

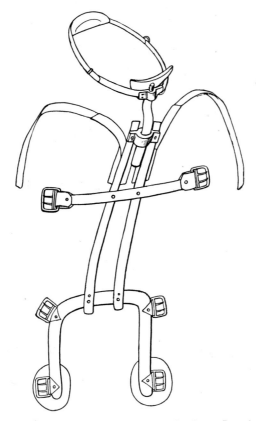

FIG. 39.—Oval Ring Head Support Added to the Antero-Posterior Support.

on the occiput. This collar has at the front a hard-rubber chin piece accurately shaped to the chin, and may have at the back a stiff piece of sole leather projecting up from the back of the ring. This steadies the head and prevents the pressure of the occiput against the back of the headpiece. This collar at the back plays on a pivot, allowing lateral motion of the head. The pivot is attached to the usual back brace, and can be raised or lowered, as it is desired to increase or diminish the upward pressure on the head. This appliance requires care and skill in application, and is useless unless properly fitted.

Other forms of head support have been tried from time to time.

A head support, devised by Goldthwait, affords good fixation, and it is serviceable in cases in which there is excessive sensi-

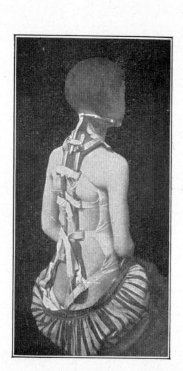

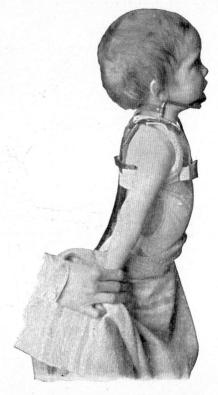

FIG. 40.—Taylor Back Brace with Oval Ring. Head support applied.

FIG. 41.—Antero-Posterior Brace with Bent Wire Head Support.

tiveness of the spine, due to cervical or very high dorsal disease.

Collars of various sorts, unattached to any other appliance, have been used, which, pressing on the chin and occiput above, and on the clavicles, sternum, and shoulders below, transfer the weight in part from the intermediate cervical vertebræ and check the forward bending of the cervical region. These collars can be made of plaster-of-Paris, but are cumbersome and unsightly. As a substitute a stiffened leather collar can be made, using sole leather stiff and stretched over a mould from a plaster-of-Paris neck cast.

In all forms of head supports, if worn for a long time, a certain amount of recession of the chin takes place, as the growth of the lower jaw is in a measure temporarily interfered with. The jaw gradually resumes its shape after removal of the head support.

When careful and skilled attention can be applied to the construction, attention, and needed alteration of a brace, it will be found of great efficiency in the treatment of Pott's disease in the convalescent stage.

The chief objection to the use of mechanical appliances as a method of treatment is that care and special skill are required, not only in the application of braces, but in the inspection and management of the cases.

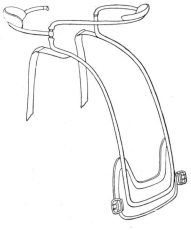

FIG. 42.—Anterior Head Support.

If the trunk is not thoroughly fixed by the straps, etc., of the appliance, the brace becomes simply a splint of steel laid upon the back, and not a therapeutic agent.

RECTIFICATION OF THE DEFORMITY (FORCIBLE CORRECTION).

Forcible correction of the deformity, with or without anæsthesia, is a method which has been recently shown to be attended with less risk than might have been supposed, has been largely discarded for methods of gradually straightening.

But although the correction of deformity by the use of violence is irrational and may be seriously injurious, the employment of moderate force in correction is frequently beneficial.

The mechanical means for rectification are those already mentioned as of use in the application of plaster jackets. Rectification judiciously applied is beneficial in all active cases of Pott's disease. Pressure symptoms will be relieved and in some instances paralysis checked.

It must also be understood that after correction a relapse of the curve will take place unless the corrected position is maintained by adequate fixed appliances until the spine is well cicatrized in the corrected position.

In favorable cases a gradual reduction of the deformity is effected by repeated application of the bandage as can be done by the proper and systematic adjustment of correcting braces.

OPERATIONS ON THE DISEASED VERTEBRÆ.

Operative measures are necessary under exceptional circumstances for the direct examination of the diseased vertebral bodies and the

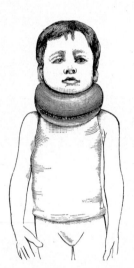

FIG. 43.—Thomas Leather Collar.

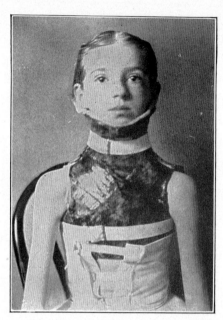

FIG. 44.—Collar and Chest-piece for Cervical Pott's Disease.

removal or drainage of the diseased bone. It must be remembered that in any event the vertebral bodies are more or less inaccessible, and that such operations are not likely to prove of benefit as routine measures.

In the cervical region the anterior surfaces of the bodies of the vertebræ may be reached either through the mouth, by a lateral incision, or by incision in the back of the neck. Through the mouth the operating space is small, the proceeding difficult on account of the anæsthetic, and the dangers of infection are evident. This method makes accessible only the second, third, and fourth vertebral bodies. The lateral method is preferable. An incision is made along the posterior border of the sternomastoid muscle; the sternomastoid and omohyoid are raised and the space made by the splenius and omohyoid is reached. The dissection is carried through the longus colli, and the vertebral arteries are avoided.

In the dorsal region exploration may be advisable in case an abscess in the posterior mediastinum is suspected. In such cases the operation of costo-transversectomy should be done. An incision at the side of the spinous processes uncovers the tops of the transverse processes and the bases of the ribs. The ribs are divided at the tuber-

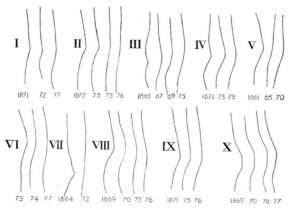

FIG. 45.—Tracings showing Results of Brace Treatment as Carried Out by Dr. C. F. Taylor. *I*, Two and three-quarters years, first and second lumbar disease, five years' treatment; *II*, eight years, eleventh and twelfth dorsal, four years' treatment; *III*, four years, first lumbar, ten years' treatment; *IV*, three and one-half years, six years' treatment; *V*, five years, twelfth dorsal, first and second lumbar, nine year's treatment; *VI*, five and one-half years, sixth and eighth dorsal, four years' treatment; *VII*, about eighteen, dorso-lumbar, eight years' treatment; *VIII*, nine years, seventh to ninth dorsal, seven years' treatment; *IX*, twenty years, five years' treatment; *X*, ten years, eight years' treatment. (Dates are given with tracings; the age given is that at which treatment was begun.)

osities and the posterior part, with the transverse process, removed. The spine is then reached by the finger.

In the lumbar region an incision is made from the twelfth rib to the ilium, two and one-half inches outside of the median line; the incision reaches to the border of the quadratus lumborum and the tips of the transverse processes should be felt. The dissection is carried down to the psoas muscle; some of the fibres of this muscle are detached with care from one transverse process. The finger introduced reaches without difficulty the anterior surface of the vertebral bodies. The finger can strip up the psoas muscle through this incision and explore the vertebral bodies. The vertebral canal should not be opened.

TREATMENT OF ABSCESS.

Abscesses may be treated by expectancy or by operation.

(1) **Expectancy.**—Under proper treatment early abscesses may subside and be absorbed without detriment to the patient.

Recumbency under the best mechanical conditions, preferably in the open air day and night, will favor the tendency to absorption.

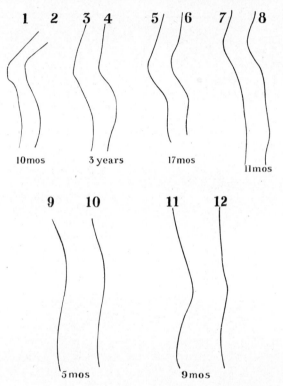

FIG. 46.—Results of Hyperextension Treatment (Goldthwait). 1, At beginning of treatment; 2, ten months later; 3, at beginning of treatment; 4, same, three years later; 5, at beginning of treatment; 6, seventeen months later; 7, at beginning of treatment; 8, seventeen months later; 9, at beginning of treatment; 10, same, five months later; 11, at beginning of treatment; 12, same, after nine months.

Aspiration will diminish the size of an abscess, but if it does not tend to absorb under the conditions mentioned, and especially if it shows a tendency to increase, it is better not to temporize, but to incise.

(2) **Operation.**—When abscesses increase rapidly, or for any reason seem an injury to the patient, incision is to be considered.

Incision of an abscess should be made under thorough aseptic precautions, and as complete drainage as possible secured; but it must be remembered that owing to the depth of the origin of abscesses in Pott's disease perfect drainage is not always as easily furnished as in more superficial abscesses. It is therefore desirable, especially in adults, to delay incision longer than would otherwise be surgically indicated.

In retropharyngeal and cervical abscesses, however, drainage can ordinarily be readily secured. In dorsal abscesses an incision in the back is frequently sufficient; but in some instances it will be necessary to perform costo-transversectomy to secure perfect drainage. In lumbar and iliac abscesses it may be necessary, owing to the depth of their origin, to incise both in front and behind, which can be done with care without opening the peritoneal cavity.

Psoas abscess may be opened in the loin or in the iliac fossa, or in both places. Drainage may be made with a strip of gauze or a rubber tube and the dressing kept sterile as long as possible. After incision curettage is not desirable, as it is impossible to remove all of the diseased material and unnecessary traumatism is to be avoided.

A *retropharyngeal abscess* is best opened by passing into the mouth a bistoury wound to within half an inch of its point with cotton, and cutting freely, using the finger as a guide. The child should be held face downward in order that the pus may not enter the trachea, and plenty of swabs should be at hand to keep the mouth clear, for the gush of pus is sometimes considerable. Such abscesses may also be opened by lateral incisions from the outside.

Treatment of Psoas Contraction.—When flexion of one or both thighs has come on it is not likely to diminish spontaneously, and if the condition is allowed to go untreated, such contractions may become permanent.

In the early stages the child should be put to bed on a frame. A light extension should be applied to the leg with pulley extension, and the pulley should be gradually lowered until the leg is straight and the flexion overcome. In cases in which the flexion has existed only a few weeks or months, this is generally easily accomplished in two or three weeks. If not, or if a more rapid method is desired in the first instance, the child should be anæsthetized and the leg straightened by force and retained by plaster-of-Paris. If this cannot be done with the use of moderate force, it is better to divide and cut the fascia and the contracted bands—an operation which cannot often be done thoroughly subcutaneously, for there are many deep bands.

TREATMENT OF PARALYSIS.

When paralysis is threatened, the patient should be put to bed on a frame so padded as to press upon the deformity and hold the vertebræ somewhat separated. In dorsal cases traction may be added. An attack may thus be averted.

When paralysis is present, a plaster jacket should be applied in strong hyperextension of the spine at the seat of the deformity (by one of the methods mentioned), and the patient should be kept recumbent until the paralysis begins to disappear.

The tendency of paralysis is strongly toward recovery under favorable conditions of treatment.

Drugs are of little or no value, and it is not possible to attach importance to the use of the cautery or of counter-irritants.

Laminectomy.—A spicule of bone or an intraspinal abscess may be the source of pressure at any stage of the disease, and in such cases, of course, operation is demanded. In cases of long standing, however, in which the paralysis has become very extensive and has involved sensation, laminectomy is of doubtful utility.

The operation consists in cutting down upon the spinous processes in the region of the deformity, the incision being slightly to one side of the centre, so that the resulting cicatrix will not be unduly pressed upon during recumbency. All the soft tissues are then stripped up with a periosteal knife, until the laminæ are exposed. The spinous processes are then removed with bone forceps over the affected area. Laminectomy forceps are then used to cut away all of the laminæ covering the cord at the seat of pressure. The dura may or may not be opened. A probe is then passed up and down the spinal canal, to be sure that all pressure is removed, and the wound is dressed. The patient should be laid on the face after operation if it is more comfortable.

The operation, however, has no place in the treatment of Pott's disease until the conservative measures have been faithfully tried over a sufficient period of time—measures which in most cases will prove efficient and successful in the relief of the paralysis.

CHAPTER III.

TUBERCULOUS DISEASE OF THE HIP.

THE term hip disease by common usage is applied to chronic tuberculous ostitis of the head of the femur or of the acetabulum.

PATHOLOGY.

The pathology of hip disease in general does not differ from that of tuberculous disease of bone which has already been referred to.

The head of the femur is the primary seat of disease, in a majority of the cases the epiphysis or juxta-epiphyseal region being the part attacked. In about twenty-five per cent of the cases the primary focus is in the acetabulum.

When once the acetabulum has become diseased either primarily or secondarily, enlargement of it is apt to take place. The irritated pelvic femoral muscles, which are in a state of tonic contraction, crowd the head of the femur against the upper and back border of the acetabulum; under this continual pressure absorption of that portion of the rim of the acetabular cavity takes place with an actual enlargement of the cavity from below upward. This so-called migration of the acetabulum is one cause of shortening of the limb, and measurement will show that the trochanter lies above Nélaton's line.

The changes in the head of the femur are chiefly the result of ostitis and pressure.

Partial destruction of the softened head of the femur may lead to a shortening of the limb and to an elevation of the trochanter above its proper level. The wearing away of the acetabulum produces the same result; but true dislocation is rare, except in the more acute cases.

A typical specimen from a fairly advanced case of hip disease shows a reddened and thickened synovial membrane, often with granulations; the cartilage is gone from the head of the femur or hangs in shreds; sometimes the whole cartilage may be lifted from the bone by a layer of granulations.

Perforation of the floor of the acetabulum may take place. Inside of the pelvis a dense wall of fibrous tissue and thickened periosteum shuts off the head of the femur or the contents of the joint from the pelvic cavity.

A natural cure results in one of two ways: by the absorption or calcification of the tuberculous tissue at an early or a late stage of

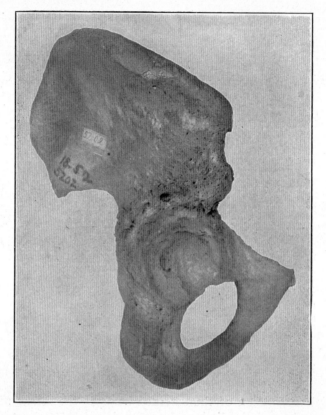

FIG. 47.—Erosion of the Upper Part of the Acetabulum. (Warren Museum.)

the disease; or by its evacuation and discharge by an external opening. The suppuration which comes later seems to be nature's effort to eliminate the diseased material, and it is the common method by which spontaneous cure results when it does occur. This late stage of the disease is characterized by malpositions and shortening of the limb and much impairment of the general condition in most cases. When spontaneous cure does occur it is usually with an ankylosed joint.

CLINICAL HISTORY.

Early Symptoms.—The beginning of the affection is most often gradual and insidious, but at times it begins so abruptly, according to

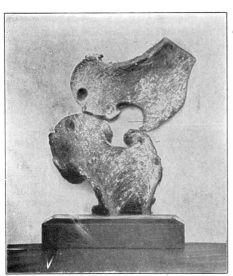

FIG. 48.—Focus in Head of Femur.

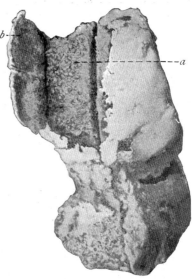

FIG. 49.—Hip. Excised head of femur. Articular cartilage turned up at one side shows tuberculous bone beneath. Primary focus was in acetabulum. *a*, Head of femur, surface tubercles; *b*, elevated cartilage. (Nichols.)

the parents' account, as to suggest a traumatic origin. The child will be noticed to limp at times with intervals of comparative freedom from lameness. This lameness increases, and it will be found that the patient is inclined to strike the ball of the foot rather than the heel in walking; although the heel can be put down to the floor, yet instinctively the knee is slightly bent and the heel raised when the weight of the trunk falls on the hip. There is a certain amount of stiffness of gait apparent in the morning when the patient first gets out of bed, and after sitting for a while; this passes away after the patient has walked or

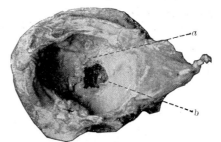

FIG. 50.—Acetabulum Seen from Outside. *a*, Tuberculous granulations; *b*, tuberculous cavity. (Nichols.)

played about. At night, as a rule, the limp is less than in the morning. The limp can perhaps best be described as a very slight stiffness and a disinclination to bear prolonged weight upon the affected limb.

If the child be inspected it will be seen that in standing the knee of the affected side is often flexed slightly, the pelvis being tipped

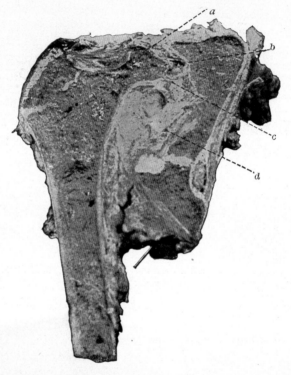

Fig. 51.—Head of Femur Eroded, Partly Destroyed, Partly Dislocated. Fibrous ankylosis. *a*, Head of femur; *b*, eroded head of femur; *c*, ankylosis; *d*, acetabulum. (Nichols.)

and the thigh slightly abducted. The tilting of the pelvis and abduction of the thigh may be so slight that it is scarcely noticeable, except by the deviation from the median line of the fold between the two buttocks. In girls the vulva on the affected side may be lower than on the other side.

Pain at this stage is very often absent, and if present is noted as night cries, to which allusion will be made.

In the early part of the disease pain at night, stiffness, and limping are the chief symptoms. Then follow malpositions of the limb, more severe disability, and perhaps greater pain and sensitiveness.

Succeeding the deformities which have just been described, one may find abscess formation and the development of sinuses; and this stage of the affection will hardly have been reached without considerable constitutional deterioration, which may become severe.

Lameness.—From being at first scarcely perceptible, the lameness increases and the limp becomes very noticeable. In very acute cases pain may become so severe that the child will refuse to use the leg,

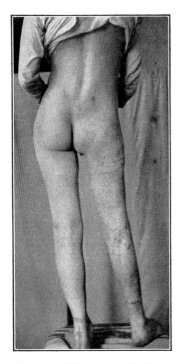

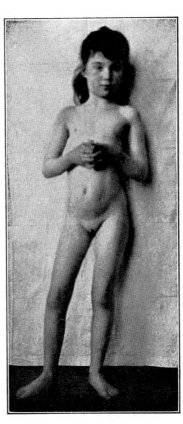

Fig. 52.—Obliteration of Gluteal Fold in Hip Disease of Right Side.

Fig. 53.—Position Assumed in Standing, with Slight Abduction of the Right Leg.

or malposition of the leg may come on rapidly and the limp may on that account become excessive; but in general the child walks without pain, though perhaps limping badly. Until the late stages of the disease lameness is not due to bone shortening.

Pain.—As the affection progresses, pain in the knee and sensitive-

ness to jarring the limb may become prominent symptoms. An unconscious protection of the joint may be noticed in the movement of the
patient; the foot of the well limb may be placed under the lower part
of the other leg when it is to be suddenly lifted by the patient, as from
the floor to the bed, or from the bed to the floor, or in moving from
one side of the bed to the other.

In manipulating the leg at this stage pain may follow the slightest
jar to the joint, or, on the other hand, the joint may be perfectly stiff
from muscular spasm and yet manipulation may be wholly painless.
In other cases motion in a certain arc is possible without causing pain,

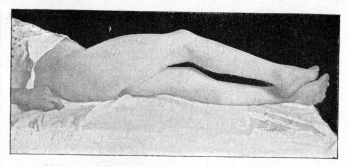

FIG. 54.—Instinctive Effort at Traction in Acute Disease of the Left Leg. (Fisk Prize Fund
Essay.)

but when the limits of this arc are reached, further motion becomes
painful or is prevented by muscular fixation. The sensitiveness of
the joint may become so great, when an acute stage supervenes, that
the slightest movement of the patient or jar of the bed or room causes
extreme suffering. This stage may come suddenly and gradually pass
away, the pain diminishing by degrees under the enforced treatment
of rest, or it may be persistent. A characteristic position is frequently
taken by the patient, who places the well foot on the dorsum of the
foot of the affected limb, exerting pressure away from the acetabulum.
*Pain may be absent at any or all stages of the disease, and is not a
diagnostic sign for or against the presence of hip disease.* Sensitiveness may be absent, upon which condition, however, at any time a
sensitive condition of the joint may supervene. The pain is often
remittent, and here, as in all the symptoms of this affection, marked
remissions may occur. The location of the pain is variable, but is
generally referred to the inside and front of the thigh near the knee
or directly at the knee-joint. The intimate relations and anastomoses

of the sciatic, obturator, and anterior crural nerves seem to furnish the best explanation of this.

Night Cries.—At an early stage of the affection the symptoms of " night cries " often appear. They occur in the early part of the night usually, and may become an annoying symptom. After the patient is asleep, and to all appearances entirely unconscious, sleep will be interrupted by a cry as if of severe pain, followed by moaning or crying for a few seconds, the child being unconscious or only half-

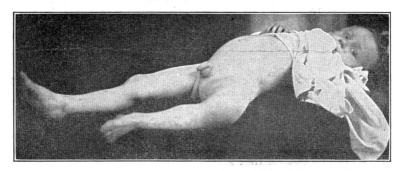

Fig. 55.—Severe Abduction and Eversion in a very Acute Case.

conscious of the cause of the pain. These do not often occur when the patient is entirely awake, and are caused by the spasmodic twitching of the muscles abnormally excitable from irritation, reflex to the inflammation of the joint. These cries may be repeated fifteen or twenty times during the night. They may be entirely wanting in the mildest cases.

Muscular fixation (muscular spasm) is always present in some degree, restricting the joint's normal arc of motion. It is due to a reflex irritability of the muscles controlling the joint, which causes them to maintain a condition of tonic spasm of greater or less degree. It disappears under full anæsthesia. Increased stiffness appearing in the course of treatment is a sign of inefficient treatment or of increase of the disease. This muscular rigidity is the most important sign of the disease, for not only is it the chief reliance in the matter of diagnosis, but it is the cause of the malpositions of the limb, of the wearing away of the acetabulum and of the head of the bone, and it lies at the root of much of the pain. It furnishes the most accurate index of the progress of the case, and improves or becomes worse as the case becomes better or worse. The importance of the recognition and accurate study of this symptom cannot be overestimated.

Atrophy.—A marked atrophy of the muscles of the thigh, hip, and leg is characteristic. It is supposed to be reflex to the disease of the joint.

Atrophy of the muscles controlling an inflamed joint begins early and may be very marked, even in simple acute synovitis. That this is something more than the mere atrophy of disuse is shown by the fact that it begins so sharply and so early, that it is greater in the diseased limb than in the well one even when the patient has been in bed from the first, and that the muscles, although atrophied, are not soft and flabby, but tense.

Diminished resistance to the passage of the x-rays in the epiphyses of the hip, indicative of greater vascularity, may be seen in the earlier stages of hip disease.

The obliteration of the fold of the buttock on the affected side is a result partly of muscular atrophy and partly of the periarticular swelling which accompanies the disease. It is a common but not a constant symptom at the early stages of the disease. It is also partly due to the flexed attitude of the limb, which naturally diminishes the prominence of the buttock on that side.

Malpositions of the Limb.—The fixation of the diseased limb in a distorted position is one of the commonest incidents of the affection. This is due to the tonic muscular contraction so often alluded to. These malpositions may hold the limb in flexion, adduction, abduction, or eversion, or in any combination of these; the cause which determines the kind of malposition in an individual case cannot be formulated. Flexion of the thigh is chiefly due to the muscular contraction, which is constant in chronic disease of the joint, and partly to an unconscious effort on the part of the patient to assume a position most comfortable for the joint and most protected from jar. These deformities generally disappear under treatment by rest or traction; but again, they reappear in cases under treatment if treatment has not succeeded in checking the progress of the disease. They often accompany a sensitive condition of the joint, which may be the precursor of abscess.

If the malposition is allowed to become permanent the final result can never be so good as when cicatrization takes place in a more normal position. The limp in ankylosed limbs depends more upon the amount of flexion and adduction than on anything except perhaps the bone shortening. It is, therefore, of much importance to diminish in all cases the amount of malposition present.

When adduction is present in both legs, as in double hip disease, and ankylosis of both hips has occurred, cross-legged progression may be necessary on account of the inability to separate the legs.

The position in standing and lying is modified by the occurrence

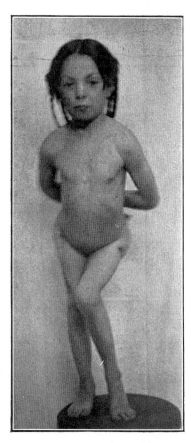

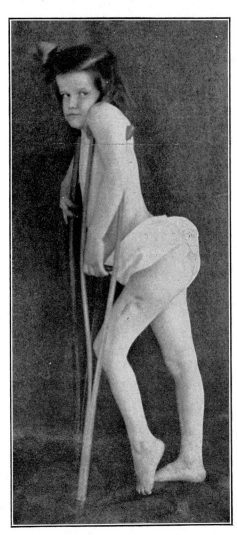

FIG. 56.—Case Showing Marked Flexion with Adduction of the Left Hip Joint.

FIG. 57.—Ankylosis of the Hip in a Position of Flexion Showing Lumbar Lordosis.

of these malpositions; abduction or adduction causes tilting of the pelvis, and flexion causes a marked lordosis of the lumbar spine in standing with the legs parallel; by standing with the diseased leg somewhat flexed the lordosis can be overcome. The same arching of the lumbar spine occurs when the patient lies on a table and the flexed leg is brought down.

Periarticular Symptoms.—An important sign is found in the thickening over the anterior surface of the joint when palpated in the groin as contrasted with the other side. An indefinite oval thickened area is felt deep down. At other times the thickening is most marked at the posterior aspect of the joint, behind the trochanter. This sign is an early one and of great value in the early recognition of the disease. A density in the superficial tissues over a diseased hip which the other side does not possess is often found at a comparatively early stage of the affection. Behind or in front of the trochanter the deep tissues are resistant and the fossa existing there is filled out, and the great trochanter feels enlarged and thicker than its fellow when grasped by the fingers deeply pressed in.

The inguinal glands of the affected side are often enlarged and they may be so much distended that they obstruct the venous return and the skin may be marbled with superficial veins. They are at times the seat of superficial abscesses. A gland lying on the iliac vessels is frequently found enlarged in hip disease and is palpated just above the ramus of the pubis. In very severe cases the upper part of the thigh and the tissues in the vicinity of the hip may become swollen generally from an œdema of the periarticular tissues. This may disappear or become localized in the formation of an abscess.

Abscess.—In a proportion of cases suppuration takes place. The site and course of the abscesses vary according to the seat and size of the original focus of the ostitis, whether in the femur or acetabulum.

Abscesses may be absorbed or may evacuate themselves spontaneously either completely or partially, the residual fluid following along the course of the sheaths of the muscles and the fasciæ, reappearing later as secondary abscesses, the same abscess causing five or six fistulous openings. These openings discharge pus and serum for months and years in most cases. These sinuses after a short time become infected with pyogenic organisms. With the bursting of an abscess and the discharge of any considerable quantity of pus the patient's condition may show rapid improvement, or, if imperfect drainage takes place, reaccumulation of the pus may occur and the patient's condition may become worse.

When the pus has left the joint it generally burrows between the thigh muscles to reach the skin, where it appears as a swelling of varying size. Fluctuation is usually marked. As the abscess invades the skin the latter becomes thin and red, and ulcerates in one or two places, evacuating the abscess. The contents of the abscess may, however, in a few instances be absorbed even at a stage when fluctuation is marked, and the swelling may disappear, perhaps leaving a depression beneath the skin.

The pus most commonly reaches the skin at the anterior border of the tensor vaginæ femoris muscles; it may, however, gravitate backward and open back of the great trochanter or at the lower border of the glutæus maximus; it may come around to the inner side of the thigh and perhaps open in front of the adductor tendons or even discharge into the rectum; finally, it may ascend the sheath of the psoas muscles and point above Poupart's ligament, or it may descend in the thigh muscles and point in the popliteal space. The seat of the primary disease cannot be inferred from the situation of the abscess.

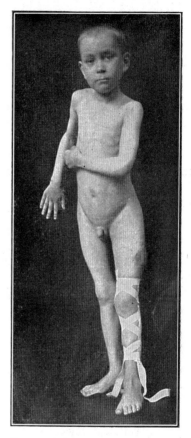

Fig. 58.—Left Hip Disease with Abscess on Outer Side of Thigh.

Shortening.—The effect of persistent muscular spasm of muscles about the hip-joint, characteristic of hip disease, is to crowd the femur against the acetabulum and to produce the enlargement of the acetabulum and the absorption of the head of the femur, with resulting shortening of the limb. Another cause of shortening is to be found in the retarded growth of the affected limb.

General Condition.—Children with hip disease are often apparently healthy at the beginning of the affection and sometimes the general condition continues good, but these cases are exceptional. More often the child is pale and the appetite fails at times; there is often loss of flesh; in some mild cases and in most of the severe ones decided constitutional disturbance results.

Double Hip Disease.—The disease seldom begins in both hip-joints at the same time, and the second joint may become inflamed while the patient is under treatment in bed for the first joint.

The course of double hip disease would appear to vary somewhat from that of single hip disease. The amount of pain suffered in the joint last affected is usually less than that of the first joint, probably because there is less jar or motion when two hip-joints are affected than when one alone is attacked.

Malpositions are more than usually troublesome and may be different in the two hips.

DIAGNOSIS.

The diagnostic symptoms in hip disease are as follows: 1. Muscular spasm (stiffness of the joint or limitation of its motion).

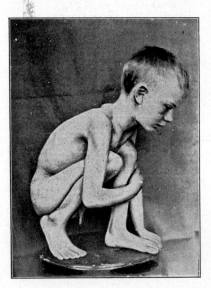

FIG. 59.—Progression in a Case of Severe Double Hip Disease.

2. Lameness. 3. Attitude of the limb in standing, walking, or lying (adduction, flexion, and abduction of the limb), and shortening. 4. Atrophy. 5 Swelling. These symptoms vary in prominence at different stages of the disease.

The early diagnosis is made chiefly by the symptom of muscular rigidity and by palpation of the joint.

I. Muscular Spasm.—The chief diagnostic sign in hip disease, upon which the main reliance must always be placed, is *the presence of stiffness of the joint or limitation of its proper arc of motion* when the limb is passively manipulated. Except in the very earliest stages there can be no hip disease without a perceptible limitation of motion, unless the focus of disease is remote from the joint. This limitation of motion is not the result of adhesions or beginning ankylosis in early hip disease, but it is the result of a tonic contraction of the muscles controlling the joint, and disappears under anæthesia in the early stages of the disease.

A comparison of the resistance of one leg with that of the other will reveal abnormal resistance. Resistance to motion in the direction

of abduction, therefore, is an early test of importance. Extreme
abduction, and rotation of the thigh flexed at right angles to the

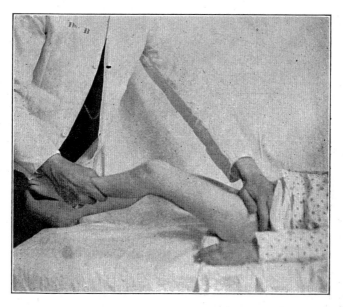

FIG. 60.—Method of Examining the Hip.

body are tests likely to reveal the smallest degree of limited motion.
In young and frightened children the tests for limitation of motion

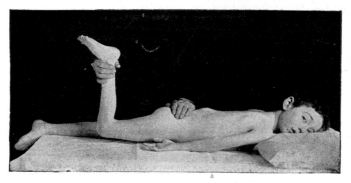

FIG. 61.—Method of Determining the Limitation of Extension in Hip Disease.

at the hip-joint are best made with the children lying on the mother's
lap or leaning on the mother's shoulder. In examining older children

for muscular stiffness, the clothes should be removed and the patient should lie upon a hard surface rather than on a bed. Attempts to move the limb should be made gradually, gently, and persistently—rough force only exciting resistance and making a delicate examination impossible. It is advisable first to put the normal leg through the same manipulations which are to be made on the affected side. The most convenient order of motion in examination is first flexion, then abduction and abducting rotation with the thigh flexed, then extension. The suspected limb should be held at the ankle or knee with one hand, while the other hand will grasp the pelvis to ascertain when motion in the joint ceases and movement of the pelvis begins. Examination under anæsthesia shows less than the examination mentioned, at the early stage of hip disease, as muscular spasm, the most important diagnostic sign, has been overcome and is absent.

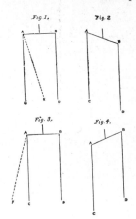

FIG. 62.—Diagram Showing Apparent Shortening and Lengthening of Leg Due to Tilting of the Pelvis.

If the limb is extended so that the popliteal space be placed upon the hard surface on which the patient lies, normally there will be no alteration of the position of the back; if, however, there is a limitation in the normal extension of the limb, the back will be arched up as the popliteal space is pressed down. This limitation of extension can also be determined by examining the patient lying upon the belly. If one hand be placed on the sacrum and the thighs be alternately raised from the surface on which the patient lies, a difference in the amount of motion at the hip without moving the sacrum can easily be determined. The limit to the amount of abduction or adduction is determined by placing one hand on the anterior superior spine of the ilium on the sound side, and with the other hand gently abducting or adducting the suspected limb; when limitation is present the pelvis, of course, moves with the diseased limb. For detecting limitation of rotation the thigh should be flexed to a right angle and rotation tested in that position. The motions most often limited in early hip disease are abduction, hyperextension, and rotation when the thigh is flexed to a right angle. The loss of motion in this group is always suggestive.

Careful inspection in the early stages of hip disease during manipulation will sometimes show fibrillary contraction of the muscles of the thigh, especially the adductors, on sudden or unexpected movement of the limb.

In the later stages of hip disease complete stiffness of the joint may be present. If this is due to muscular spasm it disappears, in

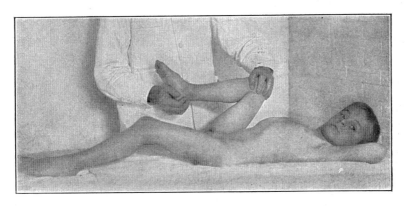

FIG. 63.—Thomas' Test for the Estimation of Flexion of the Diseased Leg in Hip Disease.

a measure at least, under complete anæsthesia. An ankylosed hip-joint is stiff under full anæsthesia.

II. Lameness.—At the earliest stages the limping may be intermittent and not constant.

III. Attitudes.—Abnormal positions of the diseased limb at an early stage of the disease are caused by the action of the muscles holding the limb stiffly in a distorted position. Neither adduction nor abduction of the limb is usually recognized by the patient as such, but the complaint is made that the limb seems longer or shorter than the other. The pelvis is tilted, which gives a practical lengthening of the limb if abduction is present, and in the same way the limb appears shorter to the patient if adducted. The tilting of the pelvis can be recognized by drawing a line from the anterior superior spine of one side to that of the other. This should normally be at right angles with the long axis of the body. In this way have arisen the terms of *apparent or practical* shortening and lengthening, which have given rise to some obscurity, being often confused with real or bony shortening.

Thomas' test for flexion is one which is sometimes of use for an estimation of the amount of flexion deformity. The patient lies on the back and the well thigh is flexed on to the abdomen and held there. This places the pelvis in the correct position, with the lumbar spine in contact with the table, and the diseased thigh is by this naturally thrown into a position of flexion if such deformity exists.

IV. Atrophy.—Atrophy is a symptom of great significance. Its absence in real hip disease is most unusual, its presence suggestive

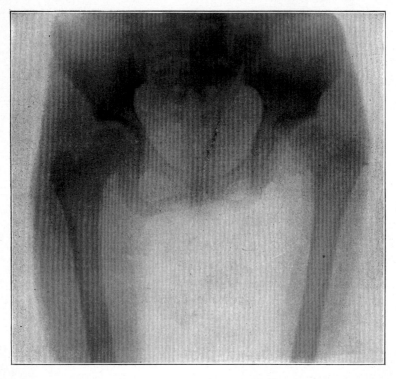

Fig. 64.—X-Ray.   Femoral disease.   Slight atrophy of femur and pubic bone.   Erosion of head of femur.   Thickening of neck of femur.

but not diagnostic, for it exists in acute joint inflammation of any type.

The measurement for atrophy is made with a tape measure by taking the circumference of both thighs and both calves at the same level on each side.   The conventional places for such measurements are at the middle of the thigh and the middle of the calf.

V. Swelling.—The existence of deep thickening over the front of the hip-joint or behind the trochanter is of importance.   It is not easily recognized.   Thickening of the trochanter major is a diagnostic sign of assistance.

DIFFERENTIAL DIAGNOSIS. *Imp* .

Some affections commonly mistaken for tuberculous hip disease in practice deserve notice.

1. **Synovitis of the hip,** of traumatic, infectious, or rheumatic origin, may present the symptoms of hip disease and an immediate diagnosis is not always possible, without close observation of the case.

As a rule hip disease is of insidious and gradual onset—with premonitory symptoms—while the reverse is true of synovitis.

2. **Lumbar Pott's disease** may have for its first symptom a limp and a restriction of motion in one leg. This is due to the descent of tuberculous detritus in the psoas muscle or to an irritation and contraction of its fibres. As a rule, this limited motion is only in the direction of loss of hyperextension, but it may take occasionally the form of a general restriction of motion and the joint may be sensitive to manipulation. The point to be determined is whether rigidity of the lumbar spine is present; if so, Pott's disease is to be suspected. But sometimes in hip disease at a sensitive stage the tenderness of the joint is so great that on attempted flexion of the spine the erector spinæ muscles are also spasmodically contracted and lead to the appearance of rigidity of the lumbar spine. The diagnosis may sometimes be a difficult one, and an opinion must be withheld and the case kept under observation until characteristic symptoms of one affection or the other develop. Later in the course of lumbar Pott's disease a psoas abscess may irritate the hip-joint on one or both sides; this may again simulate hip disease. A test of the arc of abduction of the hip is valuable in this connection, as this motion is impaired or lost at a comparatively early stage of hip disease.

3. **Chronic arthritis deformans,** morbus coxæ senilis, is an affection which would be confounded with a tuberculous affection of the hip if it were not confined to persons past middle life, when a tuberculous affection is rare.

4. **Acute Infectious Inflammation (Osteomyelitis).**—The symptoms are more acute than in hip disease, the swelling is greater, and the temperature higher as a rule. In young children the diagnosis is often obscure until operation is required by abscess. In König's collection of 758 cases of hip-joint inflammation there were 568 tuberculous cases and 110 of acute infectious coxitis.

5. **Anterior Poliomyelitis.**—At the stage of onset of infantile paralysis there may be for a short time marked pain and tenderness, with

immobility of one limb; ordinarily these symptoms are not accompanied by other symptoms of hip disease, but are accompanied by loss of power of the rest of the limb.

6. **Congenital Dislocation.**—Congenital dislocation of the hip-joint need not be mistaken for hip disease, as the clinical history of the former is of continued limp since the child commenced walking. There are no symptoms of muscular stiffness or limitation of motion of the hip in congenital dislocation; in fact, no symptoms of hip disease except the limp in gait. Patients with congenital dislocation, however, at times have slight attacks of synovitis of the hip due to the imperfect mechanism of the joint, but these symptoms subside after a short rest.

7. **Hysterical joint affections** are to be diagnosticated from organic joint disease. In nervous children at the prepubertial period a condition of joint sensitiveness with lameness and pain is observed simulating hip disease. The difference between the functional affection and the organic is chiefly that the characteristics of the former are variable in their intensity and not consistent with one another.

8. **Coxa vara,** a distortion of the neck of the femur, gives rise to shortening and limping. The trochanter is higher than Nélaton's line. There is either good motion at the hip-joint or the limitation is in the direction of abduction, while the flexion is free. The amount of limitation of motion is less than would be expected from the history of the case, which is of long duration. The diagnosis is aided by a skiagram.

9. **Knee-Joint Disease.**—Hip disease is often diagnosticated as "knee trouble," so that it seems worth while to call attention to the well-known fact that pain in hip disease is in most cases referred to the inner side of the knee. Examination will show which affection is present.

10. **Miscellaneous Conditions.**—PERINEPHRITIS AND APPENDICITIS have been mistaken for hip disease. Such an error, however, must be rare. In the chronic forms of these affections there may be slight psoas contractions and the presence of iliac abscesses. In these affections the limitation to motion of the thigh at the hip-joint is not general nor does it affect abduction, but it is most marked in the direction of limitation of extension.

PERIARTICULAR DISEASE, which has not yet attacked the joint or the epiphyses of the joint, is recognized with difficulty. Under the head of periarticular disease may be included inflammation of bursæ and lymphatic glands, psoas abscess, or psoas muscular spasm from caries of the lumbar spine.

Sarcoma of the hip may be mistaken for hip disease or hip disease for sarcoma. The x-ray may give assistance in the diagnosis and a piece of the growth should, of course, be removed for examination.

Separation of the Epiphysis of the Femur.—Separation of the epiphysis or fracture of the neck of the femur, with the resulting distortion, which may be termed traumatic coxa vara, can be distinguished from hip disease by the history aided by an x-ray examination. In acute rickets—in overgrown children—a condition, which may be considered a congestion of the epiphysis of the hip, may present some symptom resembling hip disease—limp and sensitiveness. The condition is, however, a temporary one.

PROGNOSIS.

Under favorable surroundings the disease is one which tends to recovery in a majority of cases with more or less deformity. It is the duty of the surgeon to see that the chances of recovery are as favorable as possible, and when recovery occurs that it shall result with the least deformity and the most useful limb possible.

Mortality.—The rate of the mortality due to the disease in hip disease is greater among the poorly nurtured hospital cases than where after-treatment can be carefully looked after. The rate of mortality in neglected and untreated cases is high—especially of the class placed in hospitals; with proper treatment the percentage of mortality has been much reduced.

Causes of Death.—Death may occur from (1) the generalization of tuberculosis in the form of phthisis, tuberculous meningitis, and general tuberculosis; (2) from amyloid degeneration of the viscera; (3) from exhaustion; (4) from intercurrent disease; (5) from septicæmia and exhaustion after suppuration.

Functional Results.—Spontaneous cure may result in hip disease, but as a rule with little motion and with marked deformity.

Recovery with motion after extensive tuberculous hip disease is rare, but occurs even in hospital cases. From this condition to complete loss of motion the cases range according to the thoroughness of treatment, the severity of the disease in the individual case, and the resistance of the child. The earlier that treatment is begun the better the outlook.

Length of Time for Treatment.—The early discontinuance of treatment may be a serious mistake, as relapses occur in some instances when the joint has apparently fully recovered. Treatment should be continued not only until the bone has become not only sufficiently strong to bear weight without pain and muscular spasm, but to withstand the bruises of falls or violent activity. The length of time for careful observation to insure against relapses is long. Under careful treatment recovery should take place without distortion. To secure this, mechanical treatment is needed for a long period after the cessation of active symptoms.

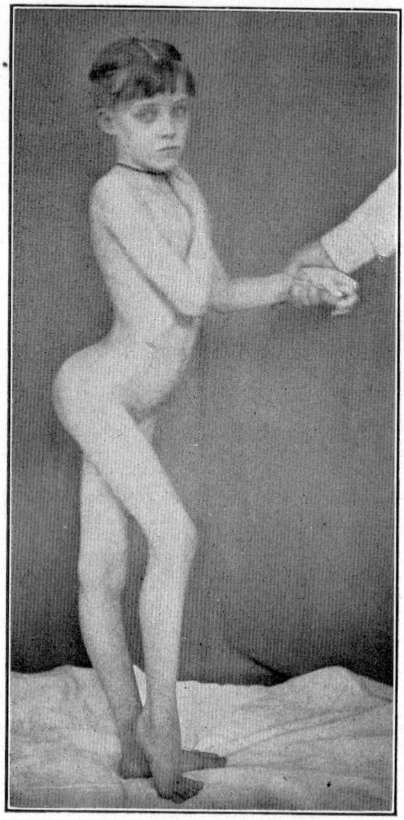

Actual shortening due to arrest of growth of the limb is beyond the control of the surgeon; but shortening from subluxation or dislocation of the head of the femur or enlargement of the acetabulum may be said to be preventable under proper treatment.

Fig. 65.—Cured Case with Marked Permanent Flexion, showing Lumbar Lordosis.

TREATMENT.

Measures of advantage in combating tuberculosis in general, fresh air and the improvement in metabolism are of importance in the treatment of tuberculous ostitis of the hip, as of other joints—but the hip-joint differs from the other joints anatomically in that it is deep-set and is surrounded by strong muscles. These, in case of acute inflammation of the joint, develop a condition of exaggerated irritability analogous to the blepharospasm in ulceration of the cornea. This condition needs surgical consideration, as unless checked it will develop deformity and destruction of the joint.

It is necessary in the acute stages to fix the joint to check or heal existing ostitis, and it is difficult to do so, as it is not easy to secure firmly the upper portion of the joint, viz., the pelvis, which, owing to the mobility of the lumbar vertebræ, is not secured by fixing the trunk; but unless reasonable fixation is secured the muscular spasm of the joint muscles will be increased by repeated jar. These muscles are in hip-joint inflammation in a state of reflex irritability or of tonic spasm, and either crowd the head of the femur against the acetabulum by a continued muscular contraction or inflict upon the joint the injury of a sudden muscular contraction of all the muscles around the hip. Adults who have experienced these attacks of muscular spasm liken the sensation to that of a blow of a sledge-hammer upon the hip.

The indications for surgical treatment in hip disease consist of the employment of such measures as will check and promote the healing

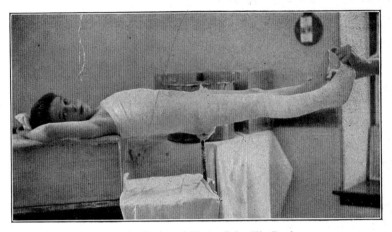

Fig. 66.—Application of Plaster Spica Hip Bandage.

of the local lesion, correct and prevent the development of deformity, and secure the best possible ultimate functional result.

As far as is possible without injury to the diseased condition of the joint, the treatment should be ambulatory, as confinement to the bed, unless necessary to check pain or conserve strength, injures the general condition.

Plaster-of-Paris Spica.—The plaster-of-Paris bandage spica furnishes a ready means of serviceable fixation of the hip. The patient, anæsthetized if necessary, is placed upon a spica stand and a moderate amount of traction is applied to the limb, which should be abducted from 20° to 30°. The skin in the perineum and over regions of bone prominence is to be protected by wadding and a smooth bandage applied in the acutest stage. It is advisable to include the well hip temporarily, removing this portion of the bandage when the symptoms of acute sensitiveness, if present, subside. The bandage should reach well up on the thorax and include the foot, if an adequate amount of joint fixation is desired. Locomotion is possible with crutches if the foot on the well side is raised by means of a raised

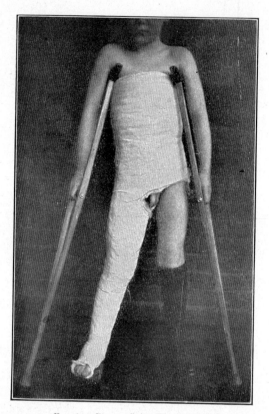

FIG. 67.—Plaster Spica Hip Bandage.

sole. A short plaster spica bandage does not fix the hip-joint, and though it checks, does not prevent the development of deformity. An effective plaster spica or its substitutes, stiffened leather or celluloid paste appliances moulded from plaster casts, if efficient, are cumbersome. They are irksome to large patients and burdensome to the very small, and lighter and equally efficient appliances are desirable.

Traction and Abduction Splint.—Various forms of apparatus have been devised for the purpose of fixing the hip by means of a traction force and at the same time overcoming the chronic muscular spasm at the hip. The one here described has demonstrated its efficiency for several years at the Boston Children's Hospital. It consists of two steel rods, longer than the affected limb, connected below by a flat bar furnished with a small windlass attachment to furnish traction, and above by a ring open in front, obliquely placed upon the rods so as to fit the buttock from the tuber ischii to above the great trochanter, as in the well-known Thomas knee splint. Attached to the ring near the top of the inner rod is welded a bent steel rod, which passes above the symphysis pubis and under the perineum of the well side, and should be long enough so that the end should not press into the buttock when the patient is seated. The upper rings are padded and covered with leather, and if properly shaped are not soiled by the feces or urine. Traction is furnished by means of adhesive plaster straps applied to the limb attached to webbing straps secured to the windlass. Circular leather straps steady the limb. It will be found that more fixation of the hip-joint is furnished than by the ordinary plaster-of-Paris spica bandage; and while the appliance is much less cumbersome, the limb is held well abducted and the tendency to the deformity of adduction checked. The appliance is light, not expensive, and requires no more skill in adjust-

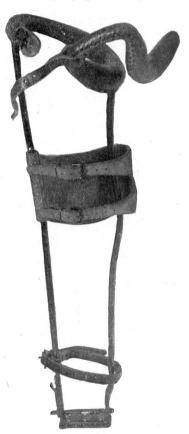

FIG. 68.—Abduction Splint for Traction in Hip Disease.

ment than is easily acquired by any one familiar with the use of appliances. Locomotion is made possible if a raised sole is applied to the well foot, but crutches are advisable in the more acute stage.

Recumbent Treatment.—In the most acute stage a convenient method of treatment will be furnished by the use of bed traction and the bed frame. The child is placed upon the back upon a frame, and the shoulders, pelvis, and unaffected leg are secured by means of straps. Traction is then applied to the length of the leg by a pulley

attached to the foot of the bed. This pulley is arranged in such a
way that it pulls upon the diseased leg in the line in which it is held
when the pelvis is placed square upon the frame. If flexion is present

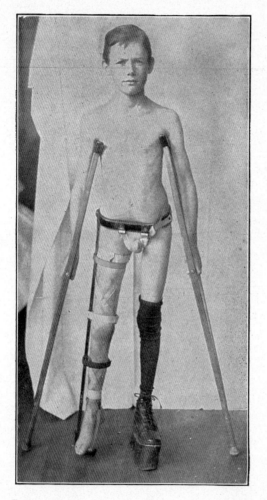 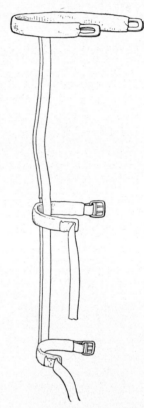

FIG. 69.—Traction Hip Splint, High Sole and Crutches   FIG. 70.—Thomas Hip Splint Covered
            Applied.   and Provided with Straps.

the pulley is elevated, and if adduction or abduction is present the
leg is pulled in or out. If the leg is pulled in a position of flexion, it
is held in position by an inclined plane or by a firm pad placed under
it. The amount of traction force to be used is a question of judgment
in each case, but as much weight should be applied as can be borne

without discomfort to the patient.   The foot of the bed should be raised to furnish counter-traction, or an attachment can be made allowing the weight and pulley to play on an attachment to the bed frame. In cases in which traction efficiently used does not afford relief, lateral traction may be added.   This is furnished by means of a cloth band passing around the inner side of the upper part of the thigh which runs straight out, and is attached to a weight hanging over the edge of the bed.   Resistance to this pull is furnished by another cloth band running around the ilium on the diseased side, passing around the patient, and over the other side of the bed to be attached to

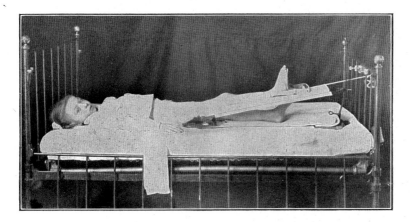

Fig. 71.—Traction by Inclined Plane.

another weight.   The amount of these weights is to be determined by the comfort of the patient.   When the acute stage has subsided and deformities have been corrected the ambulatory treatment already described can be employed.

Traction Straps.—The readiest way to obtain the hold upon the limb for an extending force is by means of adhesive plaster applied as indicated in the diagram.   It should be applied firmly to the thigh above the knee.   If applied to the leg alone, traction falls upon the knee and may cause relaxation of the ligaments of that joint.   Efficient plaster should be used, of a kind that will adhere readily without being heated.   The plasters should be changed every three or four weeks, or oftener if they cause irritation.   They can readily be removed, if the skin and plasters be thoroughly moistened with benzin or ether.   If any portion of the limb is chafed by the plaster, it may be protected by means of a cloth covered with ointment placed over

the part, and the plaster be applied over the cloth and the whole limb;
or if the chafing is extensive, the whole limb can be covered with zinc
ointment and protected by a smooth bandage, and the plaster put on
over the bandaged limb. This will require frequent renewal, but will
answer temporarily. A bandage applied over the plaster impedes the

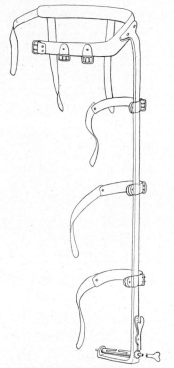 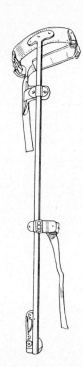

FIG. 72.—Long Traction Hip Splint. (See Figs. 119 and 122.)

FIG. 73.—Side View of the Long Traction Appliance.

circulation and increases the danger of eczema or chafing. If a
bandage is applied over the plaster and worn for a few hours after
it is first put on, sufficient adhesion of the plaster will be secured if
proper plaster is used. In certain cases an obstinate eczema is occasioned by the adhesive plaster, and it is necessary to have recourse to
some other means of extension. Substitutes for plaster are to be
found, gaiters applied to the ankle or straps above the knee. These,
however, will slip if more than a slight traction force be applied,
and are not as a rule satisfactory. Another form of traction strap
can be made in the following way: Cloth is cut to fit the thigh and

leg accurately; webbing straps and buckles or lacings are attached, which when tightened give a hold upon the thigh above the knee.

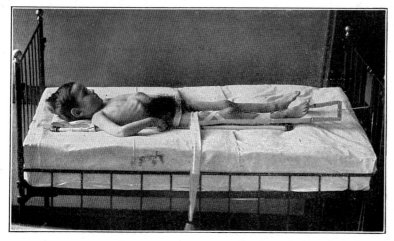

FIG. 74.—Lateral Traction in Hip Disease.

If straps are sewed to this leather or cloth legging, they can be made to furnish fairly efficient traction; but they are likely to slip, and are inferior to the simple adhesive plaster as a means of traction.

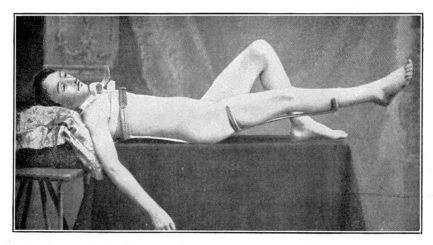

FIG. 75.—Side View of Thomas Splint Applied but not Bandaged. (Bennie.)

Crutches.—With an efficient traction splint thoroughly applied, a sufficient amount of restraint of motion at the hip-joint can be furnished to enable a patient not in the acute stage of the disease to move about with the aid of crutches, the well limb being elevated by a raised shoe. In cases with any tendency to acuteness, however, thorough traction is essential, and walking on a traction splint without crutches is liable to cause perineal chafing and less efficient trac-

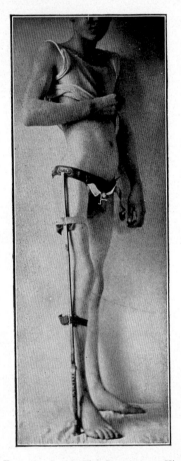

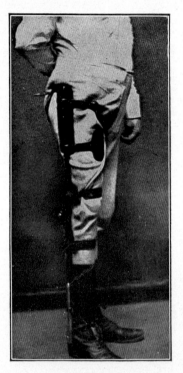

FIG. 76.—Crutch Tip Convalescent Hip Splint, Applied.

FIG. 77.—Jointed Convalescent Hip Splint, Applied.

tion, as at each step on the splint the traction force is somewhat diminished, on account of the yielding of the perineal straps. In cases in which convalescence has been established, crutches may be dispensed with and less traction exerted.

Protection.—During the stage of convalescence and in the subacute stage the exercise of care and judgment is especially needed in the treatment of a case of hip disease. The bone has healed sufficiently to permit weight-bearing without discomfort, and the natural indication is to discard all bandages or apparatus.

But unless the bone tissue is completely healed it is bruised under repeated jar incident to slight falls or constant slight injuries, and enough irritation results to cause the development gradually of deformity. At this stage the joint needs protection though it does not need fixation. Weight-bearing is to be gradually and tentatively permitted, judging each case according to its condition.

The simplest way to protect a joint is with the use of crutches, the sound limb being raised by means of a patten on the shoe of the sound limb, enabling the affected limb to swing free of the floor; but as children, if able to use their limbs without pain, discard crutches freely, and if there is no protection, no check is furnished on the tendency of the limb to flex and adduct, which tendency persists as long as joint tenderness, irritability, or congestion remains. For this reason, what may be termed perineal or ischiatic crutches are of service, permitting locomotion but protecting the joint from the injury caused by the body weight falling on the joint at every step.

A serviceable protection splint is furnished by removing from the traction splint the traction attachment, leaving the perineal ring, uprights, and foot cross bar. The apparatus should be longer than the limb, so that the body weight falls in part or in whole on the perineal ring and not on the joint. The abduction attachment can be removed or not, according to the presence or absence of a tendency to adduction. Flexion is checked by a strap securing the knee to the splint.

It is not necessary in young children that the protection splint be jointed at the knee, although this is of advantage in adults. As the patient's condition improves, the splint can be shortened and jar gradually be allowed to come upon the limb.

Relapses.—Hip disease is not ended when the acute symptoms have subsided; a process which requires so long a time for its development requires also much time for its disappearance; but after the bone is thoroughly cicatrized and the patient has developed an immunity to tuberculosis, true relapses do not occur in a healed joint. Patients, however, cured with flexed or adducted hips may suffer in later life from painful attacks from overstrain of the ligamentous attachments of the joints; this is especially true if the patient becomes heavy or muscularly weak. This painful stage yields to the treatment by rest or protection for a short time. If, however, much deformity persists, correction of the deformity is necessary.

The Treatment of Complications.

Abscess.—Abscesses due to hip disease may in the early stages be absorbed in some cases under treatment.

Incision under strict antiseptic precautions is to be advised in all cases in which absorption seems unlikely; exploration of the joint cavity should be made if the abscess communicates freely with it, and possibly softened bone may be scraped out. The abscess cavity should be examined for pockets, wiped out with dry gauze, and drained. Sinuses may persist for some time.

Where an abscess is well localized and there are no constitutional disturbances it may be treated expectantly and allowed to evacuate itself without incision. If this is done the skin before and after the evacuation should be protected by antiseptic ointment and antiseptic dressing. An incision is made if the abscess is situated where it cannot evacuate itself completely, leaving a residue.

Night Cries.—This troublesome complication usually disappears after the establishment of thorough treatment. It is indicative of an active condition of the process of epiphyseal ostitis and is as a rule indicative of imperfect fixation of the limb. In some instances it persists for several weeks under treatment. In such cases an abscess is usually developed later.

Deformity.—The deformities occurring are flexion, abduction, and adduction, or any combination of these.

Correction by the Traction Splint.—Slight cases of deformity can be corrected by the use of traction splints, which allow the patient to go about with the aid of crutches. The traction splint antagonizes adduction of the limb by its pressure on a counter-point in the perineum.

Correction by Recumbency. In the severer cases rest in bed hastens correction. If the patient is allowed to roll about in bed, or sit up, or hold the limb flexed at the knee, it is manifest that no proper traction force is being used. It is obvious, therefore, that the patient should be fastened to a bed frame and traction made in the line of deformity. As the malposition of the leg diminishes under treatment, the line of the pull is made gradually more in the long axis of the body. The ill effect of a pulling force not in the line of the deformity in the acute stages of hip disease is evident. If an attempt is made to force the limb down in a case of flexion, and a pull be made in the line of the axis of the body, the head of the femur is crowded upward to the anterior edge of the acetabulum by the force applied at the end of the lever, viz., the femur, the contraction of the flexor muscles (holding the limb flexed) furnishing the fulcrum. In milder stages of the disease this is not so important as in the acuter stages, but it is a mechanical error in any stage to attempt traction except in the line of the deformity. This error is often the occasion of increasing the pain and sensitiveness in cases of hip disease.

CORRECTION UNDER AN ANÆSTHETIC.—In cases of resistant deformity treatment by traction is tedious and in the more obstinate cases ineffectual. In cases of this character the use of judicious force under an anæsthetic is advisable. Care must be exercised not to inflict trauma upon tuberculous bone, but where resistance is firm, cicatrization of the diseased area can be supposed to have taken place, and often but little force is necessary to secure correction. Division of the contracted fascia lata and adductor muscles will be of assistance in some instances. After correction the limb should be fixed in a plaster-of-Paris spica bandage, a corrected position with slight abduction. When firm ankylosis is present manual correction will not be sufficient and recourse to osteotomy will be needed.

CORRECTION BY OSTEOTOMY.—The operation in common use was devised by Gant; in this the femur is divided below the trochanter minor. The anatomical reasons which he gave for this step were that the resistance of the psoas and iliacus muscles was set free and that a return of the flexion was not therefore to be expected, as when the bone was divided above the attachment of these muscles. He also called attention to the fact that in operating for ankylosis, after hip disease, it was desirable, if possible, to make the section through healthy bone and as far as possible from the original seat of the disease; in this way diminishing the liabilty of rekindling the old joint inflammation.

Technique of Operation.—The osteotome is a tapered chisel, which should possess a temper about halfway between that of a cold chisel and a carpenter's cutting tool, so that the edge of it will not be turned by the hardness of the bone. The cutting edge should be sharp and the width of the blade about half an inch. The blade should be marked with a line every half or quarter of an inch from the cutting edges, so that one can tell how deeply the osteotome has penetrated. A fair-sized wooden carpenter's mallet or a wooden " potato masher " used by cooks serves as a mallet.

In the performance of the operation the patient lies on the side with a sand pillow between the legs, and the skin is sterilized carefully. The chisel may be driven in through the sound skin about an inch or an inch and a half below the great trochanter, according to whether one is operating upon an adolescent or an adult. The chisel should at first be held with the blade in the long axis of the limb and

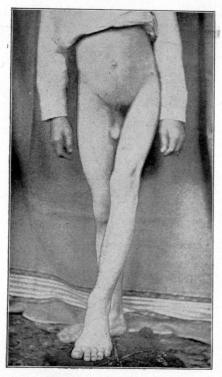 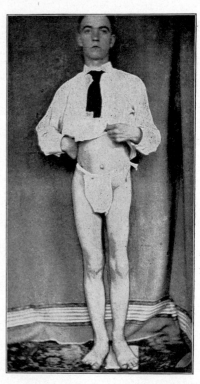

Fig. 78.—Adduction Deformity Resulting from Hip Disease before Correction. (C. F. Painter.)

Fig. 79.—Adduction Deformity Resulting from Hip Disease after Correction. (C. F. Painter.) Same patient as Fig. 78.

turned when it reaches the bone until its edge is at right angles to the axis of the limb. The osteotome should then be driven into the bone by sharp blows with the mallet, turning the cutting edge first forward and then backward, so as to cut obliquely through the whole shaft. If the osteotome becomes wedged it should be loosened by lateral motions. Any attempt at prying with the osteotome may result in breaking the blade and should be avoided. When the spongy tissue has been traversed by the blade of the chisel, it will come in contact with the opposite wall of solid outside bone and will at once be felt to be driven with greater resistance. Then the osteotome acts as a probe as well as a cutting instrument. The bone should not be entirely divided, but when it seems evident that only a shell is left, attempt should be made to fracture the femur—very little force is needed, and if the bone does not yield easily the chisel should be again driven in still farther—always loosening it after each blow of the mallet and directing the blade in a new direction.

After the bone is broken, in most cases the flexed leg can be extended and the adducted one brought straight. If the osteotomy has been efficiently performed little force is needed to correct the deformity. There is little bleeding and a small skin wound, unless it is necessary, as sometimes happens, to make a cut in the anterior surface of the upper thigh, to divide bands of contracted fascia which prevent full extension of the thigh; but under ordinary circumstances this is unnecessary if a thorough stretching is given to the limb after the division of the bones. The patient should then be fixed in a carefully applied plaster spica bandage, which should secure the hip firmly in the corrected position. The anterior spines, the patella, and the vertebral spines should be well protected by padding to prevent sloughs.

If it is desired to compensate for bone shortening it can be done by putting up the shortened leg in an abducted position. The latter will be found of assistance where the shortening is great, as the resulting tilting of the pelvis adds to the practical length of the limb. The risks attending the operation are slight.

After-Treatment.—After the cessation of bed-treatment, fixation in a plaster-of-Paris spica should be continued for at least six weeks more. If fixation in the improved position is abandoned too early the deformity may recur.

The ultimate functional results following the operation are excellent. Although there may be no motion at the hip-joint, the lumbar vertebræ are usually more movable than normal. The operation is indicated in all cases of severe deformity in which the distortion interferes seriously with locomotion, but should not be performed except upon patients in excellent condition, as the possibility of delayed union should not be disregarded. The operation should be postponed in rapidly growing adolescents.

Shortening of the Limb.—Shortening of the limb after hip-joint disease and after excision occurs in a certain number of cases from arrest of growth. Prevention of the development of the disease and such use of the limb as is compatible with the safety of the joint, inducing proper circulation in the limb, may be regarded as the only means at our command, as operative lengthening of bone, successfully done upon animals, is at present experimental surgery. It may be hoped, however, that the method may be successfully developed. The shortening due to subluxation is in a large measure prevented by efficient treatment.

Patients with much shortening of the diseased leg vary a great deal in the relief afforded by a high shoe; sometimes they find it

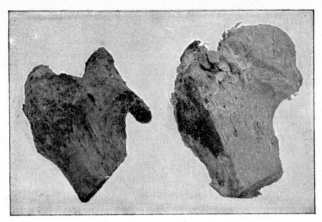

Fig. 80.   Fig. 81.

Fig. 80.—Specimen from Excision of Hip when Traction has not been Employed. Severity and duration of disease similar to that of case in Fig. 81.
Fig. 81.—Specimen from Excision of Hip Treated by Efficient Traction for Three Years. Operation done because of failure in general condition.

of the greatest possible benefit, while at other times it is a constant annoyance. The shoe can be raised by a cork sole, or more cheaply by an iron or wooden patten, or by an arrangement in which the foot, like the stump of an amputated limb, fits into the socket of a specially constructed elongated boot, which conceals the shortening.

Double Hip Disease.—During the acute stage of the disease recumbency on a bed-frame and efficient traction by weight and pulley or by two traction splints is the best treatment. After the stage of spasm has passed, the patient can be carried about in a double Thomas splint and when convalescence is established, locomotion with traction or protection splints and crutches is possible. The chief difficulty in treating double hip disease is in the prevention of deformity, not so much during the active stage of the disease, but after the convalescence has been established.

Deformity will probably not occur if patients are kept recumbent for a sufficiently long time to establish a perfect cure. If, however, they are allowed to walk or move too soon, before the joints are thoroughly strong, weight must necessarily fall upon the affected limbs in walking. If these are not sufficiently recovered to sustain the weight,

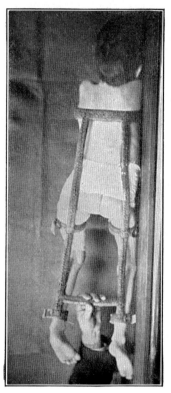

FIG. 82.—Double Thomas Hip Splint, Applied.

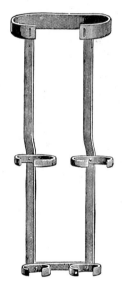

FIG. 83.—Thomas Hip Splint, Double. (Ridlon.)

deformity may ensue. The use of double protection splints is indicated at this stage. Even with very little motion in either hip-joint locomotion is often possible, although the gait is necessarily restricted.

Ankylosis of the Hip.—A firmly ankylosed hip with the limb in a suitable position gives comparatively little discomfort, but when both hips are ankylosed a formidable disability exists. Attempts to correct this can be made, with a prospect of success proportionate to the amount of bone destruction from the previous disease. The joint is cut down upon the head freed by dissection, chisel or saw, and covered by several layers of Cargile animal membrane, stretched well around it, or by a flap of fat, muscle or fascia. The wound is then closed and the limb secured in a slightly abducted position by means of a plaster spica bandage.

OPERATIVE TREATMENT.

Curetting and Drainage of Tuberculous Areas in Hip Disease.— In cases of tuberculous ostitis of the hip, when the process is limited to sharply defined foci surrounded by firm bone, the condition may be said to resemble that presented by an abscess, and drainage of such a focus is desirable. This can be accomplished by tunnelling through the healthy bone until the diseased focus is reached.

The operation is performed by exposing the part of the bone in which the focus has been located and removing it by thorough curetting. The cavity is then carefully dried and wiped out with strong carbolic acid and alcohol or a 2.5-per-cent solution of formalin, and the wound closed, with the exception of a temporary gauze wick. The operation should be performed with as little unnecessary traumatism to the joint as possible. The operation is followed by traction in the recumbent position.

Excision of the Hip-Joint.—This method of treatment is based upon the opinion that, when a tuberculous affection exists, repair is hastened by the eradication of the diseased portion. Excision is less to be advocated at the hip than at the knee or ankle, for the reason that it leaves a poor joint for weight-bearing purposes and because it is difficult and dangerous to remove the acetabulum, frequently primarily diseased in hip disease, and always involved in extensive disease of the hip. Excision of the femoral head under such circumstances is a partial operation. Excision of the acetabulum, introduced by Bardenheuer, is a possible but a dangerous operation only to be employed as a life-saving measure. The operation is performed by means of an incision made along the crest of the ilium, extending from the sacro-iliac synchondrosis to the anterior superior spine. The bone is to be cleared of muscular attachments down to the acetabulum. By means of a Gigli saw, the acetabulum is separated from the ramus of the pubis, the connection of the ilium, and the descending ramus to the tuberosity of the ischium. It is easier to remove the acetabulum without opening the joint, which can be opened later and the head of the femur saved. If the head of the femur is involved it is removed, being sawn off at the neck. The wound should be closed and traction applied to the limb, placed in a slightly abducted position.

Excision in the early cases is not justified when conservative treatment can be carried out for a sufficient time and with thoroughness. The removal of the head and neck, moreover, removes from the socket one of the supports on which the trunk rests, and the hip is more mutilated than after the cure by the natural process of gradual absorption, repair, and cicatrization, which leaves a firm though possibly ankylosed hip. The operation is therefore reserved for the cases where loose sequestra are present, as an exploratory measure where great pain is present and conservative measures have failed, and in adults where time for conservative treatment is impossible.

Method of Operation.—Of the incisions in ordinary use the straight external incision is the one most commonly used and the most serviceable.

The incision should begin at a point midway between the anterior superior iliac spine and the great trochanter, the knife being pushed directly to the bone. The cut should curve to the top of the trochanter and then downward and forward, the length of the incision being from four to eight inches.

The tissues should be incised down to the bone, the soft parts should be divided, and the capsule opened. It is best to incise the periosteum of the trochanter, and if possible with a periosteum elevator to free it with its muscular attachments from the bone. Sometimes the whole trochanter can be uncovered in this way.

After having made the cut down to the trochanter and separated the periosteum on the outer side so far as practicable, the next step is to separate the soft tissues from the bone on the inner side, stripping back the periosteum as far as it exists as such. In advanced cases of hip disease, however, it will be found that all that it is practicable to do is to clear the periosteum from the outer aspect of the trochanter and then to separate the muscular attachments from the neck of the bone, keeping the knife as close to the bone as possible. Then passing the finger around the femur and adducting the leg slightly will raise the head of the femur out of the acetabulum, and the capsule can then be divided and the head of the femur thrown out into sight and sawed off, or the section can be made by a small saw or osteotome before dislocating the bone if the finger is kept inside of the neck of the femur as a guard. If the head of the bone is dislocated, it is more easy to see the limit of diseased bone and to make the section well in the healthy tissue. The objection to dislocating the head of the bone before section is that fracture or the diseased and atrophied shaft of the femur may occur if it is done roughly, and also that periosteum may be stripped up from the inner aspect of the shaft and cause necrosis. When the head is adherent, it should be curetted or chiselled from its place.

The acetabulum should be examined and any sequestra removed and any carious surface should be scraped with a Volkmann's spoon. If the acetabulum is perforated, the edges should be chipped off until the point is reached where the periosteum lining the pelvis is attached to the bone.

After the operation a tube or a strip of gauze should be left in the most dependent angle of the wound and the rest may be sewed up if the tissues are not too much infiltrated with the products of inflammation. A heavy antiseptic dressing should then be applied and the hip should be fixed either upon a frame with light traction or in a plaster-of-Paris spica with the limb in an abducted position. As soon as it is practicable the child should be allowed to move about with crutches, wearing, as an appliance to prevent subsequent deformity, a traction splint.

Operative Dislocation of the Hip.—In the natural cure of hip disease the head is gradually pushed out of the normal acetabulum and the opposed inflamed joint surfaces freed from the irritation of mutual pressure heats.

The method of operative dislocation has been employed by one of the writers in 3 advanced cases of extensive disease when the acetabulum was involved.

One died 6 months later of amyloid disease; the ultimate result was not known in the second; the third recovered completely, and was seen 10 years later, strong and well, with a serviceable limb, with the characteristic distortion of a cured but dislocated hip, a distortion which could be corrected by osteotomy.

The operation of artificial dislocation is performed by means of the incision needed in excising the hip. The femoral head is dislocated after being freed, carious surfaces are curetted and wiped with alcohol, and ample drainage of the acetabulum provided by drainage tubes. The dislocated limb is securely flexed and adducted by a strong plaster-of-Paris spica. Ambulatory treatment is encouraged as soon as possible.

Mortality.—It may be stated then, in brief, that resection of the hip-joint as an operation is attended by an immediate fatality of about 7 per cent. The mortality of the disease after the operation cannot be estimated as less than 20 to 30 per cent, and when cases are followed up for several years it is higher still.

Amputation.—The question of amputation of the diseased limb remains for consideration. The mutilation which results is the chief objection to the operation, and is but partially met by an artificial limb. An undoubted reformation of bone has taken place in the case operated upon by one of the writers.

Absolute economy of blood—of the utmost importance in all hip amputations—is vital in cases reduced to the physical extremity seen in cases of hip disease undergoing this operation.

The limb should be elevated and stripped of blood, and an elastic bandage is doubled and passed between the thighs, its centre lying between the tuber ischii of the side to be operated upon and the anus. A pad in the shape of a roller bandage is tied over the external iliac artery; the ends of the rubber are drawn tightly upward and outward (one in front and one behind) to a point above the centre of the iliac crest of the same side. The front part of the band passes across the compress; the back part runs across the great sciatic notch and prevents bleeding from the branches of the internal iliac. The ends of the bandage are tightened, and should be held by the hand of an assistant placed just above the centre of the iliac crest.

The danger of hemorrhage may be still further diminished by transfixing the thigh from side to side above the line of incision and securing pressure with a steel skewer passing under the vessels. If rubber tubing be passed tightly around the ends of the skewer over the anterior surface of the thigh, the front vessels can be compressed and the same method can be applied to the posterior vessels (Wyeth's method). The operation in this way can be performed without the loss of any appreciable amount of blood, and there is time for due deliberation, as there is no danger of a death upon the table by a sudden gush of hemorrhage.

The operation of amputation at the hip-joint has been performed three times at the Boston Children's Hospital in extensive disease of the hip and pelvis, with operative success in all, but with ultimate death from amyloid disease in two cases. Ultimate recovery took place in one who grew to manhood and at twenty wore an artificial limb fitted to a stump in which reformation of the bone took place from the periosteum.

SUMMARY OF TREATMENT OF HIP DISEASE.

It is difficult to summarize the treatment of hip disease, for the reason that cases differ greatly in severity; some needing fixation for a very long period, owing to a severe degree of sensitiveness or to the activity of the ostitis, while in other cases ambulatory treatment with proper appliances is sufficient without recumbency.

The proper treatment of hip disease is, therefore, not the exclusive use of any method, but the use of such means as may meet the indications as they are present. During the acutest stages, the hip-joint should be fixed efficiently in bed. Thorough traction is needed to check severe muscular spasm. A long plaster spica extending well up on the trunk furnishes serviceable but cumbersome fixation. Continued confinement to bed is not beneficial to the general condition of tuberculous patients, except temporarily during the acute stage; and as soon as the acute symptoms have subsided the patient should be allowed to go about with the hip thoroughly protected against jar and spasm. This can be done by means of a traction splint, if efficiently applied, with at first the additional protection from crutches.

If the acute symptoms return under this method, thorough rest in bed is again indicated in addition to efficient traction and fixation. If the acute symptoms diminish and there is less muscular rigidity at the hip-joint, greater freedom can again be allowed, and the joint merely protected from jar. This should be continued so long as there is any danger of recurrence of active symptoms or tendency to contraction.

In brief, the hip should be fixed as long as it is sensitive, should be protected and distracted as long as there is muscular spasm, and protected until the congested and inflamed bone of the epiphysis is replaced by firm, healthy bone. Distortions of the limb should always be corrected as they occur. In many cases some motion can be saved at the hip-joint if treatment is not discontinued too soon and begun before joint destruction has become extensive and thoroughly carried out until the joint is cured.

The advantage of the employment of traction during the acute stages of hip disease has been demonstrated at the service of the Boston Children's Hospital, the ultimate results 5 years after the cessation of treatment in a series of cases having been examined. In a large number of cases, pathological dislocation, i.e., elevation of the trochanter above Nélaton's line, had been prevented in 70 per cent of the cases, while statistics of ultimate results in other clinics show pathological dislocation in all cases where traction has not been used.[1]

Abscesses can be treated on general surgical principles. Radical operative measures are needed only in exceptional cases if thorough

[1] "Traction in Hip Disease," Am. J. Med. Sciences, Dec., 1908.

conservative treatment can be secured. Out-of-door air, the best obtainable surroundings, with as much activity as the local conditions of the joint justify, stimulating the circulation by exercise, and improving the appetite and the metabolism, are the antidotes at present available to the tuberculous condition. These, if combined with such surgical treatment as will protect the affected bone from frequent traumatism, may be relied upon to effect a cure in the greater number of cases of hip disease.

CHAPTER IV.

TUBERCULOUS DISEASE OF THE KNEE.

DEFINITION.

This affection is also known as tumor albus, or white swelling.

Tumor albus in children begins oftenest, if not always, as an epiphyseal ostitis of the tuberculous type. Like other forms of tuberculous disease, it is, as a rule, limited to certain portions of the epiphysis, and either the femoral or tibial epiphysis may be attacked primarily. Cases are occasionally seen, however, in which the primary focus is in the patella or in the head of the fibula.

CLINICAL HISTORY.

The affection begins with limp and limitation of motion. The disease is usually slow in progress, but there may be periods of severe pain. Swelling of the periarticular tissues, periarticular abscess, and distortion of the limb may result, ending in flexion and subluxation of the limb with fibrous or bony ankylosis; or the affection may result in such extensive suppuration as to endanger life from septic or amyloid changes.

Swelling.—In tumor albus the knee will be seen to have lost its definite contour, the depressions on the sides of the patella have become filled out so that there is an indistinctness of outline which is as perceptible to the touch as to the sight. Most often the patella seems to be raised from its position by a semi-solid mass and the whole knee seems surrounded by a boggy infiltration. Later it assumes a spindle shape and the distention causes the skin to be somewhat anæmic in the more severe cases, whence the name of tumor albus.

The swelling at the knee, unless suppurative synovitis is present to a marked degree, differs from that of synovitis with effusion, in that the swelling is of the bone and soft periarticular tissue, and is not altogether within the joint.

In some instances, one of the condyles—usually the internal condyle—is enlarged more than the other, causing knock-knee.

Atrophy.—Atrophy of the muscles, both of the thigh and calf, is present, and reaches a serious degree in acute cases. It is more equally distributed between the muscles of the thigh and those of the leg than in hip disease. The affected limb is likely to be longer than the other, owing to the congestion of the epiphysis of the knee.

Pain.—The pain of the affection is, except during the acute exacerbations, not severe, though pain on jarring the limb is common. Night cries are much less common than in hip disease, but they occur. When, however, the patient does suffer from an acute exacerbation, the pain and tenderness are excessive. From the exposed condition of the joint jars and twists are very common, and the suffering may be extreme. Tenderness is very common, especially over the inner surface of the head of the tibia. In certain cases, however, the knee is held rigid by muscular spasm, and any reasonable manipulation fails to occasion any pain.

Heat.—Heat of the affected joint may be present in the more acute stage.

Lameness.—Lameness is a constant symptom. It varies with the sensitiveness of the joint and is much influenced by the amount of flexion present in the diseased knee.

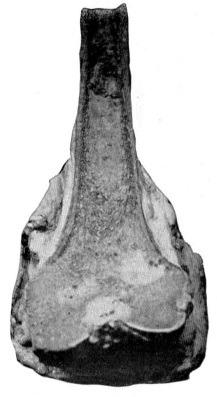

Fig. 84.—Tuberculous Knee in Adult. General synovial tuberculosis. Large irregular area of tuberculous softening in epiphyseal end of femur, extending into joint along crucial ligaments. (Nichols.)

Muscular Fixation.—Muscular fixation is a symptom of this as of all chronic tuberculous ostitis, but is less prominent than in the hip. In the early stages it may be slight. The joint may be held perfectly rigid or in partial flexion, or a certain arc of motion may be permitted. Persistent muscular spasm results in the characteristic malpositions of the affection: flexion, and subluxation of the tibia.

Deformity.—*Malpositions of the limb* result from the greater power the flexor muscles of the thigh possess in contrast to the extensors. The limb becomes gradually flexed almost from the first, and if the affection goes on without treatment, flexion may reach a right

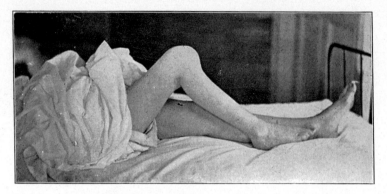

FIG. 85.—Subluxation in Tumor Albus.

angle, and this is the tendency of the disease throughout and a marked obstacle to its successful treatment.

Even when the affection is nearly cured or after a slight injury of the joint flexion may return, which is accompanied by increased heat and tenderness. Together with the flexion, and as a result also of the predominance of the flexor muscles of the thigh, subluxation of the

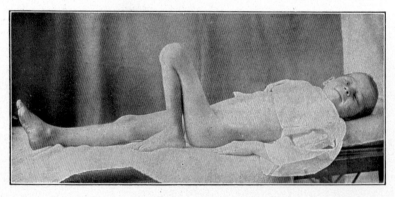

FIG. 86.—Tuberculosis of Knee-joint with Extreme Flexion Deformity.

tibia backward occurs at a later stage of the affection; this is due to the shape of the joint surfaces and the persistent contraction of the hamstring muscles always pulling the tibia backward. If the leg has assumed this distortion and is straightened without an attempt to correct the subluxation, the tibia will lie in a plane back of that of the femur, and the part of the knee formed by the femur and patella will be unduly prominent.

Another result of long-continued muscular spasm is the external rotation of the tibia upon the femur, which accompanies severe grades of flexion and persists after straightening of the leg if such is accomplished. In the same way a certain amount of knock-knee is apt to be present in the corrected limb after severe grades of tumor albus.

Abscess.—Abscess appears either as a purulent distention of the capsule, which may point at any part of the surface and discharge by sinuses for an indefinite time, or abscesses form in the periarticular tissues as in hip disease.

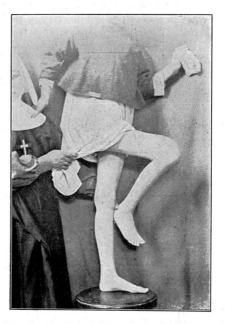

DIAGNOSIS.

The diagnostic symptoms and signs in tumor albus are an intermittent lameness; a general enlargement of the knee-joint, with a feeling of

Fig. 87.—Position of Deformity in Tumor Albus.

stiffness and pain on using the limb; heat over the joint; and the presence of local tenderness and muscular stiffness in manipulation of the joint.

PROGNOSIS.

The prognosis of tumor albus is similar to that of the same affections of the other large joints. The functional results after conservative treatment are in average cases excellent; when efficient treatment is begun at an early stage sometimes perfect motion is restored, but if the process is not arrested an incomplete arc remains and not infrequently complete rigidity may result. The earlier treatment is begun and the more faithfully it is carried out, the better is the outlook as to functional result. In advanced cases disability follows, and in neglected cases deformity of the limb, flexion at the knee, subluxation of the tibia, and the formation and discharge of abscesses are likely to occur, ending either in a complete destruction of the joint or in a cure with ankylosis.

As in all cases of epiphyseal ostitis of the larger joints, the prognosis as to the time of requisite treatment depends not only on the time needed to check the inflammation, but also for the re-establishment

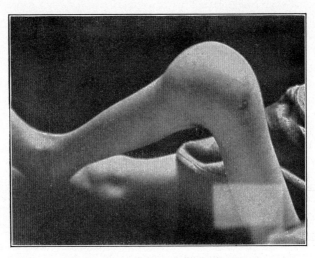

Fig. 88.—Severe Tuberculosis of Knee-joint with Marked Swelling, Flexion, and Sinus.

of sound bone tissue capable of bearing weight without danger of relapse. This in growing children demands a long time. Protection is generally necessary for from one to two years.

TREATMENT.

Conservative Treatment of Tumor Albus.

What was said in regard to the treatment of hip disease may be repeated in speaking of epiphysitis of the knee-joint. The treatment should be thorough and persistent, and should meet the indications, fixation and protection being the most important of these in diseases of the knee. The employment of protection should be continued until the epiphysis is normal in strength. Protection should be discontinued gradually and tentatively; if discontinued too soon, recurrence will take place, or deformity of the limb will develop. Fixation should be used so long as there is any activity of the inflammation.

In the acutest stage it may be necessary to keep the patient in bed, but ordinarily this acute stage is absent or is brief, and ambulatory treatment is both possible and desirable.

Fixation.—Fixation by stiff bandages is an efficient method of treatment when the bandages are properly applied. They should reach

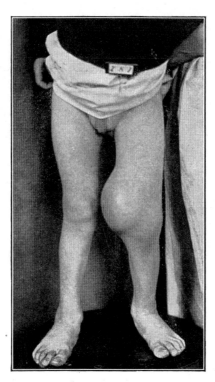

FIG. 89.—Tuberculosis of Knee-joint with Abscess.

from the groin to the ankle, in the acute cases including the foot, and as firmly as possible grasp the muscles of the limb.

Protection.—Protection from the jar of weight-bearing locomotion can be furnished by means of crutches and raising the sound limb by a thick sole which allows the affected limb to swing clear of the ground. Better protection is furnished by means of a splint with perineal support and longer than the limb, which passes below the foot so as to take the jar of locomotion.

Thomas Knee-Splint.—A simple but efficient appliance is the Thomas knee-splint, which consists of a padded iron ring fitted so as to surround the thigh at the perineum, and fastened to two rods on each side of the limb, longer than the limb and secured at the bottom to a metal plate below the foot.

The leg can be fixed by means of bandages and leather bands attached to the splint. With this splint applied, the patient sits in a

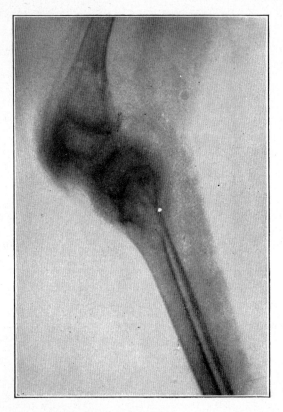

Fig. 90.—Radiograph of Old Tuberculosis of Knee-joint, Showing Destruction of Joint Surfaces and Bone, Flexion and Subluxation of Tibia.

ring supporting the perineum, while uprights run below the foot and bear the body weight.

In acute cases and cases tending to flexion the use of a plaster-of-Paris splint in addition to the Thomas splint is desirable, as better fixation is secured than by bandages alone.

The Thomas splint is slung from the shoulder by means of a strap, and the well limb is raised by means of a cork, wooden, or steel patten. Crutches are not necessary in connection with the Thomas splint.

Calliper Splint.—When the condition of the limb has improved so much that spasm and sensitiveness are absent, or in mild cases, the Thomas splint can be shortened and the ends slotted into the sole of the shoe at such a length as to keep the heel from touching the ground. In this way the patient walks about suspended by the perineal ring and bearing but little weight on the diseased joint.

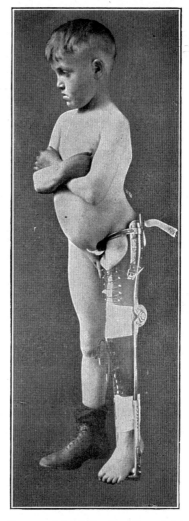

When convalescence has been further established and protected motion at the joint is possible, the knee splint may be jointed with a spring catch and check to limit the amount of motion.

The treatment by passive hyperæmia and dry heat is useful if at all in the milder and more chronic cases.

Treatment of Complications.—*Deformity.*—Flexion of the knee is commonly seen even in the early stage of the affection, associated in the early part of the disease with an acutely sensitive condition of the joint, or it may develop gradually without pain.

A flexed knee-joint may be straightened by the employment of a correcting force applied to the patient in bed; by applying a succession of plaster-of-Paris bandages, each straighter than the last; by employing force under an anæsthetic.

FIG. 91.—Jointed Traction Knee Splint Applied.

Forcible Correction of Flexion. —In cases without adhesions the knee is easily put in a correct position with the use of little or no force under complete anæsthesia. If the leg is allowed to remain in the fixed position, angular ankylosis will probably occur. When firm adhesions have been formed at the knee-joint, correction by means of appliances will be found tedious, painful, and sometimes impossible, and generally forcible correction of some sort will be necessary to break down the adhesions. One way is to break down the adhesions by forcibly flexing the leg, and then by forcible extension to straighten it. The danger of rupturing the popliteal artery, which has occurred, is in this way diminished. Many appliances have been devised to

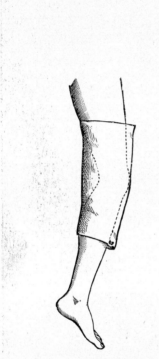

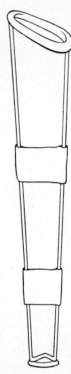

FIG. 92.—Imperfect fixation of Knee-joint by Loose Plaster Bandage.

FIG. 93.—Thomas Knee Splint with Ring Covered and Posterior Leather Attached.

give greater power in forcible correction. A procedure not requiring the use of apparatus is as follows: The patient is placed upon the floor upon the back and the surgeon stands over the patient, holding the flexed knee with both hands, the fingers being placed under the popliteal space. The whole weight of the surgeon's trunk can be thrown upon the end of the lever furnished by the patient's leg, the hands of the surgeon, pulling upon the popliteal space, furnishing resistance. After the limb has yielded and the adhesions are broken, it can be straightened if the patient is turned upon the face; a down-

CHAPTER V.

TUBERCULOUS DISEASE OF THE ANKLE AND OTHER JOINTS.

ANKLE.

THE seat of the disease may be in the articular end of the tibia or in the astragalus or in any of the bones of the tarsus. The astragalus, however, is the most common seat of disease.

Symptoms.—Pain in the joint on motion may or may not be present. Tenderness is often present over the joint capsule in front, and perhaps under the malleoli, and swelling and heat are frequent accompaniments of the affection.

Lameness is an early and a marked symptom. The swelling consists of an infiltration of the soft parts around the ankle. The depressions in the contour of the ankle in front and behind the malleoli disappear. The foot in affections of the ankle-joint usually assumes a position with the toes pointing downward, and in chronic cases with the foot slightly rolled outward (in the position of equino-valgus). This, however, is not the only malposition, for the foot may assume the position of pure talipes calcaneus.

When the disease attacks the medio-tarsal or tarso-metatarsal joints, the anterior part of the instep appears swollen and may be hot and tender. Motion at the ankle may be somewhat restricted in the midtarsus. If the os calcis is attacked primarily it is manifested by the same symptoms of local inflammation without any symptoms referable to the ankle-joint.

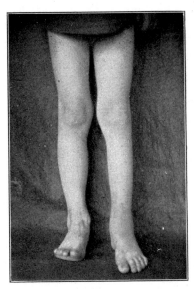

FIG. 102.—Ankle-joint Disease at an Early Stage.

Diagnosis.—The diagnosis is based on the fact that the affection is

a chronic one and is more common in children than a monarticular
" rheumatic " affection.　Swelling, limited motion, sensitiveness, and
pain are symptoms.

The *x*-ray is of value in establishing the diagnosis.

Prognosis.—Unless the disease is advanced, children who are in
good condition as a rule make good progress under conservative treat-

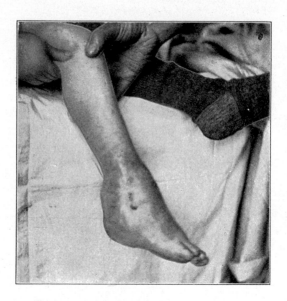

FIG. 103.—Tuberculous Ankle.　Advanced Stage.

ment.　The prognosis is somewhat better when parts other than the
astragalo-tibial joint are affected.　The prognosis in adults under
conservative treatment is less favorable.

Mechanical Treatment.—Protection from jar is indicated, as well
as fixation of the joint, when the astragalus is affected—as will be
readily seen if it be borne in mind that in locomotion the whole
weight of the body is borne at each step upon the comparatively small
surface of the upper articulating portion of the astragalus.　A plaster-
of-Paris bandage is the most convenient appliance for fixation, and
should be carried above the knee so as to fix that joint also.　Protection can be furnished either by means of crutches or, more thoroughly,
by means of a perineal support.　The Thomas knee-splint is a serviceable apparatus.

Such apparatus for fixation and protection should be worn until

the bone is sufficiently cicatrized to stand the strain incident to locomotion. If abscesses form they should be incised and traced to their
source, and if loose bone is detected this should be removed. If the
foot assumes a malposition, this should be corrected by applying
plaster bandages. The general health should be carefully inquired into
and appropriately treated. All these procedures may be grouped together and be said to complete the expectant method of treatment.

The conservative plan fully carried out is justifiable in a large
proportion of cases, and on the whole the results obtained are good.

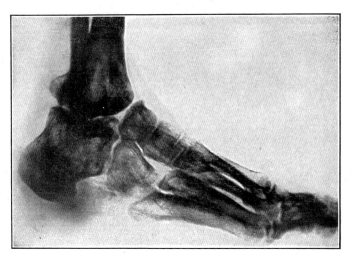

FIG. 104.—Radiograph of Ankle Ten Years after Cure following Removal of Astragalus for
Disease. (Case of Dr. A. T. Cabot.)

Operative Treatment.—When expectant treatment fails, operative
measures should be resorted to. Curettage of the small bones of the
tarsus is inadvisable when conservative treatment fails—the affected
tarsal bone should be removed entirely.

The method of choice for opening the joint and removal of a
diseased bone is as follows: The foot is held at a right angle and
a superficial incision is made along the outer border just below the
external malleolus, reaching from the tendo Achillis to the extensor
tendons. The peroneal tendons are dissected out, secured by sutures,
and then cut by a second and deeper incision. The capsule along the
anterior and posterior surfaces of the tibia is cut, the external lateral
ligament divided, and the ankle-joint thus opened freely from the
side. The foot is then dislocated inward as far as is desired, and
the joint can be inspected to any extent. After the diseased parts have

been removed, the foot is reduced to its proper position, the peroneal tendons are united, and the wound is closed. When the foot is dislocated, an admirable view is obtained of the interior of the joint.

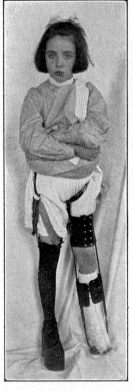

FIG. 105.—Treatment of Ankle-joint Disease by Thomas Knee-splint and plaster-of-Paris bandage on ankle.

The after-treatment of cases of ankle-joint excision is similar to the treatment of the other joints spoken of. Asepsis and immobilization in a correct position are the requirements; and to this end infrequent dressings are very desirable. Plaster-of-Paris applied outside of a heavy dressing is serviceable, as in knee-joint excision. For a time after excision the joint should be protected from weight-bearing by the application of a Thomas splint or the use of crutches.

SHOULDER.

Symptoms.—Tuberculous ostitis of the shoulder is insidious in onset, extremely chronic, and decided impairment in the motion of the joint is likely to result.

Pain, when present, is of a dull aching character, which is usually aggravated at night, and is referred either to the joint itself or to the middle of the arm near the insertion of the deltoid. In many cases this symptom is absent or very slight. Stiffness of the joint is characteristic. The patient instinctively holds the arm at rest, and attempts at passive motion provoke muscular spasm, and if the attempt is persisted in, the humerus and scapula are seen to move together. Early in the disease a change in contour of the joint becomes apparent, which is due to enlargement of the head of the humerus as well as to muscular atrophy.

Suppuration may occur. The subsequent course is slow, the result depending on the extent of the tuberculous process, which may terminate soon after evacuation of the pus or continue to complete destruction of the head of the humerus.

The possible results are: recovery with a stiff joint (ankylosis), deformity and impaired muscular power, or entire destruction of the head of the bone; and in children arrest of development of the humerus may result later.

Treatment.—In tuberculous ostitis at the shoulder-joint the indications for treatment are practically the same as those presented in other joints. Distraction is not indicated in disease of the shoulder,

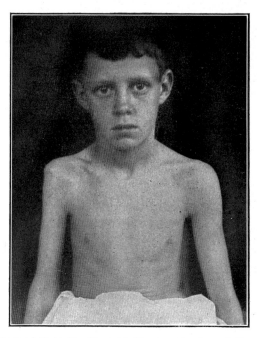

FIG. 106.—Disease of Right Shoulder-joint, Showing Atrophy and Change in Outline.

as, owing to the laxity of the joint, the weight of the dependent arm, if kept at rest, is sufficient to separate the humerus from the opposing bone surface of the scapular articulation; but in very painful cases fixation of the joint by means of a plaster bandage with the arm held abducted or fixed on a padded triangular axillary pad may be needed.

Excision of the joint may be necessary in adults, but is rarely indicated in children.

Where the joint is ankylosed in a position close to the side, functional improvement will follow operative forcible abduction of the arm, with after-treatment securing fixation of the joint, with the arm abducted.

ELBOW.

Symptoms.—The disease may begin with pain, but this is not severe and often is entirely absent. Limitation of extension of the forearm is a constant and early symptom, motion in this direction being distinctly restricted when flexion, pronation, and supination are free. A slight increase of surface temperature is usually found, but its absence does not exclude the disease. Careful examination will reveal a slight amount of swelling even at this stage of the affection,

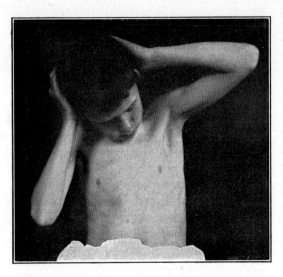

Fig. 107.—Same Case as Fig. 106. Showing limitation of abduction in attempt to raise both elbows.

shown by fulness and thickening on either side of the tendon of the triceps, and, looking at the elbow from behind, the joint appears broader than normal. As in other joints, wasting of muscles occurs rapidly. As the disease progresses the stiffness increases, motion in other directions is restricted and resisted by muscular spasm, and the joint is generally held at an obtuse angle. Starting pains may be added to the other symptoms, and become the source of great discomfort. The whole joint becomes involved in the swelling, the enlargement assuming a fusiform shape.

The swelling sometimes becomes very great. The skin may become riddled with sinuses, the tuberculous infection attacks the soft parts, and the whole elbow becomes a pulpy, granulating mass. This occurs in neglected cases of elbow disease and also as the result of relapses after excision of the joint. Tuberculosis of the head of the radius may exist, in which case limitation of rotation and local swelling are predominant symptoms.

The prognosis in tuberculous disease of the elbow is not favorable for re-establishment of motion, unless the affection is treated at a very early stage. The joint is so complicated that the disease involves a large and comparatively widespread surface of synovial membrane before its presence is discovered.

Treatment.—In tuberculous disease of the elbow fixation is demanded. This is best furnished by plaster-of-Paris or moulded leather. Excision is advisable in the more severe cases in adults where conservative treatment has failed, but it is rarely needed in children in tuberculous ostitis of the elbow.

WRIST.

Symptoms.—Tuberculous disease is characterized by swelling, heat, and stiffness. If the disease is advanced, deformity will be added

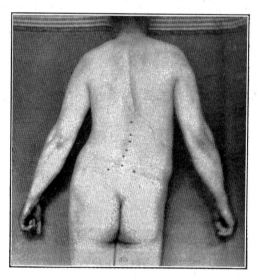

Fig. 108.—Sacro-iliac Disease (Non-tuberculous). (Dr. J. E. Goldthwait.)

to the other signs. The hand may be held flexed on the forearm at an angle of $120°$ to $130°$.

Treatment.—In tuberculous disease of the wrist-joint fixation is indicated, and it is most easily obtained by the application of anterior and posterior common wooden splints and carrying the arm in a sling. Plaster-of-Paris or a moulded leather splint forms a more permanent dressing and is equally comfortable. Compression is a valuable addition to the treatment in addition to the usual mechanical measures.

Active and passive congestion, by suction, dry heat, and artificial stasis, is of value in affections of the knee, elbow, ankle, and wrist in the less acute stages.

Excision of the joint is rarely indicated in children in the less active stage, but may be needed in adults. Other things being equal, a loose joint entails less power in the hands and fingers than a stiff one.

Here, as in other excisions, informal methods of operating may be necessary on account of the situation of abscesses and sinuses.

SACRO-ILIAC DISEASE.

By sacro-iliac disease is meant disease of the sacro-iliac synchondrosis. This affection is also known as sacro-coxitis (Hueter), sacrarthrocace, and sacro-coxalgie.

Disease of this joint is a rare condition. It is essentially a disease of young adult life, being slightly more common in men than in women. It occurs occasionally in children.

Tuberculous disease of the sacro-iliac articulation is a rare affection and extremely rare in children. When it occurs it is usually secondary to tuberculous ostitis elsewhere.

The early symptoms are limp and a peculiar attitude, the patient leaning away from the affected side; there are swelling and pain on deep pressure over the region of the sacro-iliac articulation, and some limitation in motion of the limb, but less than in hip disease. The prognosis is unfavorable. The treatment is fixation by a plaster or leather belt and the use of crutches when locomotion is possible.

CHAPTER VI.

INFECTIOUS OSTEOMYELITIS—INFECTIOUS SYNOVITIS AND ARTHRITIS.

INFECTIOUS OSTEOMYELITIS.

This process, primarily attacking the bones and at times secondarily affecting the joints, is the result of an infection by some pyogenic bacterium. It attacks preferably the diaphysis of the long bones, generally near the epiphysis, and usually one bone only is attacked. If it is confined to the shaft of the bone the joints are not involved, but when it is located near the ends of the bone the joints may be invaded.

Etiology. —The organisms found are the usual pyogenic bacilli, but the pneumococcus at times is the cause of a process indistinguishable from that caused by the streptococcus. The typhoid bacilli may cause ostitis, and secondary infections with other organisms have been reported. The femur, the tibia, and the humerus are the bones most commonly attacked.

It occurs most commonly at or shortly after the age of puberty. The affection may arise in the bone without evidence of disease in other tissues, while at other times it is secondary to a local infection in some other part of the body. The disease appears frequently after trauma, extreme fatigue, and exposure to cold and wet; it also occurs secondarily to such diseases as typhoid fever, scarlet fever, etc.

Pathology.—The bone marrow is the part primarily attacked, and the trabeculæ and cortex are at first but slightly involved. The process may spread extensively in the marrow before it pierces the cortex, where it extends and causes suppuration between the bone and periosteum and later in the soft tissues, developing an abscess which may evacuate, with the establishment of a sinus leading to necrosed bone. If the periosteum has been extensively separated from the cortex, extensive necrosis of the shaft follows, surrounded by a formation of dense cicatricial bone. As a rule the process does not extend to the epiphysis, but there may be a complete destruction of the epiphyseal line and a separation of the epiphysis. Deformities may de-

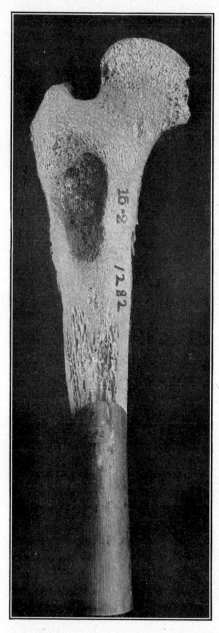

Fig. 109.—Cavity from Bone Abscess.

velop as a result of the destructive changes in the soft parts adjacent to the joint, which cause impairment of motion, ankylosis, and displacement of joint surfaces.

Symptoms.—T h e affection frequently begins suddenly with severe general disturbances, accompanied by pain in the affected bone; if in the vicinity of a joint it is held rigid on account of the pain. At other times the attack is much less severe, the general symptoms being those of a moderate general infection. In addition to the pain there are present swelling and tenderness of the parts about the affected bone, elevation of temperature of a greater or less degree, increase of pulse, and symptoms of sepsis in a degree varying with the severity of the case. Increased leucocytosis is present. The stage of onset, especially when of moderate severity, may be overlooked by the attendants of the patient, whose attention is centred on the severity of the general symptoms. If the disease is left unrelieved the condition becomes rapidly worse, in the severer cases markedly septic symptoms appearing.

Diagnosis.—The diagnostic signs of the condition are rapid onset, marked rise of temperature, symptoms of sepsis, increased leucocytosis, and signs of a severe inflammatory process over one of the long bones. In the early stage the x-ray does not afford a reliable means of diagnosis.

Prognosis.—In the severer types of this affection the condition is grave and the danger of septicæmia is considerable. The prognosis depends in a measure on the stage of the infection at which operative relief is afforded. In the less severe cases a stage of extreme pain persisting for some weeks is followed by abscess development with necrosis and the establishment of sinuses. When the affection is near the joint in young children the liability to dislocation and separation of the epiphysis is to be borne in mind. Young infants, who are frequently affected, in the majority of cases make good recoveries with early operative treatment. The motion of the joint is not necessarily lost where early operation is undertaken, but ankylosis is a common outcome of the severe grades of the condition.

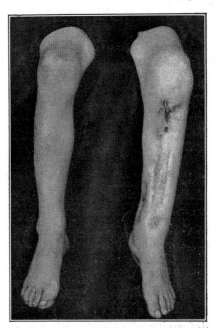

FIG. 110.—Acute Infectious Osteomyelitis of Tibia Involving Knee-joint.

Treatment.—The treatment varies with the stage of the disease. In the acute stage if the symptoms are at all severe the indication is to cut down upon the diseased area and to establish drainage. As the focus is in the marrow, the cortex of the bone is to be opened until the marrow is reached and drainage established. Where exact localization is not possible the bone can be trephined in the diaphysis near the epiphyseal line. The marrow should not be curetted. If the symptoms are slight it may be safe to delay active interference, but judgment should favor incision and drainage in all doubtful cases.

In the subacute stage it is desirable to remove the necrotic area to establish the regeneration which takes place through the periosteum. The periosteum should be separated from the bone, and in cases with extensive disease the diseased shaft removed and the inner edges of the periosteum placed in apposition, to favor the formation of new bone. The removal of this necrotic portion should not be attempted until the acute stage has passed, usually about two months after the first onset of the disease.

In the chronic stage the treatment involves the consideration not only of the removal of the sequestrum, but the filling of the remaining cavity with normal bone. As the cavity is surrounded by thick, hard bone with little vascularity, it does not readily develop new, healthy bone growth.[1] The removal of the shaft as well as the sequestrum and stitching the surfaces of the uppermost sides together is indicated in such cases. The experience of the writers has not been favorable

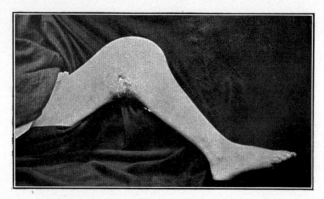

Fig. 111.—Acute Osteomyelitis of the Knee-joint.

to the use of the iodoform wax bone plug in such bone cavities and they prefer to allow the cavity to fill from clot.

When the joint is involved, in the acute stage, drainage should be established as soon as possible by free incisions. In the subacute stage where no sinus has been established the joint will need fixation and protection to check the progress of the disease and to prevent deformity. In the chronic stage with sinuses and sequestra, the treatment consists of the thorough drainage of bone with the free removal of the hardened bone. If the cavity necessary for complete drainage is a large one, it can be left to fill in with granulation or can be covered in with a periosteal flap.

The treatment of the deformities following infectious osteomyelitis is similar to that of the deformities following tuberculous ostitis.

SPINE.

Acute Osteomyelitis.—The spine is not commonly attacked by this disease. When it does occur the most common age of onset is from six to fifteen, but younger children and adults are not exempt.

[1] Journal of Amer. Med. Assn., February 13th, 1904.

The process may attack either the vertebral arches or the bodies, and is of the same general character as osteomyelitis elsewhere, modified by the peculiar structure of the vertebral column. The lumbar region is most frequently affected, but no part of the spine is exempt.

The *symptoms* are stiffness, tenderness and pain, high fever, and much constitutional disturbance as described above. Abscess occurs in practically all cases and the tissues around the abscess become œdematous. Although posterior abscesses are accessible, anterior abscesses are almost impossible to locate. Paralysis occurs in about one-third of the cases.

Deformity of the spine is not of frequent occurrence, because, although the process is rapidly destructive, the new formation of bone is rapid and the severity of the disease necessitates recumbency. The mortality is high in the more severe cases.

Direct incision to the bone, furnishing drainage, is indicated as soon as is possible. During convalescence the spine should be supported as in Pott's disease.

Typhoid Spine.—In the later stages of typhoid fever, an acute, painful condition of the spine, presenting symptoms similar to those of very acute Pott's disease, occasionally is seen. Deformity is not the rule and when it occurs is small in extent, and thickening of portions of the spinal column may be felt on palpation. The prognosis for ultimate recovery is good and the treatment does not differ from that of acute Pott's disease.

HIP.

Acute Osteomyelitis.—This location of osteomyelitis is comparatively frequent, and the process may be acute and rapidly destructive, or slower and less acute. In infants it is rather a violent process, accompanied by high fever and much swelling about the hip, and pain and constitutional disturbance are marked. Flexion of the limb and muscular spasm are pronounced and abscess occurs in most, if not in all cases. The process may cause separation of the epiphysis of the femur, destruction of the head of the femur, or dislocation of the hip by destruction of the capsule without destruction of the head. In each of these conditions the hip is found completely dislocated with perhaps grating in the joint, and this is spoken of as *floating pseudoarthrosis* or *pseudoarthrose flottante*.[1] Extensive osteomyelitis of the femur may remain after the hip symptoms have been relieved by operation.

[1] Ducroquet et Besançon: Presse Méd., No. 15, 1903.

In older children the process is less violent and bears more resemblance to tuberculosis of the hip in its clinical aspect, except that the symptoms, are, as a rule, more acute and severe. Shortening may occur rapidly and abscess is practically universal in the severer cases. In some cases the affection is less acute, and in these the diagnosis from tuberculosis often cannot be made until the abscess is opened and a culture made from its contents.

The treatment of the disease does not differ from that of osteomyelitis in other joints. The hip-joint, however, may require traction or protection after operation.

In other joints the affection presents no peculiar characteristics.

ACUTE ARTHRITIS OF INFANTS.

This condition is now identified as a variety of pyogenic joint infection, the exact pathological history of which is not known, but which is generally secondary to acute osteomyelitis. The onset is severe and is characterized by the same symptoms described above in connection with acute osteomyelitis involving the joints. Death may occur from septicæmia, and the prognosis depends more upon the performance of an early effective operation than on anything else. Treatment should consist in free incision and flushing out of the affected joint with free drainage.

INFECTIOUS SYNOVITIS AND ARTHRITIS.

An inflammation of the joints, which may be acute or chronic, serous or purulent, may occur in connection with acute infectious diseases.

Etiology.—The lesions which occur are to be attributed to the presence in the joints of micro-organisms or their products, and the organisms found in the joints are either the staphylococcus, the streptococcus, or the organism peculiar to the primary disease. An affection of the joints of a similar character is seen at times where no antecedent infectious disease can be identified. In the same connection must be mentioned pyogenic infection of the joints from wounds and similar outside sources.

In consequence of some of the above-mentioned infections there arises a chronic joint affection of another type, not to be distinguished clinically from arthritis deformans. It will be considered in that connection.

Pathology.—The affection is most often manifested by an acute

serous, sero-purulent, or purulent inflammation of the joint. The
process is generally most evident in the synovial membrane, and,
although bony involvement by extension may occur, it is not the rule.
In purulent cases there is suppuration of the synovial membrane with
loss of epithelium, and in severe cases the formation of granulation
tissue, fibrous degeneration, or even necrosis of the cartilage and
damage to the ends of the bones and destruction of the ligaments.
Spontaneous luxations may occur and ankylosis must result in the
severest cases. In a great part of the cases, however, the local process
runs its course without great local damage, for early incision is usually
resorted to before the process has accomplished extensive destruction.
Less commonly these processes are chronic or subacute.

Symptoms.—The symptoms vary according to the grade and character of the infection, from those of a simple synovitis to those of a
severe suppurative process.

Treatment.—In the milder cases the treatment is that of synovitis,
i.e., fixation, compression, hot or cold applications and dry heat. In
suppurative cases the joint should be freely opened, washed out, and
drained as soon as the existence of suppuration is recognized.

The only modification of the usual free incisions in general use
is to be found at the knee-joint, in which, in severe cases, it is advisable
to make an extensive U-shaped incision, cut the patella tendon across,
and fix the knee in a flexed position. In this way the joint is thoroughly drained. The patella tendon is sutured when repair is established.

Gonorrhœal Arthritis.

Gonorrhœal synovitis or arthritis, and gonorrhœal rheumatism are
the names most commonly applied to an inflammation of the joints
occurring in the later stages of gonorrhœa. This inflammation is
acute or chronic, and is most often polyarticular.

Varieties.—The commonest forms of inflammation are as follows:
Arthralgia, without definite lesions; acute synovitis; periarticular inflammation; tenosynovitis; and chronic synovitis.

Pathology.—The effusion, if serous, is generally thick and may
contain clots of fibrin or may be colored by blood. In the severer
cases the effusion is purulent or sero-purulent and the joint changes
may not differ from those described in the arthritis due to pyæmic
processes. Such a process shows little tendency to involve bone or
cartilage, being essentially synovial. The inflammation shows the
same tendency toward fibrous hyperplasia in the joints that it does in

the urethra, which, of course, tends to impair joint motion and ankylosis is to be feared.

Etiology.—The affection has been demonstrated to be due to the gonococcus, which are found in the joint effusion in many cases, especially the acute ones. They may, however, not be found in the effusion or in sections of the synovial membrane. A mixed infection with pyogenic organisms may be found, or, rarely, pyogenic organisms alone may be found in the joint fluid. Suppuration of the joint is not necessarily associated with mixed infection.

Men are much more frequently affected than women. The complication rarely, if ever, occurs before the third week of the disease, and occurs in about two per cent of all cases. Involvement of the joints may occur after the passage of a sound into the urethra, in the vulvovaginitis of little girls, and in the gonorrhœal ophthalmia of babies.

The prognosis can hardly be formulated. The affection is always serious and generally slow in progress and resistant to medication. In the acute stages suppuration is to be feared, and impairment of motion, perhaps ankylosis, is not unlikely to result. Simple cases often recover after a long time with practically normal motion.

Treatment.—In the acute stage the affection should be treated like other forms of synovitis, passive hyperæmia, radiant heat, and similar measures being particularly applicable. Suppuration demands incision and drainage. Convalescent cases should be treated as if convalescent from ordinary synovitis, only with greater care. The use of the anti-gonococcus vaccine is desirable before proceeding to operative measures and in obstinate cases.

Obstinate and persistent chronic synovitis, if in the hip, should be treated by protection, and perhaps traction by apparatus. Fixation by plaster bandages is to be used if the joint is painful. More accessible joints are best treated by free incision and flushing out with hot sterile water or hot weak corrosive solution in obstinate cases. Drainage for a few days should be kept up by strips of gauze, and the joint should be washed out daily in severe cases.

If operation is not practicable the ordinary measures in use for the treatment of chronic synovitis are to be used.

CHAPTER VII.

ARTHRITIS DEFORMANS.

ARTHRITIS DEFORMANS is a chronic, non-suppurative affection, which attacks the joints, at times crippling and deforming them.

It is known by a multiplicity of names, of which the following are the principal ones: Arthritis deformans, rheumatic gout, chronic rheumatic arthritis, osteoarthritis, rheumatoid arthritis, dry arthritis, and chronic articular rheumatism. The name arthritis deformans, proposed by Virchow, is used here, as it is descriptive and involves no etiological or pathological theory.

The disease is common, and varies in its manifestations, as may be inferred from the various names which have been assigned to it. Some confusion has arisen in the minds of practitioners from the terminology, which has associated the affection with rheumatism, the disease having been called chronic rheumatism, chronic rheumatoid arthritis, etc.

Many observers have noted that under the general head of arritis deformans two different clinically associated symptoms are placed. Investigations, especially the thorough and masterly research of Nichols and Richardson,[1] have demonstrated the relation of the characteristic symptoms to two pathologically distinct groups.

1. **Proliferative Arthritis.**—Characterized by primary proliferative changes in the perichondrium and synovial membrane resulting in ankylosis.

2. **Degenerative arthritis.**—With a primary degeneration of the joint cartilage resulting in joint stiffening.

PROLIFERATIVE ARTHRITIS (ANKYLOSING ARTHRITIS).—In this form proliferations develop on the surface of the synovial membrane near the cartilage and on the perichondrium of the articular cavity, combined in many cases with synchronous proliferations of the connective tissue and of the endosteum in the epiphyseal marrow directly below the joint cartilage. As a result of these changes a pannus is formed which destroys the cartilage. In many instances also a layer of connective tissue grows from the part of cartilage which is not un-

[1] Journal of Medical Research, 1910.

dermined by the pannus. Changes in the capsule and synovial membrane also take place, consisting of the development of granulation tissue with fibrous thickening. The joint is gradually disorganized, eventually terminating in ankylosis. Suppuration does not take place, and the process is not acute, although there may be acute stages. There

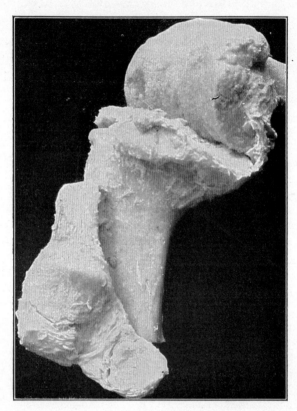

FIG. 112.—Arthritis Deformans of Knee-joint.

may be long remissions; the amount of the joint involved varies and the process may be arrested at any stage. The periarticular tissues may be swollen, but without heat or tenderness. Later the periarticular œdema disappears in part and a shrunken condition of portions of the tissues may eventually result. Disability, loss of motion, distortions, and partial dislocations finally result. As a rule there is an absence of peripheral exostosis. The bones of the affected joint show an increased permeability to the x-ray, probably from an absorption of lime salts from disease, this occurring without histological change. This form of arthritis attacks the middle-aged and the young, even the very young, but not the aged. The affection involves a single joint at first, but gradually extends to other joints, as it is characteristically polyarticular. In the severe cases a pitiable condition of stiffening distortion results, with ankylosis of all the important joints. The disease is extremely chronic. Periods of sensitiveness on the slightest jar or motion are followed by a painful stage with great disability

Etiology.—Little is known of the etiology of the affection. Adequate proof that it is a germ-caused disease is wanting, although the affection in some instances follows gonorrhœa, but in the majority of cases no germ causation is formed. The existence of some soluble irritant as yet unknown is often assumed as an exciting cause.

The prognosis is, in the middle-aged, extremely unfavorable, and very doubtful in the young, in cases involving many joints, but where in the young no more than one or two joints are affected, an arrest of the process may take place.

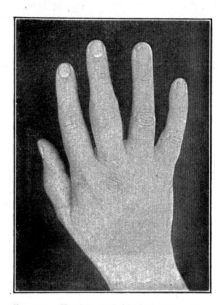

FIG. 113.—Hand in Arthritis Deformans, Showing the Enlargement at the Middle of the Middle Finger. (By the courtesy of the Department of Surgical Pathology of the Harvard Medical School.)

A diagnosis of the affection is based on its chronic character, the fact that it is polyarticular and non-suppurative with a different clinical history from that usually seen in the ordinary tuberculous joint disease.

DEGENERATIVE ARTHRITIS (STIFFENING ARTHRITIS).—In this group the primary change is the fibrillation and softening with erosion of a portion of the joint cartilage. The underlying bone becomes exposed so that the joint surface articulates with a bony and not cartilaginous surface, and with bone which becomes abnormally hard and is eburnated. The changes are not uniform throughout the joint, irregular growth of bone and cartilage takes place, often with erosion in one place and compensating overgrowth in another. There is increased perichondrial activity and new formation of cartilage and bone, with irregular increase circumferentially. The joint is irregularly enlarged; there is periarticular thickening, but, as a rule, the synovial membrane is normal, except at the periphery of the joint there may be pedunculated growth of connective tissue, which may become œdematous or infiltrated with fat, developing the so-called lipoma arborescens. There may be in these fibrous projections cartilage and bone growth, the peduncular attachment may be torn, resulting in cartilaginous bodies, often partly ossified, which remain free in the joint cavity, the so-called rice bodies or joint mice.

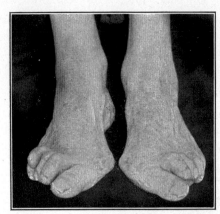

Fig. 114.—Double Hallux Valgus and Hammer Toes. Associated with arthritis deformans.

Etiology.—As the affection is almost entirely confined to the physiologically old, it may be classed generally with senile changes, e.g., arteriosclerosis or fibrous degenerations elsewhere. A toxin developed in the intestine from imperfect intestinal activity, is suggested as a probable cause, but for a satisfactory understanding of the subject, further investigation is demanded.

A similar condition is seen in the knee and hip and in some cases of tabes dorsalis, where undoubted degeneration of the cord exists, but the relation of these Charcot joints to the condition of nerve degeneration is not understood, and there is no reason to assume, in the ordinary case of degenerative arthritis, the existence of any change in the cord. The affection is monarticular, or attacks not more than two joints, except in the hands, where many of the terminal phalanges may be affected, forming what is known as Heberden's nodes. This form is more common in women.

The most constant symptom is impaired motion; the joint becomes stiffened, the stiffening being at first more marked after rest, the stiffness disappearing with use. The limitation of motion, however, increases gradually, until complete stiffness may result, with deformity and partial dislocation; there is never, however, a true ankylosis. There may be little or no pain, except the pain which comes from the distorted use of a limb.

Prognosis.—The disease is one of slow development and slow increase, with prolonged remissions and arrest at any stage.

The degenerative type is characterized by a degeneration and absorption of the cartilage of the joints, with subsequent irregular proliferation, with osseous deposits, fibrous degeneration, and

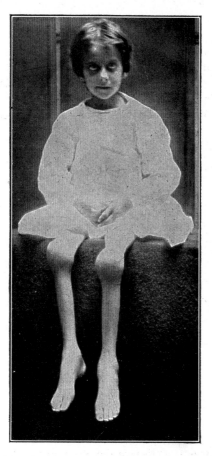

Fig. 115.—Enlargement of Knees and Ankles from Arthritis Deformans in a Child of Ten. Disease of long duration.

degenerative changes of the synovial membrane and periarticular tissue.

The disease occurs chiefly in the middle-aged and old, and is probably to be classed with the group of degenerative processes, of which arteriosclerosis is the most conspicuous example.

The cartilage may be entirely absorbed and bare surfaces of bone left. In other places there may be areas of cartilaginous thickening or hypertrophy, but where interarticular pressure occurs areas of absorption of cartilage are likely to be found.

In the marrow various changes may occur. Fatty and mucoid degeneration may follow the destruction of the cartilage, giving the bone greater translucency to x-ray illumination, and irregular formation of bone may take place in the periosteum, the fibrous attachment of the capsule, the ligaments, and the insertion of the periarticular muscles. The changes above named constitute the chief form of distortion as seen clinically. The distortion of the joint is also the result of relaxation of the capsule in places, with contraction in other places, and to the pull of the muscles from the muscular spasm reflex to joint irritation. It must be remembered that tuberculous degeneration of chronically enlarged synovial villi may occur, but it is to be regarded as a pathological process distinct from arthritis deformans.

The muscles controlling the joint become changed and undergo atrophy and fibrous degeneration. The periarticular subcutaneous tissue and the fascia in the vicinity of the joint are likely to become involved in the process, and are found to be œdematous, and hyperplasia and permanent thickening may occur. The synovial fluid in some instances, especially in the more acute stages, is increased in amount and becomes slightly turbid. Acute enlargement of the lymphatic nodes and the spleen is not often seen in the arthritis deformans of adults. The blood is normal in most cases, as to the percentage of hæmoglobin, the leucocyte count, and the differential count. The urine shows no characteristic changes.

Complications are not uncommon in advanced cases, from enlargement of the heart, chronic nephritis, and the various manifestations of arteriosclerosis.

Etiology.—The etiology of the affection is not yet definitely determined. In certain cases injury is ascribed as the exciting cause, but in a majority of cases the disease develops without obvious traumatic origin. Some disturbance of metabolism is apparently connected with many of the cases.

Symptoms.—The onset of the affection is, as a rule, gradual, and the early symptoms are most often a gradually increasing lack of flexibility in certain joints, which is followed by occasional pain after unusual exertion. Cracking of the joint is felt, which may be heard with the stethoscope. The stiffness of the joint when overused in the early stages is most evident after a period of rest, and in this early stage it may be a long period before the disease is recognized. In a certain number of cases during this early stage, before the marked appearance of characteristic changes, a slight elevation of temperature, and an increase of pulse may be observed, which may persist for some time. In addition to the general discomfort, there may be also present impairment of the general condition, and the gradual increase of the

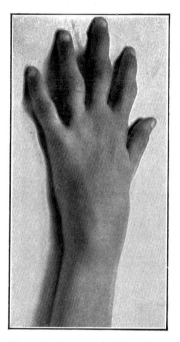

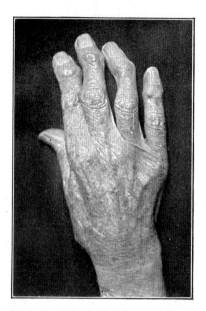

FIG. 117.—Arthritis Deformans of Long Standing (Heberden's Nodes). Marked enlargement of the distal phalangeal joints. (By the courtesy of the Department of Surgical Pathology of the Harvard Medical School.)

FIG. 116.—Hand in Arthritis Deformans in a Child Ten Years Old.

symptoms is accentuated at times by slight acute attacks. In other cases the invasion is somewhat acute, so that the affection resembles what is ordinarily known as " acute rheumatism."

Swelling.—The swelling varies greatly both in amount and in its location. In the milder cases of the most chronic type at an early stage, little swelling is present, but swelling of the synovial tissues, with perhaps synovial effusion, is likely to be recognized at a comparatively early stage of the affection, and is of importance. Later there occurs a fusiform swelling, consisting of œdematous periarticular tissues, the capsule, and the ligaments, along with some inflammation of the synovial membrane.

Stiffness.—The limitation of motion in affected joints is due partly to the mechanical obstructions to motion produced by the pathological process, and partly to muscular spasm, which, however, is a much less prominent factor than in tuberculous disease, except when the process has become extensive.

Distortion.—This swelling may diminish, leaving the joint distorted by the muscular spasm, the cicatricial contraction of some structures, and the relaxation of others, along with the periarticular thickening of the periosteum and other tissues which have become the seat of bony deposit.

Skin and Fascia.—The subcutaneous tissue and the fascia may undergo changes, which are characterized at first by swelling, which may

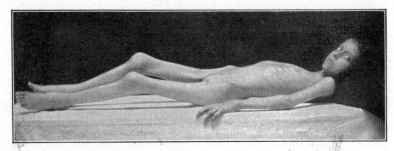

FIG. 118.—Arthritis Deformans in a Child of Ten, of Long Duration. Most of the joints affected. Showing enlargement of elbows, wrists, and ankles, and flexion deformity of knees.

be followed by thickening and contraction. In certain places in the fascia, nodules may be felt, which may be the occasion of discomfort when they occur in the plantar fascia, which is occasionally the case.

Diagnosis.—When an adult is affected with a chronic progressive affection of several of the joints, accompanied by swelling, slight pain, absence of suppuration, with an increasing deformity and an enlargement, partly of bone and partly of the capsule, diagnosis of arthritis deformans is easily made. In the less developed cases, in which the affection is monarticular or occurs in children, it is at times difficult, if not impossible, without a careful observation of the case, to determine whether the case is tuberculous or not. A diagnosis can be made by incision of the joint and inoculation experiments. In children, as well as in adults, chronic non-suppurative polyarticular affections are more probably non-tuberculous.

It goes without saying that an early diagnosis is of importance in order that the patient may be placed under proper conditions before the disease has made great progress.

Treatment.—For a consideration of the general treatment of arthritis deformans, the reader must be referred to treatises dealing with questions of metabolism and dietetics. Until the etiology of the different groups is better understood further investigation is needed, before the surgeon can find definite guidance as to general therapeutics of this class of affections. At present it is known that especial attention should be paid to the conditions affecting health. In the degenerative form it is especially important to promote normal activity of the larger intestines, and to prevent intestinal ptosis, as well as to furnish such a diet as will check or prevent fermentation in the colon and sigmoid flexure. The judicious and occasional use of cathartics, enemata, and a moderate diet, which has been found suited to the individual case, and regular exercise promoting perspiration are important. The diet for the physiologically old should differ in quantity and character from that of the vigorous. Lactic acid fermented milk is advisable where absorption from intestinal fermentation is suspected.

LOCAL TREATMENT.—The object of local treatment is to promote the circulation and to stimulate the tissues around the joints, which are undergoing a process of change, which must be regarded as a degeneration rather than an inflammation.

Rest.—When the joints are in an irritated condition, as indicated by pain, tenderness, or discomfort during and after motion, restriction of use is for a time advisable. This can be furnished by one of the mechanical appliances described for preventing joint motion in tuberculous diseases of the joints or by the application of a removable plaster or other support. Such restriction of joint motion is to be employed for as short a time as possible and to be discontinued as soon as the acute stage is past.

Exercises.—The principle of treatment is that the joints should be used within the arc of their possible motion freely, but that strain, violence, and excessive use should be avoided. Exercises for this purpose can be given in the form of passive manual manipulation or by the aid of such mechanical appliances as have been devised for the purpose of moving the joint without the use of the muscles, such as the *Zander* apparatus and others. As the joints improve, carefully prescribed active exercises can be added to and take the place of the passive exercises. Exercises, either active or passive, given for this purpose, are best done when the body weight is removed from the joint.

Hot Air. Local.—The local application of dry, hot air, carried to a point of from 300° to 400° F., has proved to be of benefit in the treatment of arthritis deformans in many instances, especially in the lighter cases, but the limb should be placed in a properly constructed oven, wrapped in flannel, and the heat raised to the highest comfortable point, and the treatment should continue from twenty minutes to an hour. In the stage of acute inflammation it is not so beneficial as at other times. The heating of the joint should be followed by rest, and, in cases that are not acute, massage following the heating may be of use.

Hot Air. General.—Hot-air baths for the whole body may be given by means of a metal cylinder lined with asbestos, which is long enough to include the body up to the armpits and is heated by gas, gasoline, or electricity. The patient lies in the cylinder and the temperature is raised to 350° or 400°.

Electric Light Baths.—The use of combined heat and light, given off by a number of incandescent electric light bulbs placed inside of a box similar to the ordinary cabinet bath, has been found of use, both as a general and local application. It is said that free perspiration is induced at a lower temperature than when the heat alone is used without the light.

Massage.—Manual massage is of assistance in stimulating the local circulation and promoting the absorption of some of the swelling. It is a remedy often of use, but sometimes exaggerates the symptoms. It should be used with judgment and the joint, if acutely irritated, should be very lightly rubbed, the attention being directed to the tissues about the joint. As the tolerance of the joint increases it may receive more massage, but many cases are rendered more acute and painful by the use of massage applied too roughly, or for too long a time. Mechanical vibratory stimulation is of use in connection with, or replacing massage. It may be given as a general treatment for purposes of stimulation, and locally it serves as a sedative to muscular irritability.

Electricity.—Electricity may be of use in the form of galvanism applied once or twice weekly, or of static electrical application made more often. The wave current and some of the high-frequency currents applied either locally or generally may be of use with these or may replace them.

Hydrotherapy.—The use of hydrotherapy in this disease is at times of undoubted benefit. The combination of a change in surroundings, careful diet, and massage, in connection with the water treatment, frequently unite in improving the patient's general and local condition. The use of warm alkaline baths may be varied by the use of baths of hot mud, a mode of treatment for which special arrangements are necessary.

Vacuum Treatment.—Placing the joint within a glass case and exhausting the air by means of a pump has been tried with benefit in some cases. It is a means of causing passive hyperæmia.

Treatment by Passive Congestion.—A local passive congestion can be accomplished in the case of the knee, e.g., by applying a bandage from the foot up to the knee, leaving the knee uncovered and applying an elastic bandage directly above the knee, sufficiently tight to cause a congestion of the joint. This congestion should not be so great as to give rise to a cold condition of the surface. The tissues should become blue and the patient may suffer some discomfort, but pain should not be experienced. This congestion should be allowed to continue for from seven minutes to half an hour, and massage should be applied to the joints afterward.

OPERATIVE TREATMENT.—When deformities exist in the lower extremity one of two things is necessary. Either the limb must be straightened by apparatus or by operative means, unless gymnastic exercises and stretching can be used for the purpose.

Mechanical Correction of Deformities.—The same methods that are used in the correction of deformities of tuberculous disease can also be applied to the deformities following arthritis deformans, with the exception that the latter occur more commonly in adults than in children and greater difficulty is met in correcting these deformities without an anæsthetic. On the other hand, greater force can be used without danger of suppuration in arthritis deformans than is possible in the tuberculous affections.

Removal of Obstructions.—The operation consists of forcible correction with or without tenotomy, after the removal of any obstructive fringes or lipomata if such interfere with the motion of the joint, or the removal of exostoses if these act as obstructions. It is manifest that when many joints are involved, operative interference is to be limited to the most important joints or the joints most important for locomotion.

The surgical treatment must necessarily be modified by the locality affected and whether the process is a proliferation or degeneration or arthritis deformans in children (" Still's Diseases ").

The arthritis deformans in children is of the proliferative type and demands the most careful treatment, as much can be done to check the progress of the affection and to limit the resulting disability.

The development of deformities must be prevented by apparatus or traction, the use of the limb promoted, and existing deformities corrected. The mechanical appliances used for the deformities of tuberculous and paralytic deformities will be often of service.

ARTHRITIS DEFORMANS IN THE LARGER JOINTS AND SPINE.

Some modification of treatment is needed where the larger joints and spine are attacked, as activity depends largely upon the freedom from disability of these parts.

SPINE.

SPONDYLITIS DEFORMANS.

Osteoarthritis of the spine, ankylosing inflammation of the spine, rigidity of the spine, spondylose rhizomélique, Bechterew's disease of the spine, Steifigkeit der Wirbelsäule, etc., are names which have been applied to the condition. The essential character of this affection is a chronic and progressive stiffening of the spine, accompanied by pain.

The spinal column is attacked by both the proliferative and the degenerative type of arthritis deformans.

Pathology and Etiology.—When the process involves the spine the same differences in types may be seen as those described. The affection may be characterized by stiffness without much bony change, or the bony change may be marked and the deformity distressingly noticeable.

In the proliferative type, the ankylosis usually also involves the costo-vertebral articulation. The process often involves the whole spinal column, but it may be limited to a portion of the spine. The affection may be associated with arthritis in the other joints, or the process may be limited to the spinal column and ribs. There is little deformity, but marked stiffness, and the spinal column may lose its physiological curves.

In the degenerative type the affection attacks regions of the spinal column. The degenerative changes already described take place, and osseous deposits and marginal hypertrophies develop, and the column becomes stiff and bowed.

The patient walks more or less bent over by the dorsal kyphosis, and in stooping the motion is entirely from the hips. In lying down the curves are not affected or obliterated in the later stages. The lower spine is generally first affected and the cervical last. In the severest cases the spine is stiff from the sacrum to the occiput, and permits no more motion than would an iron rod, and in the severer cases the ribs are ankylosed at their junction with the spine, and the

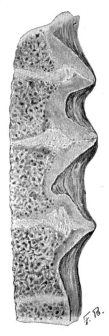

Fig. 119.—Vertical Section through Part of the Bodies of Sacral Vertebræ from a Case of Spondylitis Deformans. Drawing shows the new formation of dense bone along the anterior surface which is especially marked at the intervertebral discs. (By the courtesy of the Department of Surgical Pathology of the Harvard Medical School.)

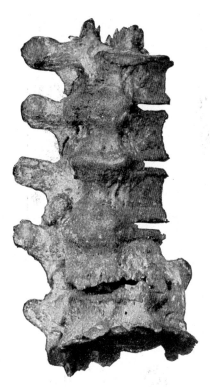

Fig. 120.—Spondylitis Deformans, Showing Deposits of Bone at the Sides of the Vertebræ. (Warren Museum.)

chest wall scarcely moves in inspiration. In less severe cases the spine is not involved to the whole extent, but marked stiffness without angular projection exists in a portion of the column. Stiffening and flexion of the hips is present in some of the cases, and leads to a most distressing gait, in which the whole body is carried bent forward.

The course of the disease is chronic in the extreme, and its duration covers many years. The bone inflammation has no destructive tendency and accomplishes nothing more than stiffening the vertebral column. The impairment of the general health consequent upon this is generally not so severe as one would anticipate.

The **diagnosis** of the proliferative type of the affection can be made by recognizing the rigidity of the entire vertebral column without the angular prominence of Pott's disease. The immobility of the ribs is a pathognomonic sign of the affection, and the involvement of other joints would merely confirm one's opinion of the character of the disease. A diagnosis of the degenerative type is made by the deformity and increasing stiffness.

Prognosis.—It need hardly be said that the prognosis is unfavorable as to complete recovery. Early cases may pass into a quiescent stage by means of proper treatment and the pain subsides. Most cases are improved by support and fixation.

Treatment.—The general measures likely to be of use have been described. In the acute stage the use of fixation is indicated. A plaster or leather jacket, applied without suspension, or some form of supporting corset are the best means of obtaining this. As the acute symptoms quiet down, massage is of value.

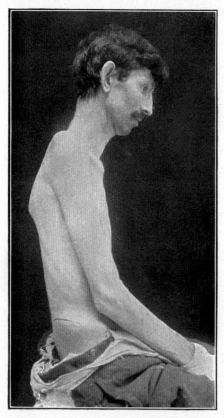

FIG. 121.—Arthritis Deformans Following Gonor-rhœa Involving Spine and Many Other Joints. Spine perfectly rigid except upper cervical region. (By the courtesy of the Department of Surgical Pathology of the Harvard Medical School.)

The spine should be protected by a support so long as it is painful and irritable. The use of manipulation to ward off the approaching ankylosis is harmful and undesirable at all stages of the affection.

HIP.

Arthritis deformans of the hip-joint is an affection which is not uncommon in patients above the age of forty-five. It may occur as

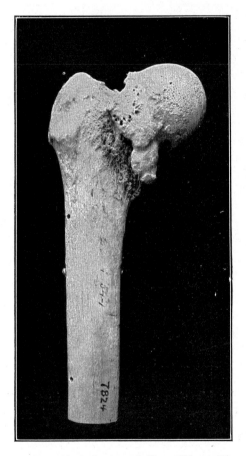

Fig. 122.—Arthritis Deformans of Hip. (Warren Museum.)

a monarticular affection or in connection with a simultaneous affection of some of the other joints.

Pathology and Etiology.—When affecting the hip the disease has been known as senile coxitis, malum coxæ senile, etc. It begins in many cases insidiously, while in others, and especially monarticular cases, it follows after a fail upon the trochanter. The affection may occur in adolescents and children.

Symptoms.—The affection begins with pain in and about the joint, often shooting down the course of the sciatic nerve at the back of the leg instead of down the front, as in epiphyseal ostitis. Movements of the joint beyond a certain arc are painful, and a noticeable limp is present. Muscular atrophy of the limb comes on and the nates of the affected side are flaccid and flattened, and apparent shortening

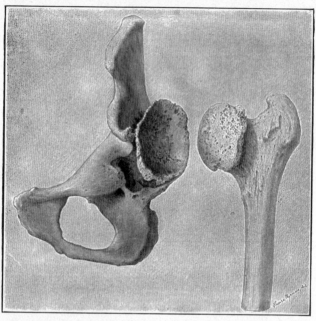

Fig. 123.—Arthritis Deformans of Hip-joint, Showing Shortening of Neck of Femur. Broadening of head and broadening and loss of depth in acetabulum. (Warren Museum.)

from flexion and adduction may be present in the diseased limb, as well as true bone shortening. Muscular fixation is at first not a prominent symptom, except in very sensitive conditions of the joint, but the arc of motion gradually diminishes, until finally the joint may become entirely stiff in perhaps a normal position, or perhaps adducted or flexed.

Diagnosis.—The affection is likely to be confused with other forms of inflammation of the hip-joint.

Treatment.—Arthritis deformans of the hip demands treatment, first to relieve the pain, and secondly to correct the deformity. The symptom of pain is rarely so great as to cause disability. In such cases hot baths, massage, galvanism, hot packs, and the other measures mentioned are often of use. The use of crutches and canes will often be needed. The deformities which follow this affection are usually those seen in hip disease, but they are more gradual in development. Joint irritation from overuse is to be met here as elsewhere by rest to the joint. The use of the protection splint described in hip disease may temporarily be necessary when the joint is acutely irritated.

More is to be gained ordinarily by gradual correction by mechanical means than by forcible straightening in this class of affections of the hip.

KNEE.

The knee is one of the large joints most frequently attacked by this affection.

Symptoms.—Pain, irritability, and a sense of stiffness, especially after sitting a while, are the most frequent early symptoms. After walking a while the knees feel freer, but they stiffen up after rest and are also painful in the morning on waking. Going up- and down-stairs is difficult and irritating. The discomfort is increased by cold and wet and by overuse, and acute attacks of pain and swelling may occur.

In some cases the affection progresses insidiously and gradually, without acute attacks. On examination in the early cases the synovial membrane is somewhat thickened and the surface depressions of the knee are filled out, and the movements are almost always attended by a more or less marked grating.

In the progressive cases and in those of longer standing the painful symptoms are more marked, and heat and tenderness are prominent, according to the acuteness of the symptoms.

At times there is on walking a sensation of catching in the knee, as if something had been squeezed between the bones. This points to an hypertrophied condition of the synovial fringes. The first limitation of motion is a resistance to complete extension, and the tendency to a flexed position is marked, favoring ankylosis in this position.

In general, the tendency of the affection is toward greater and greater impairment of the joint motion, with wasting of the muscles and atrophy of the skin, so that in the advanced stages one can see a stretched and shining skin tightly drawn over the deformed and distorted joint.

The **prognosis** depends largely upon the degree of change in the joint surface when treatment is begun. If it is slight, as shown by moderate thickening and soft grating on motion, much is to be expected from the prevention of overuse and the regulation of the circulation in the knee. If the changes in the joint are advanced, and especially

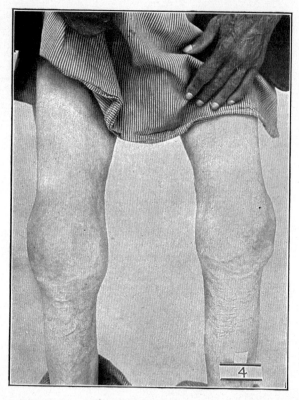

Fig. 124.—Arthritis Deformans, Bony Enlargement of Knees with Effusion. Palpable fringes. Limitation of motion. Crepitus and pain on motion. (By the courtesy of the Department of Surgical Pathology of the Harvard Medical School.)

if other joints are showing signs of a progressive involvement, the outlook is unfavorable.

Treatment.—When pain is present rest is very strongly indicated. During the quiescent stage, the local measures described above should be used.

When ankylosis of the knee in a faulty position has resulted from arthritis deformans, brisement forcé is to be tried for its rectification. It is not, of course, to be expected that motion will be present in the joint in its new position, yet some motion may be preserved in the joint.

CHAPTER VIII.

OTHER AFFECTIONS OF THE BONES AND JOINTS.

SPRAINS.

THE name sprain is used to designate a common condition caused by wrenches and twists, and occasionally by blows to the joints. The injury may be most marked: (1) in the ligaments; (2) in the synovial membrane, which may become the seat of an acute synovitis; (3) to the tendons surrounding the joint. Any one of these or any combination of them may exist in a given case.

The *symptoms* consist of pain, more or less severe, and tenderness, localized at the point of the chief injury; in the more superficial joints ecchymosis of the subcutaneous tissue appears, followed by swelling. A period of greater or less disability follows, during which the symptoms diminish in severity, and in favorable cases entirely disappear.

The *diagnosis* from fractures is important and is to be made with great care. In this the *x*-ray is of much use.

The *prognosis* is favorable and progress is hastened by treatment.

When the injury to the tissues is severe and tissues are torn, a period of fixation of the joint and compression are advisable by means of a plaster-of-Paris bandage or a light splint.

Such fixation should be temporary, and measures to stimulate the circulation undertaken as soon as possible—massage, electricity, dry heat, douches, and graduated use.

In less severe cases adhesive plaster strapping affords relief, especially at the ankle. In many cases, where the ligaments are not torn, dry heat and massage should be begun at once and hyperæmia used.

Sprain Fractures.—In many injuries classed as sprains, an *x*-ray will show the existence of complete or incomplete fractures of the articular ends of the bones, often involving the articular surface. The treatment of such injuries is that of fractures.

Epiphyseal Strains.—In the case of children or adolescents whose epiphyses have not yet united, injuries and strains to the joints may be complicated by a strain or partial displacement of the epiphysis on the shaft, resulting in congestion of the epiphysis manifested by pain and tenderness often prolonged. The *x*-ray may fail to show any gross displacement, but the long continuance of the joint symptoms in such cases should excite suspicion, and treatment should be prolonged until such symptoms have disappeared.

SPINE.

Sprains of the Spine.—After a severe wrench or twist of the spine or after some accident causing extreme motion in one or another direction, a condition of pain and disability ensues, presenting much the same symptoms as those accompanying sprains in the other joints.

Stiffness, pain on motion, and perhaps lateral deviation of the spine occur in the severer cases. In the milder cases the patient should avoid actual exercise and movements which are painful. In the severer ones, the back may be supported by adhesive plaster strapping or plaster-of-Paris jackets, while in the severest class recumbency is necessary.

HIP.

Sprains of the hip are manifested clinically as synovitis of that joint and are described in that connection.

KNEE.

On account of the strength of the muscles and ligaments controlling the joint, gross ligamentous or muscular injury are rare at this joint, the results of trauma being generally expressed as synovitis.

Lesions of the tubercle of the tibia are seen [1] in which, after a sudden strain falling upon the partially extended knee, or after no assignable strain, swelling and tenderness of the tubercle of the tibia have followed, associated with pain on complete extension of the leg. The condition is seen chiefly in boys at or about the age of puberty.

The condition would seem to be due in some cases to an inflammation of the bursa under the patella tendon,[2] and in others to an injury of the partly ossified and vascular epiphysis of the tubercle of the tibia. X-ray appearances are apt to be misleading, as during the normal ossification at this age the tubercle appears to be torn loose from the tibia below. Only when there is a marked difference in the radiographs of the two knees and the tibial tubercle is displaced

---

[1] R. B. Osgood: Boston Med and Surg. Journal, January 29, 1903.
[2] Lovett: Report Boston City Hospital, series viii., 1897, p. 345.

upward is one justified in diagnosticating any displacement of it by force. The treatment consists of fixation when necessary, but in the milder cases restricted use is sufficient.

ANKLE.

On account of its flexibility and its constant liability to twists, the ankle is the commonest location of sprains. The location of the tenderness, swelling, and pain on manipulation will serve to identify the anatomical location of the injury.

The treatment consists either in fixation in a stiff bandage or, what is in most cases advisable, in immediate massage or hot-air baths, or both.

Chronic Sprain.—In many cases the treatment is too soon discontinued after sprains, and a tenosynovitis or subacute inflammation of part of the synovial sac may persist and be accompanied by local heat and tenderness. In other cases fixation has been continued too long, and wasting of the muscles and disturbance of the local circulation and innervation have induced a condition of irritability. The treatment consists of measures to stimulate the local circulation and the careful and graduated resumption of use with the treatment of any static error in the foot.

The sprains of other joints do not require especial mention.

CHRONIC SYNOVITIS.

Chronic serous synovitis is also known by the names of dropsy of the joint, hydrarthros, hydrarthrosis, etc.

Apart from the cases in which chronic serous synovitis is (1) merely the continuance of the acute condition, its cause is to be sought (2) in the presence of some mechanical irritation (such as hypertrophied synovial fringes, loose bodies, etc.), (3) in the presence of some infectious process (such as gonorrhœa or syphilis), or (4) in connection with some general disturbance (such as arthritis deformans, hæmophilia, etc.). Intermittent synovitis should be mentioned as not coming under any one of these heads.

The pathological changes in simple chronic synovitis are represented by increase of vascularity and thickening of the synovial membrane, with hypertrophy of the synovial villi. The subsynovial tissue thickens in cases of long standing along with the capsule, and the ligaments may become weakened and stretched.

Intermittent synovitis, also called intermittent hydrops, is a well-recognized but rather infrequent affection, accompanied by no definite pathological changes, except perhaps a little laxity or thickening of the joint capsule. The knees are most often affected. No etiology has been formulated for the condition, the sexes being equally affected and the cases pretty evenly distributed through adult life. The characteristic of the affection is a non-inflammatory serous effusion occurring at more or less regular intervals, lasting a few days and disappearing spontaneously, to return again and again.

No satisfactory treatment has been formulated.

HIP.

Synovitis of the hip may occur in children or adults. It may follow any of the causes producing synovitis, but the common clinical antecedents are either trauma, rheumatism, or gonorrhœa. Its importance clinically is its resemblance in children to tuberculous hip disease.

After a fall or during a " rheumatic " attack, pain, lameness, muscular spasm, flexion deformity, night cries, and muscular atrophy may be present for a while. These symptoms may disappear so rapidly that one is led to infer that synovitis has been present rather than tuberculosis or acute osteomyelitis.

In children the diagnosis of synovitis of the hip-joint should be made only when recovery has occurred in a few weeks and has proved permanent.

Treatment.—In children cases of synovitis of the hip-joint are to be treated in the same way as cases of tuberculous ostitis.

Cases in adults, which are clearly to be recognized as synovitis, should be treated by rest to the joint, including, if necessary, either traction or protection by apparatus, followed by massage and stimulation of the local circulation.

KNEE.

Chronic Synovitis.—Chronic serous synovitis is at times the sequel of an acute or subacute attack. In such a case the acute symptoms gradually subside, leaving a joint somewhat thickened and containing fluid. If the condition persists, the muscles become weakened and relaxed, and lateral mobility may be present. The weakness of the muscles is itself a source of a vulnerable joint. At other times the chronic synovitis is the result of an irritation caused by loose bodies in the joint, displaced semilunar cartilages, hypertrophied synovial fringes, or lipoma arborescens. The continued strain on the knees induced by flat-foot is at times a cause of chronic synovitis. At other times it exists in connection with constitutional disease, such as syphilis and gonorrhœa, and the intermittent form must be mentioned.

The treatment of the chronic form which has lasted over from the acute stage consists in fixation, if heat, pain, and tenderness are present, along with compression by bandaging or strapping over the front of the joint with adhesive plaster. This fixation should be followed by massage, hot-air baths, and douches to restore the circulation and to improve the muscular condition along with the gradual resumption of use.

If the synovitis exists as the result of mechanical irritation, the irritating cause should be removed by operation. If flat-foot is present it should be corrected.

As a symptom of constitutional disease, treatment of the systemic condition is indicated. In resistant cases in which the diagnosis is not clear, the joint should be opened, explored, and any irritating cause removed.

Hypertrophy of the Synovial Villi.—As the result of a synovitis, or in connection with continued strain of the knees as in flat-foot, or in arthritis deformans, hypertrophy of the synovial fringes occurs to an extent that makes of them foreign bodies. The symptoms caused by them are pain, effusion varying at times, creaking, occasional catching, and some swelling of the joint membrane, with perhaps tenderness.

The treatment at first should consist of fixation in the severer cases, and compression by plaster strapping over the front of the joint in the milder cases. Douches, massage, and the measures suited to the treatment of chronic synovitis should follow. Flat-foot should be corrected and the knee in general placed under the most favorable mechanical conditions possible. If this does not control the affection, the joint should be opened by an anterior incision on one or both sides of the patella, the interior of the joint inspected and explored, and the projecting fringes removed with sharp scissors or a knife. The joint should be fixed for two or three weeks, after which passive motion and graduated use are begun.

Loose bodies in the joints are found most often in the knee, but occasionally in other articulations. They can be divided into classes, according to their structure, as follows: fibromatous, lipomatous, chondromatous.

Loose bodies lie free in the joint or are attached by a slender pedicle. They may vary in size from that of a small pea to that of a horse chestnut, and are of all shapes. Sometimes they are facetted and crowded together like the carpal bones, and again they are mulberry-shaped or pyriform. In one joint they may appear singly or in great numbers.

They are often found in connection with the changes known as arthritis deformans, and also in joint disease of various types. They may be found in connection with joint tuberculosis. In certain cases no cause can be assigned for their occurrence.

In a majority of cases the first intimation to the patient that anything is wrong is that while in the act of walking or stooping he is seized with such agonizing pain in the knee that he may fall to the ground, in many cases overcome with the sensation of faintness and sickening pain, and such an occurrence is apt to be followed by an attack of synovitis lasting several days. These attacks are likely to be repeated without any assignable cause. On manipulation of the joint with the fingers it is often possible to detect a loose body, which shifts its position and is found first in one part of the joint and then in another. The most common spot where they can be detected externally is in the pouch over the external or internal condyle of the femur, and when one of these substances has been found it is desirable to see if others are present in the joint.

With repetition of attacks the joint becomes more tolerant and the synovitis less severe.

Finding a movable body which can be slipped from place to place by manipulation establishes the diagnosis. In cases in which the loose body cannot be found, one must depend largely upon the history, making, however, frequent examinations under different conditions with the hope of ultimately detecting the foreign body. The x-ray may be of use.

The diagnosis between loose bodies, hypertrophied synovial fringes, and dislocation of the semilunar cartilage is often a difficult one to make, and dependence must be placed chiefly upon tenderness in a very small spot over the head of the tibia as establishing the probable occurrence of dislocation of one of the semilunar cartilages. Diagnosis has sometimes to be made by exploratory incision.

Treatment.—In cases in which the loose body gives but little inconvenience and is kept from passing between the ends of the bone by a knee-cap, it may not be advisable to undertake operative treatment. In other cases, especially in arthritis deformans, the joint may have become so much impaired by the disease that even if a foreign body were removed little would be gained.   In the great majority of cases, however, inasmuch as the disease occurs in otherwise healthy persons, mostly young adults, the operative removal of the foreign body is advisable.

Lipoma.—Fatty growths may form in the joints, acting as foreign bodies and causing chronic or recurrent attacks of acute synovitis.

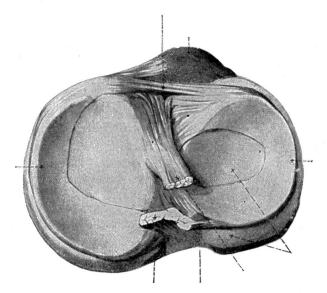

FIG. 125.—Tibial Joint Surfaces of Knee Seen from Above, Showing Semilunar Cartilages. (Fick.)

Although other joints are not exempt, the common seat of occurrence is in the knee.

The lipomata vary in size, being sometimes as large as an egg, and attached to the synovial membrane by a pedicle.   In shape they may be regular or irregular and are studded with small tabs of fatlike tissue.   Once formed, such a mass acts as a foreign body, and clinically a swollen joint is found with little or no effusion.   The function is imperfect and pain may be present, and the joint is liable to lock in partial extension.   The swelling is chiefly noted at the side of the patella tendon.   The treatment consists in the removal of the mass.

Dislocation of the Semilunar Cartilages (Hey's Internal Derangement).—The affection is nearly always traumatic in origin and consists in the tearing loose from its tibial attachment of the internal

or external semilunar cartilage.   The internal is the one most frequently displaced.

The *symptoms* are in a measure similar to those caused by loose
bodies, and similar to, but generally rather more than, those caused
by hypertrophied synovial fringes and the like.   The patient, by some
violent muscular effort or by some sudden twist, as in dancing, tennis,
kicking football or falling from a horse or carriage, wrenches or
twists the knee and finds it impossible to extend it fully, and walks
with it bent in the way described, suffering much pain, and a sharp

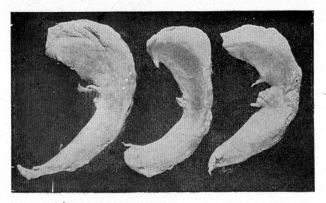

FIG.   126.—Three Right Internal Semilunar Cartilages, Showing Fracture Opposite Internal
Lateral Ligament, Upper Surface.   (Tenney.)

attack of synovitis follows.   On examination one may find a protrusion
of one of the semilunar cartilages, which establishes the diagnosis.

In some instances much tenderness can be found over the internal
cartilage at the front of the joint where none is present over the
outer.

The affection is masked in many patients by the severity of the
acute synovitis which follows the injury, and the true character of the
accident may not be learned for a long time afterward.   One occurrence of the accident predisposes to subsequent attacks.   Lateral
mobility of the knee is likely to exist in cases of long standing.   This
dislocation affects, for the most part, persons between twenty and
fifty years of age, and men are much more frequently affected than
women; it rarely occurs in children.

Patients who are liable to the displacement soon learn the manipulation of reduction themselves.   The knee should be bent to its fullest
extent; the tibia should then be drawn away from the femur as far
as possible, to separate the joint surfaces, at the same time rotating

the tibia inward or outward as the internal or external cartilage is displaced, and then the leg should be extended quickly but not forcibly to its fullest extent, while the surgeon manipulates with the thumb the situation of the semilunar car-

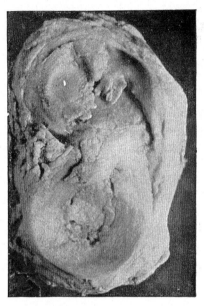

tilages, especially if any undue prominence should be felt. An anæsthetic may be necessary.

The cartilage, after reduction, may become united to the tibia by its former attachments or it may remain loose, to cause further attacks; or, less commonly, entire detachment of the torn piece may occur, in which case it becomes a loose body of the cartilaginous class.

The treatment after the original accident is reduction of the displaced cartilage, followed by the usual treatment for the acute synovitis which ensues. If the attacks recur, especially on slight cause, it is likely that the cartilage has been permanently loosened from its attachments and will in

Fig. 127.—Semilunar Cartilage of Right Knee, Showing Effects of Long-Continued Friction. (Tenney.)

all probability become a source of further trouble. The treatment may under these circumstances be mechanical or operative.

1. *Mechanical Treatment.*—Although the use of knee-caps with pads beside the patella, elastic bandages, etc., may prove of use in preventing in part future attacks, they are to be regarded as palliative rather than curative.

The apparatus advocated by Shaffer for this condition consists of an outside upright attached to the boot and reaching to the upper part of the thigh, and an inside upright reaching from the upper thigh to the upper part of the calf, with a pad placed over the inner aspect of the knee. The apparatus is jointed at the knee, but the joint is arranged to prevent full extension of the knee. The object of this treatment is, by preventing harmful motions and positions for some months, to produce a reunion of the cartilage to its proper attachments and a return of the ligamentum patellæ to its proper length.

2. *Operative treatment* is, as a rule, surer, quicker, and more ac-

ceptable to the patient. The joint is opened inside or outside of the ligamentum patellæ, according to the cartilage displaced, by a vertical incision. The joint should be explored and the loose part of the cartilage removed. The joint capsule should be stitched and the wound closed. Fixation should follow for two or three weeks, after which passive motion and massage should be commenced.

Cysts of the Knee-Joint.—Cystic swellings in connection with the larger joints, especially the knee-joint, occur at times. These swellings are found from time to time in the neighborhood of the knee-joint, generally in the popliteal space. Such cysts, as a rule, connect with the joint. The affection is found most often in early and middle adult life. The diagnosis from bursitis is often difficult. If such cases are troublesome, extirpation of the sac is the only treatment likely to be of use.

Trigger Knee.—The so-called trigger knee, described also as *genou à ressort* or *schnellendes Knie,* is characterized clinically by a disturbance in extension of the leg, which is normal until about 160° is reached, which is then completed with a snap and forcible jerk, during which there is also outward rotation of the tibia. It is not connected with any disease of the knee-joint nor any obvious abnormality save looseness of the ligaments. The prognosis in children is good, depending upon tightening of the ligamentous structures with or without treatment. Mechanical treatment is apparently not necessary, at least in children.

Chronic synovitis of the ankle-joint has been considered under Chronic Sprains.

SHOULDER-JOINT.

Chronic synovitis of the shoulder is an affection existing either as a sequel of an acute attack, the result of some injury, or as a slow, persistent process, beginning with slight symptoms easily disregarded. The earliest symptom to attract notice is stiffness, observed particularly in forced movements, as in placing the hand on the head, etc. Pain is a variable symptom. A slight fulness about the joint may be detected at this time. As the disease progresses, motion becomes more restricted, swelling increases, and atrophy of the deltoid and scapular muscles gradually occurs.

Tenosynovitis may exist and simulate closely chronic synovitis of the shoulder.

Bursitis of the shoulder is most conveniently spoken of in this place, and replaces largely the old term " periarthritis," loosely used to describe various painful conditions about the shoulder. When the subdeltoid bursa is involved, there are local tenderness, pain in motion, and limited abduction. Stiffness of the joints in an adducted position comes on early, and the condition is accompanied by atrophy of the shoulder muscles. Bursitis of the subcoracoid bursa is accompanied by tenderness over the bursa, pain in motion, especially in abduction and rotation, and by the same general symptoms described.

These affections may result from injury or come on without apparent cause, in some instances being vaguely classed as " rheumatic." The diagnosis of these conditions from synovitis and from muscular strain is not always easily to be made. The tendency of all these affections of the shoulder is toward a chronic course, in most instances.

Treatment.—In these conditions, the indication is first for rest and fixation. These are readily secured by means of a sling and a bandage securing the arm to the side. It is important to mention that the weight of the arm dragging upon the joint structures may be a factor in keeping up the pain and irritation. Compression will be needed if there are swelling and effusion. Traction may be required in the severest cases. Fixation should not be continued longer than there is subacute inflammation, and can be gradually discontinued; first discarding the bandage and retaining the sling, which can be discontinued later. So long as muscular irritability exists, rest is indicated. In these cases an increased arc of motion and diminished sensitiveness will usually follow a few days' rest of the joint, and permanent ankylosis is rendered less likely by the application of timely immobilization. But in all cases fixation should be promptly followed by measures to restore motion and to stimulate the circulation.

The question of the use of passive motion in the convalescent stage does not differ essentially from the same question in other joints, except that it comes up oftener. If the stiffness is due to adhesions, manipulation under an anæsthetic, followed by massage, etc., may be of value; but in the majority of light cases gradual passive exercises will suffice. Gentle, graduated, passive motion carried to the verge of being painful is of great advantage in many cases of shoulders stiffened from a slight degree of chronic inflammation. If the stiffness above alluded to is the result of the fixation due to muscular spasm, forcible passive motion will be of no use, as the reflex spasm will reappear after the effect of the anæsthetic has passed away, as long as the disease of the joint remains.

In bursitis of the subdeltoid bursa, if fixation of the arm in the ordinary position does not afford relief, a splint may be applied to

—— the arm at right angles to the long axis of the body; that is, with the humerus horizontal in the standing position. Removal of the bursa may be required in the most resistant cases.

ELBOW-JOINT.

Chronic synovitis may appear in this, as in other joints, from the usual exciting causes, and presents the same characteristics. What is popularly spoken of as a " *tennis elbow* " is a chronic synovitis and irritability, in which injury to the ligaments, especially to the internal lateral ligament, is a marked feature. Its treatment does not differ from that of a similar condition in other joints.

WRIST.

Chronic synovitis may occur under the same conditions existing in other joints. *Tenosynovitis* is characterized by pain on the motion of certain fingers, with, perhaps, a sensation of rubbing or creaking in the affected tendons, and tender points are present in the course of these tendons.

The synovitis of other joints does not require especial mention.

BURSITIS.

Hip.—Inflammation of the bursæ about the hip-joint must be recognized as a condition likely to give rise to symptoms possibly resembling hip disease. This inflammation is most often traumatic, but may be tuberculous. Suppuration and the formation of fistulæ may occur. According to the location of the inflammation the symptoms will differ. The treatment consists of the temporary use of crutches and incision in the severer cases.

Bursitis of the Knee.—The various bursæ about the knee may become inflamed and give rise to disability, often of an obscure nature.

HOUSEMAID'S KNEE.—The most common seat of this affection is in the prepatellar bursa which lies over the patella and part of the ligamentum patellæ.[1] This affection is found chiefly in persons whose occupation leads them to spend much time in kneeling. The affection is characterized by slight swelling, sensitiveness on pressure, and discomfort in flexing the knee, which is localized at the site of the bursa. Palpation shows a more or less distinct swelling, which lies over the patella and which is rendered more tense by the flexion of the joint.

[1] Bize : Journ. d'Anat. et de Phys., Paris, xxxii., 1896, p. 85.

In the acute stage it is likely to be mistaken for synovitis of the knee-joint, but the patella does not float. The chronic enlargement of the bursa is generally the outcome of a series of acute attacks. Fluctuation is clearly present, and the swelling is more sharply localized to

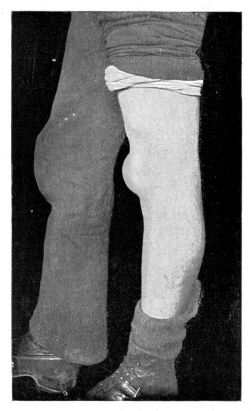

Fig. 128.—Prepatellar Bursitis.

the region in front of the patella than in synovitis. In the chronic stage of the affection, heat, sensitiveness, and discomfort are ordinarily absent.

Although the acute affection shows a tendency toward recovery under rest, the chronic affection does not have this tendency and is likely to continue unabated, while suppuration sometimes occurs. The inflammation of the bursa occasionally is found in connection with gout, rheumatism, or syphilis.

Treatment.—The acute affection ordinarily yields readily when the limb is placed in the extended position upon a ham splint and the constant irritation of walking is avoided. If suppuration occurs, incision affords the only hope of relief. In chronic bursitis the most satisfactory treatment is to lay the entire bursa open by a crucial incision and dissect out the tough fibrous sac.

BURSITIS OF THE DEEP PREPATELLAR BURSA.—This bursa lies beneath the ligamentum patellæ next to the tibia,[1] and the symptoms of its inflammation are pain in complete extension of the leg, referred to the tubercle of the tibia; pain and tenderness, referred to the patella tendon; apparent enlargement of the tubercle of the tibia, and bulging at the sides of the ligamentum patellæ. The affection may be mistaken for inflammation of the superficial pretibial bursa. Careful examination will usually differentiate it from synovitis of the knee-joint. Tuberculosis of this bursa may occur.

The treatment does not differ from that of housemaid's knee.

The inflammation of other bursæ about the knee-joint presents no peculiar symptoms, and the existence of the affection is made evident by the presence of a fluctuating swelling at the site of a bursa.

FRACTURES AND FISSURES IN THE VICINITY OF JOINTS.

Besides fractures directly into joints, disabilities and deformities may result from these injuries and from epiphyseal separation and fissures in the close vicinity to joints. The planes of the joints being altered and the elasticity of the joint capsule and periarticular tissues being impaired by trauma and fibrous cicatrization and thickening.

This condition is met not only by the careful apposition of the parts in case of fracture, but also by the securing of the limb in such a position as will furnish useful function in case of stiffness and by the avoidance of too long fixation, early active motion being permitted, at first under careful direction.

In injuries of this sort in the vicinity of the shoulder, care should be taken to secure the arm at first in a slightly abducted position by an axillary pad. Marked abduction is necessary in such injuries of the hip. In the elbow, the position of forced flexion is often desirable for the first two weeks following injury (except in cases of fracture of the olecranon), followed by fixation in the right-angled position. Front foot drop is to be prevented in injuries of the ankle. Flexion in injuries near the knee is to be prevented.

Passive motion is sometimes needed, but it should be borne in mind that the purpose of passive motion is to break up adhesions. It

[1] Lovett: Boston City Hosp. Reports, 8th series, p. 345.

is not serviceable in restoring elasticity to previously torn ligaments. This is to be accomplished by gradually increasing active exercises, practiced daily, either free or with mechanical aids, the simplest of these being weight and pulley appliances.

Bursitis of the shoulder has been spoken of under synovitis of that joint.

ANKYLOSIS.

Ankylosis is the name used to characterize the persistent stiffness of a joint. This may be " complete " when all motion is lost, or " partial " or " incomplete " when some part of the normal motion

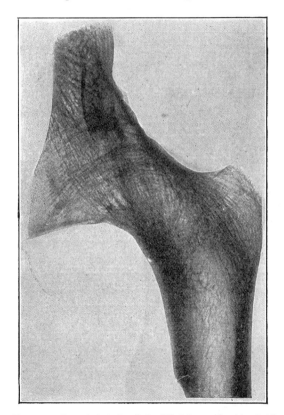

Fig. 129.—True Ankylosis of the Hip-joint. (Joachimsthal.)

remains. It is also classified as " bony " or " fibrous " ankylosis, according to the character of the tissue binding together the joint surfaces. False ankylosis, pseudo-ankylosis, etc., are terms used to designate a condition of joint stiffness in which the restriction of joint motion is due, not to destruction of the joint surfaces, but to other causes, such, for example, as the development of osteophytes and the like around the edges of the joint occurring in arthritis deformans,

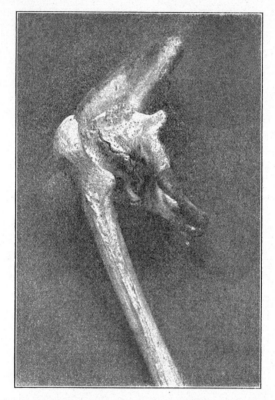

Fig. 130.—Pseudo-ankylosis of Hip-joint Due to Arthritis Deformans.   (Joachimsthal.)

the contraction of the joint capsule, etc.   The name ankylosis should not be applied to the stiffness of joints due to the tonic muscular spasm of acute or chronic joint disease.   This disappears under anæsthesia, whereas ankylosis is not affected by it.

The pathology of ankylosis is the pathology of the affections which cause it.   It represents in general the end result, the cicatrix, of an acute or chronic joint inflammation or of a more or less severe trauma.

The causes of acquired ankylosis are therefore to be found in acute or chronic joint inflammation, in the ankylosing form of arthritis deformans, in fractures involving the joints, in trauma of various kinds, and in periarticular suppuration and trauma. The fixation of normal joints for any reasonable time does not cause true ankylosis. The position in which ankylosis occurs is of great importance, as the usefulness of a limb in cases of irremediable ankylosis will depend on stiffness in a useful position.

The desirable position for ankylosis of the hip is in a few degrees of flexion with no adduction or abduction.

In the knee the useful position is with the leg nearly straight.

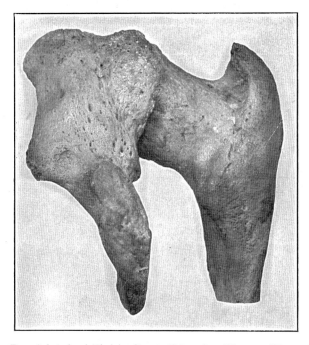

Fig. 131.—True Ankylosis of Hip-joint Due to Tuberculous Disease. (Warren Museum.)

In the ankle the desirable position for a stiff joint is with the foot at a right angle to the leg.

In the shoulder the arm is most useful if slightly abducted and a little flexed.

With a stiff elbow the only useful arm is obtained with the forearm at a right angle to the arm.

The *diagnosis* of ankylosis is made by the absence or limitation of motion. It is not diminished by anæsthesia, and in true ankylosis the x-ray shows the disappearance of the line between the bones and the continuity of bony structure in bony ankylosis. The prevention of ankylosis, therefore, consists in the efficient treatment of the affections likely to cause it.

The *treatment* of ankylosis when the union is not bony, naturally differs from that when the ends of the joint are connected by bone. In the latter case non-operative treatment is useless.

In incomplete ankylosis an attempt may be made to stretch the connecting structures and thus increase the amount of motion.

Manual Stretching.—This may be done by gradual manual stretching, in which gentle manipulative force is used at short intervals and repeated daily. If too much force is used, inflammatory reaction will be started in the joint, and the condition will be made worse. The use of a proper degree of force should be followed by a daily increase of joint motion without great pain. This is especially the case after fractures involving the joints.

Mechanical Correction.—The attempt at stretching may be made by means of a *pendulum* apparatus, in which a carefully controlled rhythmical movement is exerted to any desired extent, by the *Zander* apparatus, or by the use of manual force.

Bier's congestive method, hot-air baths, massage, and vibratory massage are often of use in connection with the measures described, and are especially suited to the stiffness following fractures and joint injuries, the loss of motion in arthritis deformans, and after non-tuberculous inflammations in and around the joints.

Forcible Stretching.—In case these measures prove ineffectual the patient should be anæsthetized and the arc of motion of the stiffened joint increased by the use of moderate force to stretch or break the adhesions existing. This should be followed by rest to the joint for one or two days, followed by the resumption of the gentle measures described. The injudicious use of force, as a rule, does more harm than good by exciting inflammation and causing new adhesions. After the use of manipulative force the joint should be fixed in the position of greatest usefulness, described above.

In *bony ankylosis*, if the ankylosis has occurred in a position of deformity, the joint should be corrected by osteotomy or excision and the limb placed in a useful position, or the operative attempt should be made to form a new joint.

Osteotomy is, as a rule, linear, and is generally performed just above or below the joint surface. Wedge-shaped osteotomy inevitably shortens a limb, but may be required in cases of extreme deformity.

Excision may be done at the site of an ankylosed joint, not with a view of restoring motion, but to correct deformity. The planes of the resected ends of the bones should be so placed as to give the desired position of the joint after union.

Formation of New Joints.—In bony ankylosis the formation of a new joint at the site of the former one may be attempted. The method of interposing a layer of fascia, pig's bladder, several layers of Cargile membrane, or other foreign substance between the resected ends of the bone in cases of true bony ankylosis has been described and successfully carried out with marked success by certain surgeons.[1] The hope of success in the operation depends upon the fact that aponeurosis attached to fatty tissue when subject to pressure tends to form an hygroma or bursa. If, then, the line of union where the joint formerly existed is chiselled or cut through in approximately the original joint plane, and aponeurotic, or muscular, and fatty tissue is interposed, there is hope of a restoration of joint motion in place of the former bony ankylosis. The capsule and synovial membrane, if the latter remains, are extirpated and only essential bands of ligaments are left. Bony outgrowths are removed, adherent tendons freed, cicatricial contractions cut out, and a flap of the desired tissue is taken from the neighborhood and turned in between the ends of the bones. This flap should be secured to the edges of the capsule and is left attached by its base. Use of the limb is at first painful, and passive motion under anæsthesia may be required. The hip and elbow are the most favorable joints for this operation, and the knee, on account of its flat articular surfaces, the least favorable.

Numerous miscellaneous joint affections remain for consideration which do not lend themselves well to classification. They will therefore be considered in this place.

Bone Defects.—The filling of cavities and defects in bone due to various causes (congenital or from osteomyelitis) with a solid substance, or one which becomes solid, is a problem which has for a long time attracted the attention of surgeons. Of the many measures tried, a few are worthy of consideration.

Antiseptic Wax.—This method is as follows: Equal parts of oil of sesame and spermaceti are sterilized in a water bath, and later 60 parts of this are mixed with 40 of iodoform, which gives a yellowish, brittle wax, melting at about 50°. When it is to be used it is heated just above the melting point and constantly stirred.[2]

[1] Murphy : Trans. Am. Surg. Assn., xxii., 315 (with literature). Hoffa : Zeitsch. f. orth. Chir., xvii. Baer, Am. Jour. Orth. Surg., vii., 1, i.

[2] Simmons : Annals of Surgery, January, 1911.

This depends for its success on the thorough asepsis of the part filled, and is not suited to bone still retaining in its tissue septic germs; it is more suited to small cavities with firm walls.

When the cavity is a large one and the defect due to an inflammatory process, the best proceeding is to remove the whole diseased portion of the bone, including the hard cortical involucrum, if such exist, leaving the periosteum. This should be carefully cleansed and wiped with alcohol and the opposing walls stitched and pressed together. New healthy bone will, under favorable circumstances, develop, furnishing a useful limb.

Where a congenital bone defect is present in one of two adjacent bones, a portion of the bone can be separated from the normal bone and inserted into the defect. This can be done in either one of two ways.

1st. One portion of the bone may at first retain its original connection, while the other portion is secured by periosteal suture, in its new position. Subsequently, after union of the part, the portion where circulatory connection is still retained is separated and secured in its new position.

2d. By the complete separation of a portion of bone from any part of the skeleton and insertion to fill a defect, the transformed portion is secured in its new place by bone plates or ivory plugs.

As has been demonstrated by clinical experience and laboratory experiment under favorable conditions, firm bone is secured by this procedure.

Bone Sinuses.—The successful treatment of these depends upon the condition of the original source of origin of the sinus.

When a tuberculous or septic ostitis is present in a bone, the resulting sinus is a channel of drainage and cannot heal as long as discharge comes from the original source. If the discharge is scanty the sinus may heal, but as the discharge accumulates a fresh sinus forms.

The cure in this condition consists, when this is possible, in the treatment of the original ostitis, either by drainage with disinfection or removal of dead bone.

In some instances the sinus remains unhealed, owing to the infection of the walls of the sinus after the original ostitis has healed. This condition can be relieved by dilatation of the sinus and the disinfection of the walls by antiseptic injection, iodoform bougies, or bismuth paste. Another method is to secure complete drainage of the sinus by applying suction cups daily and thereby promoting complete evacuation and healing through the cohesion of the sinus walls.

Fragilitas ossium.[1]—Idiopathic osteopsathyrosis and osteogenesis imperfecta, also known as fragilitas ossium and brittle bones, are conditions in which multiple fractures occur in young children, and sometimes in such cases persist through life. The condition is at times inherited and its etiological relations are obscure. Union as a rule occurs readily and pathological investigation has shown the conditions to be apparently distinct from rickets and chondrodystrophy. No satisfactory treatment has been formulated.

OSTEOMALACIA.

Osteomalacia is a process somewhat similar to rickets in causing softening of the bones, the etiological and pathological relation of which to rickets is at present much discussed and very imperfectly formulated, but the pathology of which is different from that of rickets. There is absorption of the lime salts, beginning in the marrow of the bone and affecting first the spongiosa, and the resistance of the bone is so impaired that it bends or breaks. The disease is most prevalent among the lower classes, affecting certain localities more than others, and females are attacked more often than males. The affection as described affects adolescents and adults rather than children.

The symptoms consist of dull pain and perhaps tenderness in the affected parts, hyperæsthesia of the skin, and discomfort in walking or sitting. This is followed or accompanied by yielding of the bones and fractures, complete or incomplete.

The treatment of the disease must be directed to the relief of the symptoms and must be conducted on general principles.

CHONDRODYSTROPHIA FŒTALIS.

Achondroplasia (fœtal rickets).—Although this condition is described frequently under the name of " fœtal rickets," it is essentially a different pathological process. Clinically the children at birth seem to present the signs of a severe grade of rickets which has run its course. The head is large and the bridge of the nose depressed. There is beading of the ribs and perhaps flattening of the sides of the chest, and the long bones of the extremities are shortened and perhaps bowed and enlarged near the joints.

The essential pathological process is, however, a disturbance of

[1] Maier: Zeitsch. f. orth. Chir., xxvii., 1 and 2, 145.

the normal process of ossification of the primary cartilage. The cartilage atrophies and the process of ossification takes place abnormally early. In true chondrodystrophia the bones will remain distorted, the joints will probably be limited in their range of motion, and the general growth of the body retarded, resulting in dwarfism. The milder cases may reach adult life. The treatment can only be palliative.

HABITUAL OR RECURRENT DISLOCATIONS.

Patella.—Dislocation of the patella or slipping patella is like to occur either spontaneously or for very slight cause in certain young girls with lax muscular fibre and a feeble development. Boys are only exceptionally attacked.

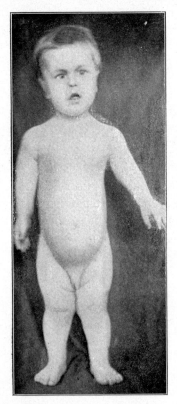

FIG. 132.—Chondrodystrophia Fœtalis, "Congenital Rickets."

In consequence of some slight twist of the leg, as in dancing, rising from a chair, going upstairs, or some similar motion, an excruciating pain is felt in the knee, and the person either falls in consequence of faintness or finds herself unable to use the leg. The patella is found almost always dislocated outwardly, sometimes twisted so that its lateral edge rests against the front of the femur. The reduction of the dislocation is very simple and is very soon learned by the patients themselves. The leg is fully extended and the patella gently pressed back into place until it assumes its proper place with a click, or often it slips back of its own accord when the leg is straightened. An attack of synovitis follows, as in the case of loose bodies, but the joint soon acquires a tolerance so that each succeeding attack of synovitis becomes less. The cause of the affection seems to be, in most cases, the lack of tonicity in the extensor muscles of the thigh, or the elongation of the ligamentum patellæ.

After many attacks of dislocation the patients complain of a cer-

tain sense of insecurity in walking, which in severe cases may amount
to a distressing disability, limiting the patient's ability to walk or
engage in active occupation.

Mechanical Treatment.—If an elastic knee-cap is split in front and
furnished with lacings or straps, and if felt pads are sewed upon
the sides of the cap at such places as would exert pressure upon the

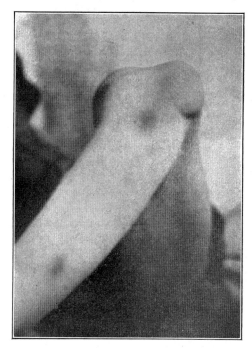

Fig. 133.—Dislocation of Patella.

sides of the patella, an arrangement is furnished which, when properly
adjusted, will give a serviceable support in lighter cases, allowing
motion at the knee.

Some retentive apparatus, along with the use of massage and
exercise, may effect a cure, especially in rapidly growing girls.

Operative Treatment.—In resistant cases, or those unable to follow out proper mechanical treatment, operation will be required.[1]

This consists in the removal of an elliptical piece of the front of
the capsule of the joint internal to the extensor tendon and a stitching
together of the edges of the opening, thereby tightening the inner

[1] Bade : Zeit. f. orth. Chir., xi., 3, 451 (with bibliography).

part of the capsule.[1] In resistant cases a vertical incision outside of the patella tendon must also be made to allow the patella to be pulled into place by the tightening of the capsule on the inner side. The tubercle of the tibia may be transplanted [2] farther in on the tibia, or the patella tendon may be split longitudinally and the inner half carried under the outer and attached to the tibia outside of the tubercle.[3]

Habitual or recurrent dislocation of the shoulder becomes at times an affection requiring orthopedic treatment.

The causes of the condition may be formulated as follows: 1. Laxity of the capsule of the joint. 2. Partial fracture of the head of the humerus. 3. Partial fracture of the glenoid cavity. 4. Tearing away of muscular insertions and rupture of tendons. 5. Abnormality in the shape of the head of the humerus not demonstrably due to fracture. It would seem as if in certain instances the cause of the recurrence of the dislocation was insufficient immobilization of the arm after a primary dislocation. Reduction is as a rule easy, and inflammatory reaction in the joint is notably slight or even wholly absent after reduction.

Prognosis.—In a shoulder-joint in which a dislocation has twice occurred, the second time from insufficient cause, it is not likely that the liability will become less frequent as time advances if no treatment is undertaken. As a rule, the dislocations will occur with greater frequency and from slighter causes as time progresses.

Treatment.—The methods of treatment are:

By apparatus; by massage and exercises alone; by temporary fixation and massage; by operation.

The use of apparatus confining the arm to the side is to be condemned.

Fixation for some time is called for when a second dislocation has occurred from slight cause. The arm is lifted by applying a sling, which supports the forearm and point of the elbow. The arm is held to the side by a swathe, thus preventing all motions of the joint. This removes as much weight as possible from the joint capsule.

Such cases have been operated upon successfully by reefing the anterior part of the capsule of the joint through an anterior incision.[4]

[1] N. Y. Med. Record, April 20, 1895.—Trans. Am. Orth. Assn., vol. viii., p. 227. —*Ibid.*, vol viii., p. 237.

[2] Annals of Surg., 1899.

[3] Goldthwait: Am. Journ. Orth. Surgery, vol. i., No. 3.

[4] Burrell and Lovett: Am. Jour. Med. Sciences, August, 1897.

Sacro-Iliac Articulation.—This articulation, although a true joint under ordinary circumstances, is firmly held in place, but is relaxed in pregnancy, and in some instances the relaxation may persist after confinement, giving a marked disability in locomotion.

Under normal conditions pronounced violence is needed to inflict an injury upon the articulation.

The joint, like the articulation of the symphysis pubis, is rarely affected primarily in the rare tuberculous arthritic process to a recognizable degree, but it is not improbable that when the lumbar spine is involved in an extensive degenerative arthritic process the sacro-iliac articulation may also be involved, and in the destructive purulent ostitic processes this region may be involved.

Symphysis Pubis.—*Relaxation* of the joint in the symphysis pubis occurs rarely during pregnancy, at times affecting also the sacro-iliac joints, so that walking becomes difficult or impossible. After delivery the abnormal condition may disappear or may persist as a source of disability. It is best treated by a leather or plaster jacket fitting tightly over the sacrum and ilia, along with as much limitation of walking as may be necessary.

TUMORS OF THE BONES AND JOINTS.

Primary tumors of bone belong to the group of connective-tissue tumors. The periosteum and bone marrow form the matrix for their development. These tumors correspond to the various types of connective tissue, fibrous, mucoid, cartilaginous, and osseous. Among primary tumors are to be classed sarcomata. Secondary tumors of any kind may occur, among the latter being carcinoma. Angioma, hæmatoma, echinococcus cyst, and aneurism must be mentioned as other possibilities.

MALIGNANT DISEASE OF THE SPINE.

Sarcoma and carcinoma of the vertebral column are occasionally met. Carcinoma has been noted following similar disease of the breast and testicle, and less frequently of the stomach. The disease usually begins as an infiltration of the spongy tissue of the vertebral bodies, which is gradually replaced by the malignant growth. There may be but little change in the appearance of the bodies, but these will be found converted into a soft, friable mass. Destruction of the bone substance with deformity may occur. The most frequent site of malignant disease is in the lumbar region, and the next commonest location is in the dorsal vertebræ.

The symptoms are similar to those of Pott's disease, pain being very prominent, with frequently paralysis.

When deformity occurs it will be found to present a more rounded prominence than is usually seen in Pott's disease. When following malignant disease elsewhere, which can be recognized, the diagnosis should present no special difficulty, but in other instances it is usually hard or even impossible. The prognosis needs no comment.

Malignant Disease of the Hip.

The variety of tumor which most often affects the head of the femur in young children is a round-cell sarcoma of the periosteum, but the epiphysis is rarely the seat of the tumor.

The early symptoms in cases in which the head of the femur is not primarily involved are very slight, and consist chiefly of a swelling which is painless and not fluctuating; limp and slight restriction of motion may be present. Soon, however, it becomes evident that the enlargement is predominating over all the other symptoms and the swelling progressively increases, suggesting perhaps hip abscess. Fluctuation, however, is absent and the swelling embraces the whole circumference of the limb. There is an enlargement of the superficial vessels and the swelling later becomes enormous. The patient becomes emaciated and wastes away. The affection may be very painful or again it may be attended with very little suffering. According to the histological character of the tumor the treatment would consist in the removal of the growth, followed by the use of toxines or in amputation at the hip-joint. The statistics are not favorable to amputation as a means of cure.

SYPHILIS.

Our knowledge of syphilitic affections of the joints is unsatisfactory and inexact. The following facts seem well substantiated.

In *acquired syphilis* arthralgia without objective symptoms may occur early in the secondary stage. Simple serous synovitis, associated with pain, redness, and swelling, may accompany the secondary symptoms, and this condition may pass on to a chronic hydrops. In the tertiary stage chronic serous synovitis may be present.

These and other processes may be the result of gummata of the ends of the bones, or in the periosteum, or situated about the joints.

Secondarily to these periosteal and bone lesions come the capsular and synovial thickening and the cartilage degeneration.

Hereditary syphilis is proportionately more often attended by joint complications than is acquired syphilis.

The most characteristic form of joint disease in hereditary syphilis in children is the *osteochondritis* of Parrot. This consists in a broadening of the cartilaginous layer of the epiphysis next to the diaphysis, with irregularity of the zone of ossification. At the same time there occur thickening of the epiphysis and a growth of granulation tissue, sometimes breaking down in the medullary cavity. Secondary synovitis may accompany this process. The clinical symptoms of this osteochondritis are thickening of bone at the epiphyseal line, tenderness, and joint inflammation, secondarily with lameness and even uselessness of the limb for a time. It may involve several joints. The affection is sometimes spoken of as syphilitic pseudoparalysis of infants.

Later hereditary syphilis may show a somewhat similar affection, due to overgrowth of the epiphysis and spoken of as " chronic osteoarthropathy of hereditary syphilis " or " false tumor albus." The thickened and deformed epiphyses form a mass which appears as a spindle-shaped swelling, most often at the knee. There is typically no muscular spasm, although marked atrophy of the muscles is present. Pain is generally absent, although rarely there may be some tenderness and local heat. What inflammation of the joint is present is secondary and not characteristic. It is favorably affected by the usual treatment for syphilis.

Syphilis of the Spine.—Syphilitic destruction of the bodies of the vertebræ must be regarded as possible and not unlikely, but the recorded cases of this sort are not in general satisfactory as proving pathologically that such a condition has existed. The presence of syphilis in a patient with a knuckle in the back does not prove that tuberculosis is absent or that the vertebral destruction is of a syphilitic character. The diagnosis of syphilitic spondylitis in most cases has rested on the slenderest clinical evidence.

GOUT.

The joint affection, which is the manifestation of the constitutional malady known as gout, ordinarily begins as an acute attack, and is followed by a chronic inflammatory process, increased by constant exacerbations. The synovial membrane first presents the appearances of acute inflammation; the cartilage also shows a tendency to inflammatory degeneration and erosion, and on its free surface and in its tissue, as well as in its capsule and periarticular structure, there appears a deposit of acicular crystals of urate of soda, which localized deposits are known as "tophi." There is a permanent thickening of the synovial membrane. There is but little tendency to suppuration, unless the calcareous deposits ulcerate through the skin by pressure and so open the periarticular tissue. The common seat of the affection is the metatarsophalangeal joint of the great toe (podagra). The joints of the hands, and the knee- and elbow-joints are also often affected.

OSTITIS DEFORMANS.

Paget's Disease.—This name designates a deformity affecting the long bones, chiefly in their diaphyses, causing them to bend.

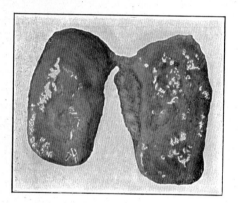

It most frequently attacks the lower extremities first, also involving the spine and the skull. The upper extremities are at times curved. The process consists of a thickening and curving of the affected bones, the bone hypertrophying as a whole and its curves increasing, while the external surface is roughened. In most cases the enlargement takes place by the expansion of the cortex; in other cases the spongy part of the bone is extended. The skull shows marked thickening and enlargement.

FIG. 134.—Knee-joint Surfaces in Gout, Showing Deposits.

Microscopic examination shows appearances of absorption and new formation, and the proportion of mineral salts in the bones is diminished.

Etiology.—In the matter of etiology nothing definite has been established. The disease attacks men in middle adult life more frequently than women. The relation of the disease to arteriosclerosis is obscure, some writers claiming that pathologically they are identical. This point of view cannot yet be regarded as established.

Symptoms.—The affection is generally ushered in by a long period of pain described as "rheumatic," and perhaps by headaches.[1] Some cases are, however, practically painless. The general condition of the

[1] Wollenberg: Zeitsch. f. orth. Chir., xiii., 1.

patient is often not seriously affected. The attitude is characteristic; in advanced cases the patient stands with the legs bowed and the spine bent in a gradual backward curve; the body may be carried forward

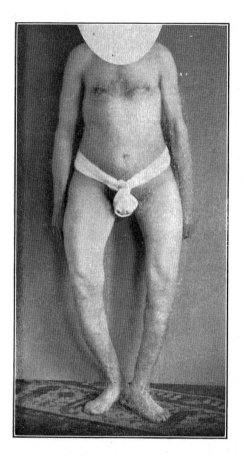
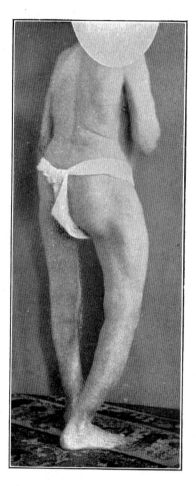

FIG. 135.—Ostitis Deformans. Male, age fifty-four. First definite signs seven years before photograph. Present involvement most marked in cranium, clavicles, right ulna, left radius, pelvis, tibiæ, and fibiæ. (R. B. Osgood.)

bent at the hips, the skull may be greatly enlarged, and the spine lose its flexibility. In such cases the body is shortened in the erect position. The diagnostic symptoms are the occurrence of bow-legs beginning in the latter half of life, the bending backward of the spine, the hypertrophy of the bones, and especially the great thickening of the skull. Fractures occur rarely, and in cases observed have united readily.

Prognosis.—The prognosis of the affection as far as life goes is not unfavorable, and death generally occurs from intercurrent affections. No satisfactory treatment has been formulated. Protective apparatus in the severer deformities may be necessary, but they increase muscular weakness and are to be avoided if possible.

PATHOLOGICAL CONDITIONS OF THE NERVOUS SYSTEM.

Charcot's joint disease, spinal or neuropathic arthropathy, neural arthropathy, tabetic arthropathy, etc.

A destructive form of joint disease may be associated with locomotor ataxia, syringomyelia, Pott's disease, acute myelitis, injuries of the peripheral nerves, cerebral apoplexy, tumors of the cord, crushing of the spinal cord, progressive muscular atrophy, and anterior poliomyelitis.

The pathological process is in many respects similar to that in arthritis deformans, except that the destructive process is more rapid and the formative activity less. This process may result in spontaneous luxation in severe cases. Synovial effusion may be present, and suppuration may occur. The essential character of the affection is the rapid melting away of cartilage and bones, and the joint changes may be present at an early stage of the nervous disorder.

The affection is most often monarticular, and adults are generally affected. The joints are affected in approximately the following order of frequency: knee, hip, shoulder, tarsus, elbow, ankle, wrist, jaw, and spine.

Swelling, effusion, disability, and sometimes pain are the first signs of the joint involvement. Spontaneous arrest of the process may occur, and ankylosis may rarely result, but more commonly the joint is disorganized to the point of luxation. The diagnosis is often difficult, especially in the early stages.

The treatment does not differ essentially from that of inflamed joints in general. Although excision of the joint has been successfully done under these conditions, local operative measures are not, as a rule, to be advised. In cases in which syphilitic history is present, proper treatment should be given.

Arthropathy of the vertebral column has been rarely observed in tabes. It is manifested by a deformed position of the column, shown by scoliosis and backward bending of the spine.[1] Partial relief may be afforded by fixation.

Arthropathy of the Hip.—As in most other instances, Charcot's disease of the hip simulates very closely arthritis deformans of the ordinary type. The changes in the joint are, however, much more

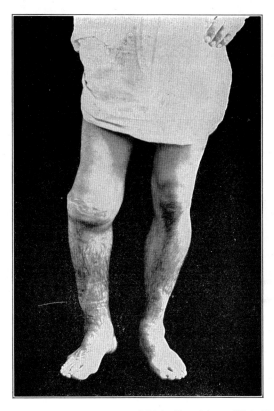

Fig. 136.—Charcot's Disease of Right Knee-joint. (Weigel.)

acute and extensive than those with which we are familiar in arthritis deformans. Rest is indicated for the joint, with traction if it gives relief.

HÆMOPHILIA.

Hæmophilia is accompanied at times by characteristic joint lesions, which in their clinical resemblance to tuberculosis are worthy of no-

[1] Spiller ; Am. Medicine, November 1, 1902, p. 701 (with bibliography).—Graetzer: Deutsch. med. Woch., December 24, 1903.

tice.[1] The knee is the joint most frequently affected. Like other manifestations of this diathesis, joint affections occur most often in male children or young adults, decreasing in frequency with increasing age. The hemorrhage may be intraarticular or periarticular. After repeated acute attacks of hemorrhage into the joint, chronic joint changes are likely to ensue. There is an overgrowth of brown-stained synovial tufts. The cartilage may degenerate, and sharp-bordered defects in it are frequently found. Adhesions, contractions of the capsule, and bony displacements may occur. Erosion of the ends of the bones may take place along with a proliferation at the edges not unlike arthritis deformans. Rheumatic pains are a common clinical accompaniment of the affection, and its character is essentially chronic. Swelling and muscular spasm are present during attacks of irritation, and the diagnosis from tuberculosis is to be made more from the history than from any characteristic features.[2]

General treatment offers but little hope, although the use of gelatin by mouth, in doses of six or more ounces daily, has been found of use, and thyroid extract has been reported as controlling hemorrhage in such cases.[3]

Protection to the diseased joints is of more use than any other one measure, but the prognosis as to recovery is doubtful at best. Aspiration with a small needle may be safely done for purposes of diagnosis. Fatal hemorrhages have occurred as the result of operation on these supposedly tuberculous joints.

SCURVY.

Joint affections in infantile scurvy are not uncommon, and simulate closely epiphysitis. The enlargement may be confined to one of the bones forming an articulation. The thickening is due to periarticular or rather subperiosteal hemorrhage, and the joint itself is not usually affected, though hemorrhage may occur. Such joints yield readily to the usual treatment of infantile scurvy.

SECONDARY HYPERTROPHIC OSTEO-ARTHROPATHY.

This is the name given to a condition occurring sometimes in connection with chronic pulmonary disease, in which the fingers are clubbed and stiffened, the shafts of the bones are thickened, and the spine is bent forward in a kyphosis. It occurs sometimes in connec-

---

[1] Carless (with analysis of 253 reported cases): Practitioner, 1903, lxx., 85.
[2] Gocht: Münch. med. Woch., 1899, February 21, 271.
[3] J. T. Rugh : Ann. of Surg , May, 1907.

tion with Pott's disease. The relation of the affection to acromegaly and osteomalacia is not clear.[1]

ACTINOMYCOSIS.

Actinomycosis is a specific infectious disease occasionally attacking the bone secondarily, and is caused by the streptothrix actinomycotica (ray fungus). The process in the bone is a destructive one.

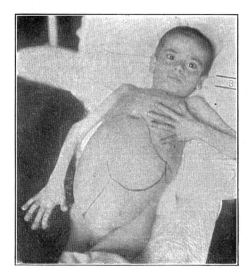

Fig. 137.—Secondary Osteo-arthropathy Due to Pott's Disease, Showing Enlargement of Liver and Spleen.

The spinal column, ribs, and sternum may be attacked, but the maxilla is the bone most frequently affected, and the involvement of bone being only secondary and incidental.

Actinomycosis of the spine is rare, but few cases having been reported. In the cases seen by the writers it has resembled Pott's disease very closely. In one case the diagnosis was made from a microscopic examination of the discharge from the sinuses.

The treatment consists in the administration of iodide of potassium.

Echinococcus cysts of the spine have been observed.

[1] Whitman: Pediatrics, 1899, vii., Nos. 4 and 5 (with bibliography).—Janeway: Am. Jour. Med. Sci., October, 1903 (with bibliography.)

MYOSITIS OSSIFICANS.

This affection in its symptoms is closely enough allied to those caused by certain joint diseases to require mention. The affection seems to be roughly divided into 2 types: (1) a multiple affection involving various parts of the skeleton spoken of as myositis ossificans progressiva and apparently constitutional; (2) a form dependent on single or repeated trauma (traumatica). The pathology is unsettled and may be studied in the references.[1] The characteristic of the affection is, in the first form, the occurrence of multiple bony tumors in connection with the muscles. Such cases begin generally in childhood. The muscles are tender to pressure and deformities may result from the presence of masses of bone in abnormal situations. No satisfactory treatment of this variety has been formulated. The traumatic form results in a persistent thickening at the site

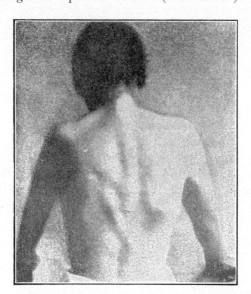

Fig. 138.—Myositis Ossificans.   (Michelson.)

of some injury, which impairs the muscle or muscles involved, and there may be found by the x-ray even a few days after injury plates of bone in intimate association with muscle tissue. In some instances this is undoubtedly merely periosteum torn from the bone; in other cases this explanation does not hold and one must assume the independent formation of bone in muscular tissue.

If such formations do not absorb sufficiently to prevent proper function of involved parts they should be removed by operation.

[1] Bocker: Zeitsch. f. orth. Chir., 1908, xxii. 1–3.—Jones and Morgan: Archiv Röntgen Ray, etc., 1905–6.

CHAPTER IX.

THE DEFORMITIES OF RICKETS.

THESE deformities result from the inability of the bone to sustain without bending the weight or pressure or strain which comes upon it from the muscular action, constituting assumed attitude or locomotion.

These deformities follow a pathological condition existing in the bones in early childhood and in adolescence.

Definition.—Rickets is a constitutional disease which affects young children. In the osseous system there is a local or general disturbance of the normal process of ossification, as a result of which the epiphyses become enlarged and the affected bones become soft and pliable; growth is delayed and deformities of a serious character may arise. The affection itself does not belong to the category of surgical diseases; but the resulting deformities demand strictly surgical treatment.

Ossification after the rhachitic process is over may become excessive, making the bone more firm and dense than normal. Infractions or partial fractures, with the break on the concave side of the long bones, may occur before curative ossification has been established. The ligaments become relaxed and stretched and the muscles flabby from disuse.

Occurrence and Etiology.—Rickets is an affection occurring commonly during the first dentition. Cases of rickets, however, occur during adolescence and a condition resembling rickets is at times congenital and has been discussed under the heading of Chondrodystrophia Fœtalis.

The rickets of adolescence, or late rickets, is a disease which affects persons at about the age of puberty. The physical signs are the same as in the rickets of early life, except that the epiphyseal enlargement is generally not so great. Boys and girls are about equally affected.

Causation.—Rickets is an affection of faulty nutrition. It is much more prevalent among the crowded poor of the cities than in rural communities, and certain races seem to be more subject to the affection than others. The children of the negro, Italian, and Portuguese poor are more frequently afflicted than the Irish in our Atlantic American cities.

Changes in the Bones.—Enlargement of the epiphyses appears, especially at the wrists, ankles, and anterior ends of the ribs. These

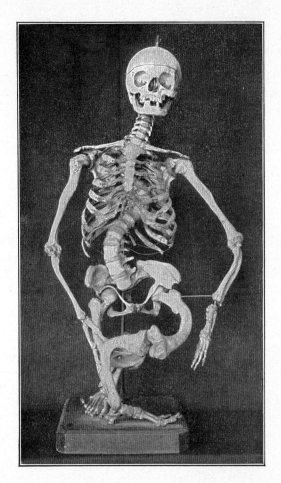

FIG. 139.—Skeleton in Rickets. (Warren Museum.)

enlargements do not involve the joints. At the ribs one finds the "rosary," a series of bead-like enlargements easily felt at the junction of the cartilages and the ribs, and a small degree of epiphyseal enlargement is easily detected here, and is not likely to be mistaken for anything else. When these changes have occurred, the bones have already softened and curvatures of the long bones may have begun.

The forces that work to produce deformity in the softened bones are muscular action, gravity, pressure from weight, atmospheric resistance, and the pressure exerted on bony structures by growing organs.

The typical *head* of rickets shows a high, square, prow-shaped forehead, with a decided prominence of the lateral parts of the frontal bones (frontal eminences) and sometimes the parietal eminences as well.

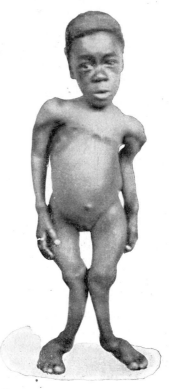

The *anterior fontanel,* which should normally close at about the eighteenth month, remains widely open and does not ossify until perhaps the third year, or even later. The *posterior fontanel* sometimes remains open for months.

Deformities of the *chest* are among the most common produced by rickets, and they occasionally exist without any well-marked signs of rickets elsewhere. It is not unusual to see young girls about the age of puberty who have discovered some inequality in the chest or prominence of the lower ribs, perhaps, but who present no other signs of rickets. In these cases it seems reasonable to assume that a slight degree of bone softening existed in childhood.

In a typical rhachitic chest the clavicles are shorter and more curved than they naturally should be. The chest is narrow and prominent in front; it shows the effect of lateral compression, and the sternum projects so prominently that the

Fig. 140.—Extreme Deformity from Rickets.

name of pigeon breast, or pectus carinatum, is commonly given to it. A transverse depression in the chest, known as Harrison's sulcus, also occurs in the typical cases, which is most evident just below the nipples. The prominence of the abdomen is almost universal in well-marked rickets. Rhachitic children, as a rule, learn to walk late.

A very common deformity of the *spinal column* due to rickets is a posterior bowlike curve (involving the dorsal and lumbar regions).

It is a uniform curve of a part of the column, and is most prominent at the junction of the dorsal and lumbar regions. This attitude seems the result of a long-continued seated position, with a weakness of the muscles, which fail to hold the spine in the erect position. The curve is usually rounded rather than sharp, and the prominence is

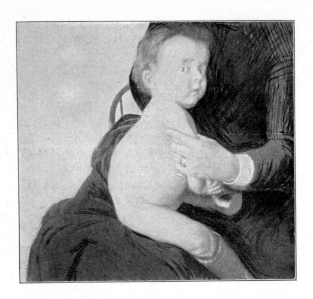

Fig. 141.—Deformity of Spine in Rickets.

not limited to one vertebral spinous process, as is the case in early Pott's disease. The rhachitic curve of the spine is, as a rule, flexible if the child lies upon its face and is lifted by the legs. In the acuter stages and after marked bone changes have taken place marked stiffness may be seen.

The *attitude* of a child affected with well-marked rickets is characteristic. It exists in most marked cases of knock-knee and bowlegs, and sometimes in a less degree with milder grades of the affection. The child stands with the legs apart, the thighs flexed, and the knees bent, the back is arched, and the shoulders are thrown back.

Deformity of the *pelvis* may be induced by rickets, the body weight being borne by a bony arch which causes it to bend under weight, and deformities may result, which may be of importance in childbirth.

Except in very severe cases, the *arm* bones are not seriously curved.

The curvatures follow no special rule, but generally they are an exaggeration of the normal curves of the bone. The curvature of the arm bones may be due to creeping, or to lifting the child continually

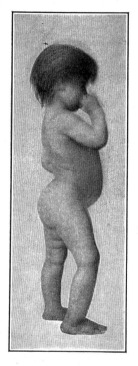

FIG. 142.—Attitude of Severe Rickets, Showing Lordosis and Rotation of Pelvis.

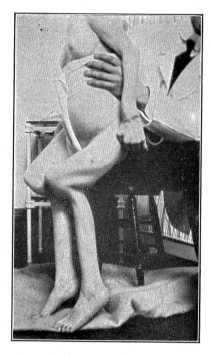

FIG. 143.—Case of Osteomalacia in a Girl of Fifteen Years, Showing Deformities of Legs and Arms. (C. F. Painter.)

by taking hold of the forearm in one place, but often apparently is the result of muscular action.

The rhachitic deformities of the legs are of such importance that they will be considered separately.

Flat-foot is a very common accompaniment of rickets. The affection is considered under flat-foot.

In general, the skeleton is not only deformed but stunted, and persons who have rickets severely in childhood do not reach average size in adult life, as a rule. The osseous deformities, in most cases, persist to a certain extent through life. Notably is this true of the shape of the skull and the chest.

Diagnosis.—The diagnosis in fully developed rickets is simple; but when the affection is beginning, its recognition may be attended with difficulty.

In beginning rickets, suggestive symptoms are restlessness and sweating at night, and universal tenderness in acute cases. In cases where the disease is more fully developed the diagnostic points are, the epiphyseal enlargement of the ends of the long bones, especially the wrists and the sternal ends of the ribs; the prow-shaped head; the deep, small chest; the big belly; delayed dentition; delayed walking, and an anterior fontanel open long beyond the proper time. If the disease has advanced still further, one often finds curvature of the bones of the legs and arms.

Prognosis.—When the disease is left to itself it generally runs its course, and after a decided degree of bony deformity has occurred the process of bone softening is spontaneously arrested, and the bones harden in their deformed condition. Spontaneous arrest of the disease may take place at any stage without treatment, but, as a rule, in severe cases not before a serious degree of bony deformity has been produced. When the disease is treated efficiently, the prognosis as to life is always favorable, and the disease is, as a rule, easily amenable to treatment.

The kyphosis above alluded to disappears or diminishes with the growth of the child under proper treatment. Lateral curves, however, are more permanent.

Treatment.—The treatment of rickets consists, first, in the proper feeding and hygiene of the child. Drug treatment is manifestly secondary in importance to careful regulation of the diet and hygiene.

The discussion of the operative and mechanical treatment of rickets will be taken up under the head of knock-knee and bow-legs.

KNOCK-KNEE.

Knock-knee, or *genu valgum,* is the name applied to an internal angular prominence of the knee, in which the bones of the leg form an abnormal lateral angle with the bones of the thigh, and this angle opens outward.

Occurrence and Etiology.—The deformity is one of common occurrence, and about half as common as bow-legs. Both deformities affect boys more often than girls.

Knock-knee is a deformity which appears for the most part shortly after the children learn to walk, but it occurs occasionally at the time of adolescence.

Knock-knee occurring in the first period named is almost always associated with general rickets, and is sometimes called *genu valgum rhachiticum*, to distinguish it from the form occurring at puberty, which is spoken of as *genu valgum staticum* or *adolescentium*.

Mechanical Production of Knock-knee.—The chief cause of the deformity seems to be a static one, due to the superimposed body weight, pressure from faulty position, and abnormal strain, acting upon soft bones.

As the normally formed human being in the upright position stands with a certain amount of knock-knee, it is evident that the external condyle of the femur and the corresponding facet of the tibia transmit more body weight than do the corresponding internal articular surfaces.

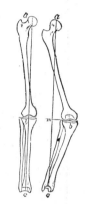

Three bony deformities are likely to be found in cases of knock-knee, viz.:

(*a*) Difference in the size of the condyles of the femur.

(*b*) Inequality in the articular facets of the tibia.

(*c*) Bending of the diaphyses of the bones above or below the joint. The first named one being the usual and commonest variety.

The patella lies farther outside than it should do, and the knees are laterally loose. The leg is rotated outward on the thigh in the more marked cases, and this is sometimes so marked

FIG. 144.—Axis of a normal leg, and of one affected with Knock-knee.

that a sort of compensatory inversion of the front of the foot has been acquired almost to the condition of varus to aid in keeping balanced, while flat-foot exists in other cases.

Symptoms.—Children and adults tire more easily than they should when they have knock-knee, and occasionally pain and sensitiveness are complained of over the internal lateral ligament of the knee; as a rule children with knock-knee are clumsy and have a poor sense of balance. In the standing position it is noticed that the knees are unduly prominent on the inside aspect of the leg, and that the tibiæ diverge so that the feet are perhaps only an inch or so apart, or, again, in severe cases, a considerable distance. In cases in which the angular deformity is very great, the patients find the easiest position for standing is with one knee behind the other, so that in this way the feet may be brought together with one knee generally a little hyperextended.

The gait of a patient with double knock-knee is a rolling one, consisting of a series of slight lurches, which are, however, not nearly so marked as in bow-legs or congenital dislocation of the hip; while what is particularly noticeable is the outward throw of the leg when it is being brought forward. " Toeing in " is common, especially

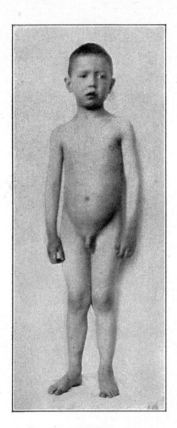
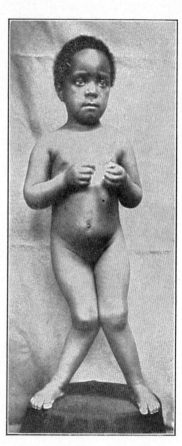

FIG. 145.—Slight Knock-knee.   FIG. 146.—Moderate Knock-knee.

in the slighter grades, and slight knock-knee is the most common cause of the toeing in, noticed in young children.

The angular deformity disappears when the knee is flexed to a right angle, except in cases in which the chief deformity is in the tibia.

As the deformity is most severe when the leg is in the extended position, all mechanical treatment applied to the correction of knock-knee must be to the fully extended leg. When the leg is fully flexed any inequality in the length of the condyles is most evident, as seen in outline from the anterior surface of the thigh. This may be registered by shaping a lead strip to the lower surface of the femur when

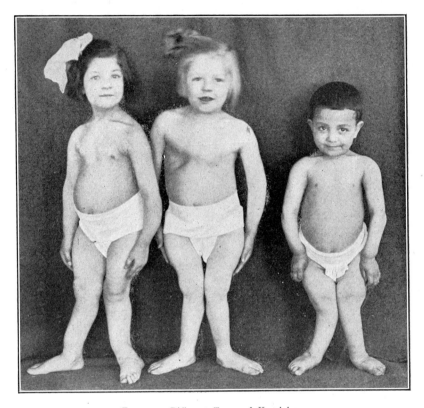

Fig. 147.—Different Types of Knock-knee.

the knee is fully flexed, and drawing an outline on paper from the lead strip.

Occasionally one sees a combination of knock-knee and bow-legs in the same subject.

Loose Knees.—In young children beginning to walk, who have grown rapidly or who have perhaps the mildest degree of rickets, there is often developed a laxity of the knee-joint which may require treatment. Such children stand with the knees prominent inward, but the deformity disappears on lying down and no overgrowth of the internal condyle is to be found. The knees can easily be hyperextended and are abnormally movable laterally, and such children are unsteady on their feet. The treatment consists of the measures to be described in speaking of the mildest cases of knock-knee.

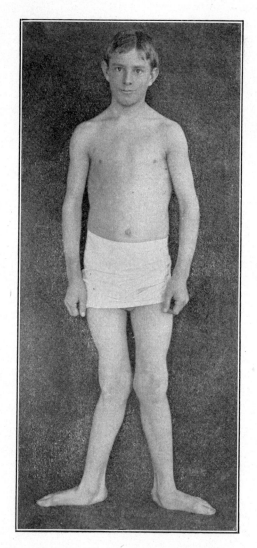

FIG. 148.—Severe Flat-foot Associated with Knock-knee.

Measurement of the Deformity.—The simplest and most reliable method of registration is to have the patient sit upon a sheet of brown paper with the legs extended and the feet pointing upward; and then, with a pencil held perpendicularly to the paper, to trace the outline of the legs.

Diagnosis.—The diagnostic points which mark the affection known as knock-knee are an inward angular deformity at the knee, which disappears on flexion of the leg upon the thigh. There is also in the

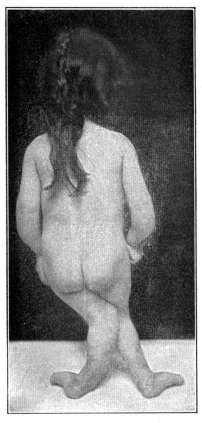

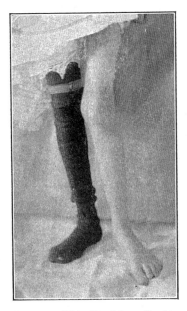

FIG. 149.—Severe Knock-knee due to Rickets. Seen from behind.

FIG. 150.—Slight Knock-knee Resulting from Tuberculous Disease of the Left Knee. Now cured.

latter position to be noted a relative prominence of the internal condyle of the femur in nearly all cases. The x-ray is of use in defining the chief location of the deformity when necessary.

Prognosis.—In severe cases spontaneous improvement is not to be expected. Children with a slight degree of knock-knee which is not progressive will probably outgrow it without any treatment if in vigorous health. If the deformity is moderate or severe, the chances are strong that the affection will remain stationary, or more probably will become worse as time goes on, unless active treatment is begun.

Treatment.—The treatment of knock-knee falls into three divisions: I. Expectant. II. Mechanical. III. Operative.

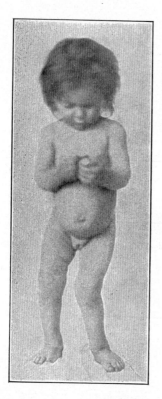

FIG. 151.—Bow-leg of Right Leg, Knock-knee and Flat-foot on Left.

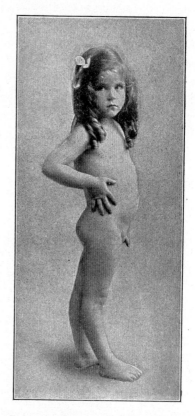

FIG. 152.—Hyperextended Position of the Knees, Frequently Seen in Connection with Knock-knee or Loose Knee.

I. The *expectant method of treatment* relies upon nature's efforts to repair the deformity; efforts which are aided on the part of the surgeon by keeping the child off of its feet to a greater or less extent, and by constitutional treatment and by massage and corrective manipulation.

When the expectant method is chosen in rhachitic knock-knee, the child should at once be put under the best possible conditions as to hygiene and diet.

The legs should be rubbed and manipulated each night, and the manipulation, in cases of knock-knee, should be directed to the gentle

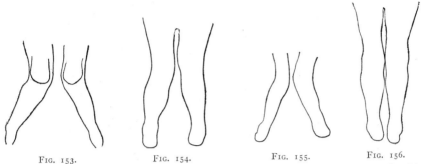

Fig. 153.   Fig. 154.   Fig. 155.   Fig. 156.

FIGS. 153 and 154.—Knock-knee. Mechanical treatment for one and one-half years.

FIGS. 155 and 156.—Knock-knee Cured in Three Years by the use of Simple Outside Upright. A good average result.

correction of the deformity by repeated mild manual pressure. With one hand the manipulator presses the knee outward, while with the

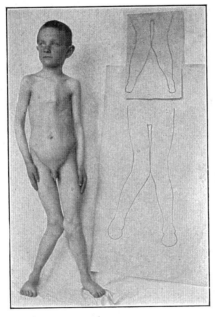

FIG. 157.—Case of Knock-knee, Showing also the Tracings of the Legs at an Interval of Four Years with no Treatment.

other he presses the lower part of the tibia inward. Even with a very slight degree of force a certain yielding can be felt in the direction of improvement, and then the pressure should be relaxed and the limb allowed to resume its first position. This manipulation should be repeated gently many times, continuing each pressure only a few seconds.

Tracings should be regularly taken to determine whether the deformity is improving or is stationary.

It is advisable in early knock-knee to raise the inner border of the boots one-quarter of an inch in order to bring the line of weight bearing at the knee as far outside as possible.

II. *Mechanical Treatment.*—Treatment by apparatus aims at the gradual correction of the deformity, commonly by making counter-

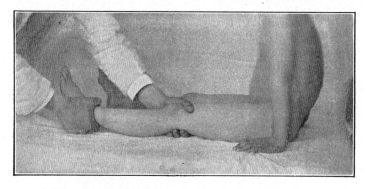

Fig. 158.—Manipulation in the Treatment of Knock-knee.

pressure against the internal condyle to prevent the further giving way of the knee and to pull it outward to a fixed point furnished by an outside upright. Mechanical treatment is to be used up to the age of 4 and osteotomy from 4 upward.

In the ambulatory treatment of the affection, a form which has been in use for some years at the Children's Hospital has proved itself efficient in practical use. It is a light steel rod attached below to a steel sole plate and jointed at the ankle. It runs up the outside of the leg as far as the trochanter, and then the rod is bent backward and upward, to lie against the upper part of the buttock and to serve as an arm by which the legs can be everted if the child toes in in walking. The knee is drawn upon by a square leather pad, pulling from the shaft opposite the knee.

III. *Operative Treatment.*—The modern operative treatment of knock-knee is comprised under the simple operations of osteotomy and osteoclasis.

Osteotomy.—The operation consists in the division of part of the bone by the chisel, and the completion of the procedure by fracture of the partly divided bone.

The operation is performed as follows: The patient's leg is rendered aseptic and the patient lies on his side with the leg extended, the outer side of the knee resting on a sand-bag.

The osteotome is inserted as near to the joint as is practicable without injury to the joint. The osteotome is inserted on the inner side

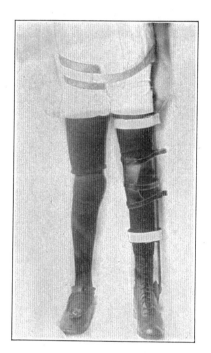

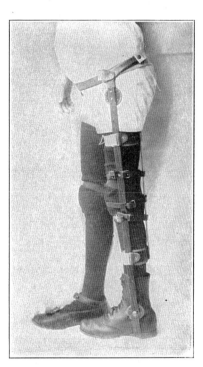

FIG. 159.—Knock-knee, Irons Applied.
Front view.

FIG. 160.—Knock-knee, Irons Applied.
Side view.

of the femur just above the adductor tubercle. The osteotome, which is driven through the sound skin without an incision, is at first placed with its blade parallel to the long axis of the limb and driven to the bone by light blows of the mallet. When the bone is reached the blade is turned so as to be at right angles to the long axis of the femur, and by successive blows with the mallet the operator cuts nearly through the whole thickness of the bone. The osteotome is likely to become wedged very firmly unless the precaution is taken to move the handle laterally after each blow. In this way alone can one cut from the front to the back of the bone, for driving the chisel straight through in one line accomplishes but little. When the osteotome has disappeared to a depth indicating that three-quarters of the bone has been divided, it should be withdrawn and an attempt made to fracture

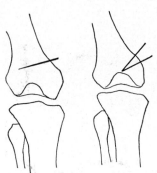

Fig. 161.—Line of Cutting in Osteotomy for Knock-knee. The picture on the left is the ordinary Macewen operation. The one on the right shows the removal of a wedge of bone required only in the severest cases.

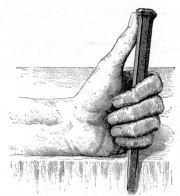

Fig. 162.—Proper Position for the Hand and Osteotome in Performing Osteotomy.

the thigh by bending. If this cannot be done, the osteotome should cut further, for the common mistake is a failure to divide the anterior and posterior borders of the femur.

When the bone has broken, unnecessary manipulation should be avoided, but the limb should be put in a slightly over-corrected position, and, after an aseptic dressing has been applied, a plaster-of-Paris bandage should be put on to hold the leg in this position. But little pain follows the operation. No change of dressing is needed; the plaster may be removed in three or four weeks, another reapplied, and in six weeks or more the patient allowed to stand on the limbs. Sometimes, when the deformity lies chiefly in the head of the tibia, the operation of osteotomy may be performed there either alone or in connection with femoral osteotomy. The removal of a wedge of bone is rarely necessary from either the femur or tibia in cases of knock-knee, except in very unusual cases. However, the operation described above is the one to be performed. *Osteoclasis* is less suited to the correction of knock-knee, because it lacks the precision of the osteotomy, and where a fracture near the joint is required the definite location of the fracture is desirable, which is to be accomplished best by the cutting.

BOW-LEGS.

In bow-legs the legs are most often bowed with convexity outward. This deformity is the reverse of knock-knee, and is termed *genu varum*. It is single or double, generally the latter, and may exceptionally exist in one leg when knock-knee is present in the other.

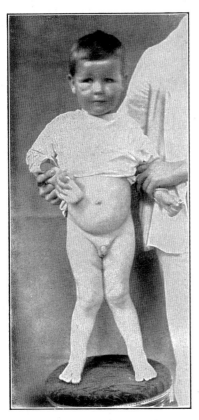

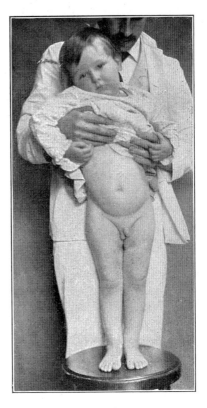

FIG. 163.—Moderate Knock-knee Before Operation.

FIG. 164.—Same Case After Macewen Osteotomy.

The curve is most often a gradual and uniform bowing of the femur and tibia, so that with the feet together the outline of the legs forms an oval which in severe cases approaches a circle. A second class of cases presents a bowing chiefly in the lower third of the tibia which is more angular in character, and the femurs are practically normal; a third class presents, either alone or in conjunction with the other deformities, a bowing forward of the tibia and sometimes of the femur also.

Occurrence.—The anatomical changes found are those of rickets. The bending of the bones is in most cases, like the other deformities

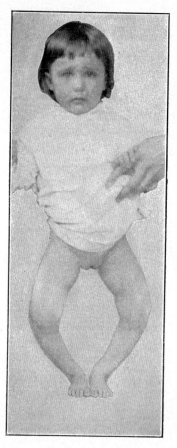

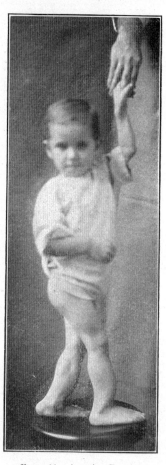

FIG. 165.—Bow-legs. Curve Involving Whole Leg.

FIG. 166.—Anterior Bow-legs.

of rickets, a simple yielding, without fracture, except in rare instances, where infractions as spoken of may be present.

Causation.—Bow-legs is essentially a rhachitic deformity in children, and true bow-legs can occur only in a child whose bones are soft enough to bend easily. It occurs in the first three or four years of life, and ordinarily in connection with general rickets; sometimes, however, other rhachitic manifestations cannot be detected.

Bow-legs of a marked type is seen in children who are too young ever to have borne their weight upon their legs. Early walking, so much talked about as a cause of bow-legs, is not to be accounted a factor of any importance in their production unless rickets in some

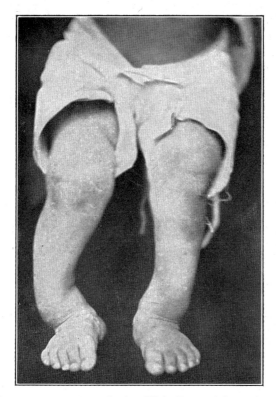

Fig. 167.—Bow-legs Affecting Chiefly Bones of Lower Leg.

degree is present. Why the bones should bend outward as they do is a question which is by no means settled.

Anterior curvature of the thigh and the leg bones is manifestly the result of body weight coming upon a flexed limb, conjoined perhaps to the action of the most powerful muscles in the body (the flexor muscles of the thigh) pulling in the same direction.

The child walks with a distinct waddle and generally with the feet wide apart and a tendency to invert the toes.

The deformity is almost always more conspicuous in the standing position, both because these children stand with the legs so far apart to secure a good balance and because the knee-joints generally yield somewhat in a lateral direction when the body weight is superimposed.

An inward rotation of the lower part of the tibia exists in bowlegs which causes " toeing in " in walking, the correction of which is important after operation.

Diagnosis.—The condition of bow-legs is evident on inspection.

It is often difficult to determine how much of the deformity lies in the tibia and how much in the femur. If the legs are crossed until

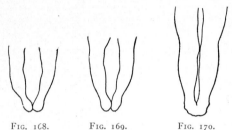

FIG. 168.   FIG. 169.   FIG. 170.

FIGS. 168, 169, and 170.—Case of Bow-legs. Progress in three years under expectant treatment.

the insides of the knees are together when the child is in a sitting position, it will be seen whether the femurs include an oval space between them or are parallel to each other.

Prognosis.—The prognosis in outward bow-legs is favorable in young children, in anterior bow-legs less favorable under expectant or mechanical treatment, but in young children rational mechancial treatment of ordinary outward bowing offers almost sure relief. Operative treatment can ameliorate almost any condition of deformity and often entirely rectify it. When the deformity is extreme or the bones are eburnated, it is not, of course, likely that the child will outgrow the bow-legs.

Treatment.—The treatment of bow-legs, like that of knock-knee, is to be considered under three heads: I. expectant, II. mechanical, III. operative.

I. The *expectant treatment* is suited to a large percentage of cases of the deformity in young children. In general, when the curve is uniform, involving femur and tibia alike, the chances are more favorable for spontaneous cure than if the deformity is localized in the tibia and more angular. During expectant treatment the general condition should be most carefully attended to. The child should be encouraged to be off of his feet as much as possible, and the legs should be massaged and manipulated each night, being gently bent toward a straight direction.

In all cases tracings should be taken at least once each month, and if after two or three months no improvement is evident, mechanical treatment should be begun.

In the case of babies the expectant plan of treatment is the one to be followed at first.

II. *Mechanical treatment,* which is to be pursued up to the age of four years, is based upon the principle of drawing the knee inward to a rod which has counter-points for sustaining outward pressure at the upper part of the thigh and at the ankle. Here, as in knock-knee, traction from a rigid rod is more definite and more satisfactory than from an elastic one. The form of apparatus used is of little consequence so long as it answers the indications and holds the knee extended.

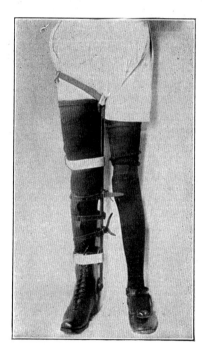

The apparatus shown is the one generally in use at the Children's Hospital in Boston, and is serviceable. It consists of a steel upright, which is attached below to the sole plate of the shoe. It runs up nearly to the origin of the adductor muscles, but it must fall a little short of them or it will excoriate the skin in walking. The upright is then bent forward and upward, and curved to fit into the groin and come up as far as the posterior part of the dorsum of the ilium. In this way a lever is provided with which to evert the feet to any extent by altering the curve of these arms and strapping them together behind. Pads for the outside of the legs are made of leather and buckled by two or three straps to the upright, opposite the greatest convexity of the curve.

FIG. 171.—Bow-leg. Brace Applied.

Anterior tibial curves are not susceptible of improvement or cure by mechanical treatment except in slight cases in which the bones are soft.

III. *Operative Treatment.*—**Osteoclasis.**—Mechanical fracture is made feasible by the use of osteoclasts, of which the one of Rizzoli

is the simplest and illustrates the principle. There are more modern
and more rapidly acting instruments, which will be found described
in the treatises on Orthopedic Surgery. The instrument is applied
to the bared limb, the padded rings being adjusted as far as is possible

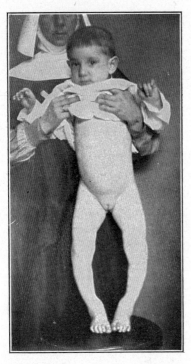 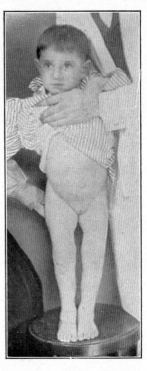

Fig. 172.—Bow-legs of Moderate Degree   Fig. 173.—Same Case After Osteo-
Before Operation.   clasis.

from the point at which fracture is desired, and the breaking pad
where the fracture is to be located. In placing the rings of the osteoclast on the limb, care should be taken not to put them too near to the
joints of the ankle or knee, as the epiphyses might be separated by
carelessness. Pressure is increased until fracture of the bones takes
place. The fracture of the bones is evidenced by a loud snap which
can be heard anywhere in the room.

After the bone has been broken, the osteoclast should be removed,
the fragments placed with the hands in a somewhat over-corrected
position, especial care being taken to correct the rotation of the tibia.
Sheet wadding is carefully placed around the leg, and the limb fixed

in a plaster bandage. The bandage should reach from the toes to the hip, and the limb should be held in the corrected position until the plaster has hardened thoroughly. Experience has shown that the procedure is ordinarily free from risk, and in properly selected cases the danger of non-union after fracture may be disregarded. The limb should remain in a fixed bandage for six weeks or more, and no appliance is needed as an after-treatment.

The amount of force required for the fracture of an adult bone

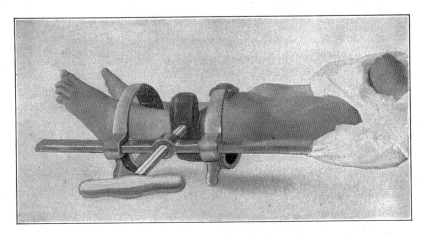

FIG. 174.—Method of Applying Osteoclast.

is very great, so much so as to make osteotomy in most instances a preferable procedure.

Cases should not as a rule be operated upon until the rhachitic process has been arrested, or recurrence of the deformity may take place.

Osteotomy should be employed in place of osteoclasis in cases of bow-legs (1) when the curvature is so near the joint that osteoclasis is not practicable; (2) when the bone is so strong that osteoclasis is not desirable on account of the contusing of the soft parts; (3) when several curves exist in the same leg; (4) sometimes when the curvature is anterior; (5) in cases of bow-leg in which the distortion is largely in the lower epiphysis of the femur; (6) in cases in which it is desired to locate the fracture very accurately, as in badly united fractures of both bones of the leg with displacement.

Osteotomy for bow-legs is a similar operation to that for knock-knee; the division of bone is made wherever it appears most necessary.

In young children the fibula need not be cut with the osteotome, but can be broken manually.

Anterior Bow-Legs.—In the treatment of anterior bow-legs, i.e., where the curve is forward and not to the side, the tibia may be broken by the osteoclast applied in the usual way, and after the fracture has been loosened by the hands the leg may be set straight. Tenotomy of the tendo Achillis aids this attempt and is often necessary. Osteotomy, however, as a rule, is more satisfactory in these cases. In anteriorly curved bow-leg in children, a linear osteotomy can be employed dividing the posterior two-thirds of the tibia and using the anterior portion as a hinge with the interlacing broken fibres and uninjured periosteum to promote healing. The osteotome is inserted in the side of the tibia. By this procedure the shortening caused by removing a wedge is avoided. Considerable manipulation is necessary after the osteotomy to free the fragments from the shortened posterior tissue, which is necessary to give a corrected position. In older cases a wedge-shaped incision may be necessary.

Cases will be met where several curves are present, and the judgment of the surgeon will be exercised in a choice of what bone is to be attacked and if more than one shall be operated upon at one time. The surgeon's purpose should be to correct those deformities which most interfere with normal gait, and leave others to the correction of growth or to a second operation.

RHACHITIC CURVES IN THE UPPER EXTREMITY.

These rarely present themselves for treatment, and but little further need be said except that by means of osteotomy the curves of the upper extremity can be treated as readily as those of the lower.

The methods described can be applied in the correction of improperly united fractures of the upper and lower extremities. The principles of treatment for the correction of these curves, in the main, are those considered in the treatment of rhachitic curves.

CHAPTER X.

COXA VARA.

THE name coxa vara is applied to a condition in which the neck of the femur becomes more horizontal than the normal angle of

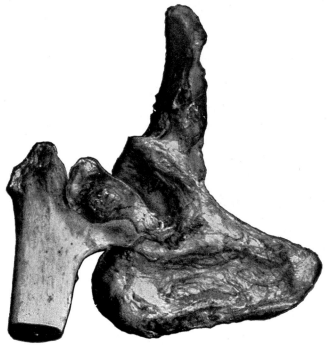

FIG. 175.—Specimen of Coxa Vara, no Clinical History. (Warren Museum.)

120°-140°, which it makes with the shaft. This bending of the neck may reach in extreme cases an angle less than 90°.

Etiology.—The affection is rarely congenital, but more often acquired, and in its purest form appears in adolescents as an affection apparently primary, being called in this case " static " coxa vara. In such cases one must assume a diminished resistance of the bone, but evidences of general rickets may be absent. The deformity also occurs in connection with general rickets in children, in osteomalacia, and after destructive diseases of bone, such as tuberculosis, osteomyelitis, arthritis deformans, ostitis fibrosa, etc. It also arises after fracture of the neck of the femur in adults and children and after

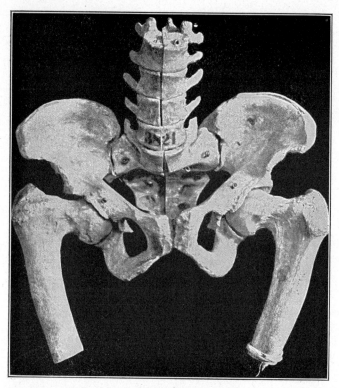

FIG. 176.—Specimen of Severe Double Coxa Vara from an Adult Female (No. 3821 in the Vienna Pathological Anatomical Museum). (Albert.)

epiphyseal displacements in children, in the latter instances being called "traumatic" coxa vara.

The affection may be unilateral or bilateral, and affects males more often than females.

The neck of the femur not only yields downward, but is apt also to rotate on the long axis of the femur. The most common twist of this sort is backward, which causes eversion of the foot and leg, although inversion of the foot and leg is sometimes present from the reverse twist. There may, however, be a simple downward displacement without any appreciable twist. Exceptionally there may be bending outward of the upper part of the femur, which gives rise to a deformity similar to that caused by the bending of the neck of the femur.

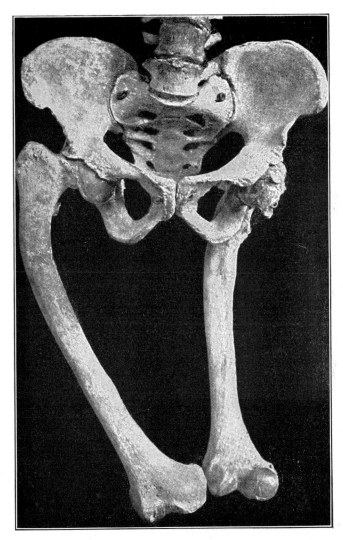

FIG. 177.—Coxa Vara and Bending Outward of the Upper Shaft of the Femur.   (Albert.)

In *traumatic coxa vara* a fall in a child may be followed by a temporary lameness in one hip, which later shows the signs described above, or such a fall is followed immediately by pain, shortening, eversion, and limited abduction of varying degree. An *x*-ray shows either an epiphyseal displacement or an impacted fracture or infraction of the neck of the femur. Such cases are frequently unrecognized until marked changes in the neck of the femur have taken place. Again, after recovery from a fracture of the femoral neck, walking may be begun before complete consolidation has taken place, and a yielding of the neck of the femur may occur later.

Symptoms.—The symptoms of coxa vara are discomfort and irri-

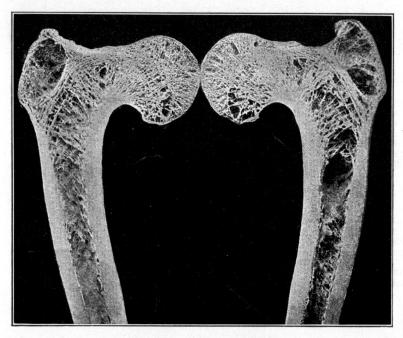

Fig. 178.—Sagittal Section of Coxa Vara, Showing Rearrangement of Trabeculæ to Compensate for Cross Strain. (Abbott.)

tability in the affected joint on walking with characteristic limitation of motion in abduction due to the altered relation of the trochanter and head of the femur, the trochanter impinging on the pelvis in abduction. In periods of joint irritation this limitation may extend to other joint motions. Lameness is present, and in bilateral cases the gait becomes a waddling, restricted gait.

Shortening of the affected limb is present, with generally some muscular atrophy; the trochanter is found above Nélaton's line and unduly prominent, and flexion of the thigh is generally made in an abducted plane. In severe double cases the thighs may be crossed on the abdomen in extreme flexion. The x-ray shows a diminished angle of the neck of the femur with the shaft.

Diagnosis.—The recognition of coxa vara is not always easy. The signs on which reliance must be placed are shortening, elevation of the trochanter, limited abduction, and prominence of the trochanter. If the child stands on the affected leg the buttock of the well side will not drop (Trendelenberg's sign), which is the case in congenital dislocation of the hip. An x ray is of assistance in establishing the changed relation between the neck and shaft of the femur.

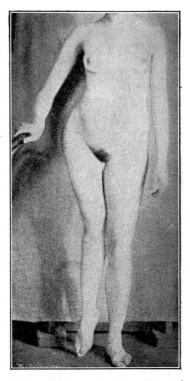

The condition most likely to be confused with coxa vara is hip disease, but in the former, generally abduction is the only motion limited and joint restriction is rarely extreme; shortening is present to a degree which would only exist with much destruction of bone in tuberculosis, and the x-ray is of much value.

In young children it is sometimes difficult to discriminate between this condition and congenital dislocation of the hip. In both the trochanter is prominent, and above Nélaton's line, shortening is marked and limitation of joint motion comparatively

FIG. 179.—Traumatic Coxa Vara of Right Leg, from an Accident Occurring when Patient was Four Years Old. (Hoffa.)

slight. In dislocation the head of the bone can generally be felt under the fingers and can be slipped in and out of the socket, but in some cases this is not easy to detect, and the x-ray alone will at times establish the diagnosis.

Diagnosis.—The diagnosis is generally to be made by the signs given above, aided by the x-ray, and the conditions most likely to be confused with coxa vara are congenital dislocation of the hip and hip disease.

Prognosis.—In the coxa vara of young children accompanying general rickets, it seems likely that the deformity is in many cases at least outgrown from the rarity of severe coxa vara in adults, who have had rickets in childhood. In other cases there seems no reason to look for spontaneous cure.

Treatment.—The treatment of coxa vara is to be classed as conservative or operative.

Conservative Treatment.—In the stage when the bone may be regarded as congested and therefore unfit to bear weight-bearing strain, crutches, or some apparatus forming a perineal crutch (the Thomas knee-splint and the convalescent hip-splint) may be used. With restricted walking and standing, such treatment may be regarded as likely to quiet joint irritation and as a check to the increase of the deformity. If sufficiently long continued it should influence growth toward the normal. Massage is a useful addition to such treatment in stimulating the local circulation. Traction in bed in an abducted position is desirable in acutely irritated cases.

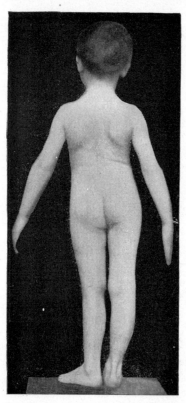

Fig. 180.—Fracture of Hip Four Years after the Accident. Shows Eversion. (Whitman.)

Operative Treatment.—If conservative treatment has failed to give relief, or if the case is already well marked, some more active treatment is desirable. If there is reason to suppose, from the history, the symptoms, and the *x*-ray, that the bone of the femoral neck is still soft, the patient should be anæsthetized, and the leg forcibly abducted with the idea of bending the neck. It is not desirable to produce a loose fracture. Following this the leg is fixed in an abducted position by a plaster-of-Paris spica for two months, after which protected use (by means of a perineal crutch) may be begun.

Osteotomy.—In cases where there is no reason to suppose that the bone is still soft enough to bend, and where operative correction

seems advisable, osteotomy of the neck or shaft of the femur affords
the best means of relief.

The method generally advisable is to divide the shaft of the femur
transversely below the trochanter minor by an osteotome, and after

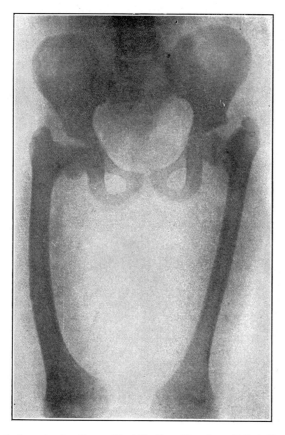

Fig. 181.—Radiograph of a Severe Rhachitic Coxa Vara in a Patient Six Years Old.
(Joachimsthal.)

correction of the rotation of the femur to abduct the leg and fix it
in a position of marked abduction in a plaster-of-Paris spica.

A wedge-shaped osteotomy at the same level may be performed
in cases where no rotation of the leg exists, and has the advantage of
leaving a hinge of bone at the inner surface of the femur so that no
slipping by of the fragments will occur; but it is generally more difficult to perform than a linear osteotomy, in addition to which it
increases shortening.

An osteotomy of the femoral neck through an anterior incision attacks more directly the seat of the deformity, but this operation requires a rather deep incision; drainage of the wound is poor, and the method offers in most cases no marked advantage over the one advocated.

Traumatic Coxa Vara.—In cases seen long after the accident the treatment is the same as that described above. In recent cases force should be used to correct the diminished angle of the neck and the limb fixed in abduction. Unprotected use of such a leg should not be allowed for many months after the correction.

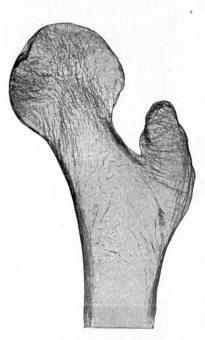

FIG. 182.—Radiograph of a Sagittal Section of a Specimen of Coxa Valga, Amputation of the Thigh having been Done in Childhood. (Turner.)

COXA VALGA.

Coxa Valga [1] is the name applied to the condition which is the reverse of coxa vara, and which has been extensively studied in the last few years. In this the angle between the neck and the shaft of the femur is increased above 140°. In connection with this deformity also twists of the neck of the femur may occur.

The causes of the deformity are as follows: trauma probably resulting in defective epiphyseal growth, osteomalacia, rickets, osteomyelitis of the pelvis, infantile paralysis, and amputation of the leg causing disuse, multiple exostoses, genu valgum, and congenital dislocation of the hip. Congenital cases have been described,[2] and some cases arise in which no cause can be assigned.

The symptoms are pain and irritability of the affected hip, with a limp caused largely by the abducted and lengthened leg on the side affected. The leg is generally rotated outward, is longer than the

[1] Drehmann : Zeitsch. f. orth. Chir., xvi., 1-2.
[2] Galeazzi : Am. Journ. of Orth. Surg., iv., 240.—Young : Am. Journ. of Orth. Surg., iv., 256.—Mauclaire and Ollivier : Arch. gén. de Chir., 1908, i., 1.

other, and is carried in a position of abduction. The trochanter is less prominent than normal and is generally below Nélaton's line;

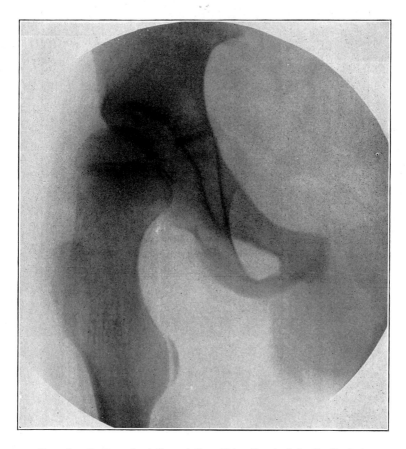

FIG. 183.—Radiograph of Case of Coxa Valga Due to Infantile Paralysis.

abduction is free and adduction restricted at the hip-joint. The diagnosis is greatly aided by a skiagram.

The affection has been too recently recognized and studied to enable one to speak definitely as to the treatment yielding the best end results. Excellent immediate results have been reported from each of the following methods of treatment: (1) Exercises and massage [1]; (2) forcible adduction and retention in plaster-of-Paris in a

[1] Stieda : Arch. f. klin. Chir., 87, 1, 243.

position of extreme adduction [1]; (3) osteotomy of the neck of the femur and allowing the shaft to slip upward on the neck by dimin-

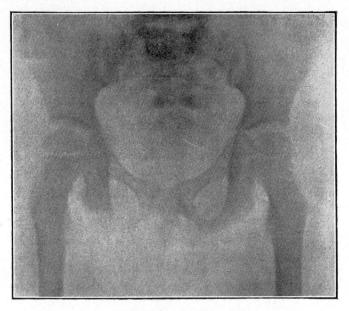

FIG. 184.—Radiograph of a Case of Coxa Valga. (David.)

ishing traction in the after-treatment [2]; (4) subtrochanteric linear osteotomy [3]; subtrochanteric wedge-shaped osteotomy.[4]

[1] Kumaris : Arch. f. klin. Chir., 1908, 87, 3, 625.
[2] Galeazzi : loc. cit.
[3] Allison : Am. Journ. of Orth. Surg., v., 228.
[4] Tubby : British Med. Journ., 1908, 2482.

CHAPTER XI.

LATERAL CURVATURE OF THE SPINE.

DEFINITION.

By this term is understood a constant deviation of the spinal column, or a portion of it, to either side of the median line of the body, with a resulting distortion of the trunk. The affection is also called scoliosis.

Lateral curvature is either congenital or acquired.

FREQUENCY.

The affection is a common one, but its prevalence can only be estimated, as statistics gathered vary apparently according to the standard of the observer; but it is probable that lateral curves of a grade need ing treatment will be found in from 20 to 30 per cent of our school children.

The distortion is seen more frequently in girls than in boys, but statistics as to the comparative frequency of the deformity in females as compared with males vary.

Age.—Although it is probable that the distortion exists to a slight extent at an earlier age, the majority of cases brought to the surgeon for treatment are from ten to sixteen years of age.

PATHOLOGY.

The pathological changes in acquired lateral curvature are not those resulting from destructive disease of the vertebræ, but are the alterations of bone induced by abnormal pressure and strain.

The spinal column, as a whole, is bent and twisted, and the individual vertebræ are in places altered in shape as well as misplaced from their normal relation to the vertical plane of the trunk. The ribs and pelvis may be altered in shape. The muscles and ligaments are altered in their tonicity and length, and internal organs may be displaced.

Characteristic of the deformity is the combination of a side curve of the spinal column with a twist, the spinous processes pointing

away from and the vertebral bodies being turned toward the convexity of the curve. This rotation is the result of the structure of
the spinal column, which cannot bend to the side without twisting.

The changes seen necessarily vary according to the stage of the
affection and the degree to which the deformity has developed.

In the earliest stage of scoliosis slight if any anatomical change
will be found in the bones, ligaments, or muscles; but in the later
phases of the affection, marked distortion of the whole spinal column,
as well as the individual vertebræ, is to be observed.

Wherever a side curve with rotation of the spine has taken place,
the bodies are crowded together on the concave and separated on the
convex side of the curve, and the vertebral bodies become thicker on
one side than the other, and changes in shape of the articulating and
transverse processes and intervertebral disks also take place. The
ribs follow the transverse processes, and show a characteristic projection on one side and flattening on the other. The projection of
the ribs is naturally more noticeable than the projection of the transverse processes without ribs, so that in the lumbar region the rotation
seems slight when compared with that of the dorsal region.

If the column is curved laterally in two or three directions, rotation necessarily takes place in different parts of it in opposite directions.

The intervertebral cartilages necessarily twist with the vertebræ
and are compressed on one side more than on the other in cases of
marked curves; in severe cases they will be found on measurement
thicker on the side of convexity than of concavity, so that instead of
being flat they are wedge-shaped from side to side. In some cases
the rotation is more marked than the curve, the line of the spines being
nearly straight, while the bodies are found badly out of line, the axis
of rotation being near the spines.

The ribs project backward at the angle on the side of the convexity of the curve and forward on the side of the concavity, and the
contour of the thorax is changed from the altered shape of the ribs.
Cross sections of the thorax shows an alteration of the diagonal
axes of the chest, and the section on the convex side is smaller than
that on the concave side, owing to the flattening of the ribs. The
vertebral bodies are also crowded into this half of the thorax, so
that there is less room for expansion of the lung on that side than on
the other side. In the severest cases of distortion, the lower ribs on
one side may rest upon the crest of the ilium or sink into the pelvic
cavity.

The muscles of the spinal column in an early case of lateral curvature are unaffected, except in cases of a purely paralytic nature; but in advanced cases the muscles are degenerated.

In advanced cases of lateral curvature, the ligaments on the con-

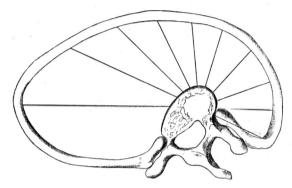

FIG. 185.—Transverse Section of a Scoliotic Thorax.   (Albert.)

cave side of the spinal column are shortened and those on the convex side are elongated.   This is the result of adaptive shortening, and is not found in the early stages of the affection.

The pelvis is not necessarily distorted in lateral curvature of the spine, but the bones of the pelvis may, if not sufficiently unyielding in their structure, become altered by abnormal pressure or strain.   The

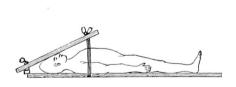

FIG. 186.—Method Used for Producing Deformity of Head by Flat-Head Indians.   (From Sketch from Lewis and Clark.)

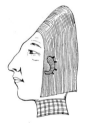

FIG. 187.—The Flat-Head Indian.   An old man.

pelvis may assume the appearance of obliquity from a prominence of one hip due to the uncovering of the crest of the ilium by the overprojecting ribs, but true obliquity is exceptional.   When there is irregularity in the length of the legs, obliquity of the pelvis necessarily exists.   The spinal cord is not affected by lateral curvature.   The spinal nerves, in consequence of the large size of the foramina, are not liable to suffer compression, but symptoms of nerve-root pressure are at times observed in advanced cases.

The abdominal viscera are less likely to be displaced than the thoracic organs, though the liver may be out of place and altered in form, the spleen may suffer some compression, and the aorta is necessarily displaced, but to a less degree than in Pott's disease. The lung on the convex side of the curve is much more compressed and flattened than on the other and the heart is generally found displaced toward the concavity of the curve in severe cases.

It is known that bone, like other portions of the human frame, muscle, and skin, adapts itself to conditions, being changed in shape and strength under pressure and strain, as is shown by the Flat-headed Indians, whose skulls were distorted by pressure mechanically applied for a long period in infancy. The foot of a Chinese lady is another illustration.

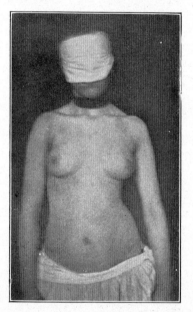

Fig. 188.—Front View of Lateral Curvature, Showing Prominence of Left Mamma in Right Dorsal Convex Curvature.

ETIOLOGY.

The phenomena of lateral curvature, curve and rotation, have been produced experimentally on the cadaver of infants, and in animals by securing for six months the spine of growing dogs by a stiff bandage in a bent position. Growing children, obliged to retain an abnormal position through paralysis, often acquire scoliosis, and the Siamese twins, prevented from normal attitudes, developed lateral curves.

To explain the development of scoliosis it is only necessary to assume the existence of a constantly applied force exerted upon the spinal column in abnormal directions. As the resistance offered by the bone differs in different portions of the spine, and, as individuals differ, similar distorting conditions do not produce the same deformity in different individuals. Of the factors favoring abnormal distribution of superimposed weight, the following may be mentioned as being the most common:

1. Faulty attitudes in standing or sitting.

2. Inequality of the length of the limbs, pelvic asymmetry, or other causes tilting or twisting the pelvis.

3. Abnormal attitudes due to occupation, to defective eyesight or hearing, to torticollis, muscular weakness, or paralysis.

4. To contractions following empyema.

5. Congenital defects, absence or defects of the ribs or vertebræ.

The primary curve may be followed by secondary distortions due to abnormal muscular pull of the thoracic and abdominal muscles upon

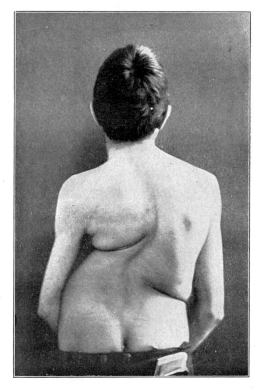

FIG. 189.—Right Lateral Curvature.   (Weigel.)

the ribs and vertebral column in the patient's attempt to establish proper poise. These distortions vary according to the variations in abnormal strains and the abnormality in tissue resistance at different thoracic levels.

Lateral curvature is naturally favored by causes which will diminish the resistance of bone to abnormally applied weight. Apart from disease of the structure of bone, these are: (1) rickets and osteo-malacia; (2) abnormal lack of bone resistance of the spinal column, from rapid, excessive, or ill-nurtured growth.

SYMPTOMS.

Early History.—The deformity of scoliosis is developed during the growing years, becoming arrested, as a rule, at the end of the period of growth.

The affection is ordinarily discovered by the patient's mother at the age just previous to puberty, although it is developed earlier than

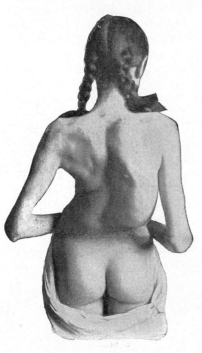
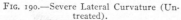
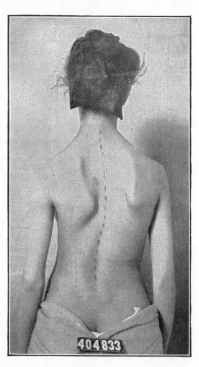

FIG. 190.—Severe Lateral Curvature (Un-treated).

FIG. 191.—Right Dorsal, Slight Left Lumbar Curve.

this in a majority of cases without being recognized, except in the severe cases. The patient suffers no inconvenience in this early stage, and as the child is at an age (five to ten) when the figure is not care-fully scrutinized, little attention is paid to the slight elevation of the shoulder or projection of the hip. Upon superficial examination but little else is to be seen, and these symptoms disappear on recumbency or suspension. A careful examination often discloses a curve of the spine to the side.

In a majority of cases, however, when the surgeon is consulted, well marked development of the distortion has already taken place.

The muscular system may or may not be well developed, but in

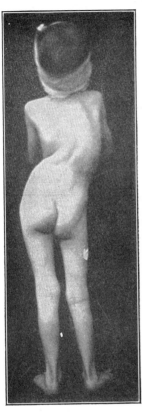

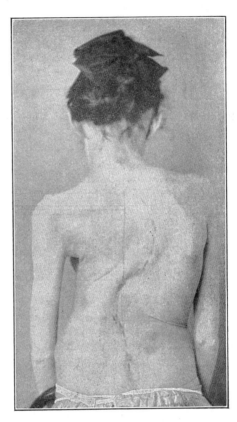

FIG. 192.—Lateral Curvature due to Infantile Paralysis of Muscles of Trunk.

FIG. 193.—Severe Right Dorsal, Left Lumbar Curve Showing Marked Lumbar Rotation on the Left.

a majority of cases the muscles are not large or strong. In a few instances of growing girls with marked impairment of strength some thoracic pain may be felt, and fatigue on exertion in walking or standing. But cases of severe curvatures will be seen in which development has slowly continued during the years of younger adult life. In the severe cases seen in early or middle childhood the deformity will generally prove to be due to congenital defects, rickets, empyema, or infantile paralysis.

Spontaneous arrest when adult life is reached takes place in a very large number of the slighter cases, without further development of the deformity. Even in many of the severer types of the deformity, patients will be observed who apparently go through adult life without increase of the deformity.

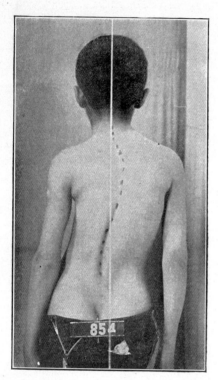

FIG. 194.—Right Dorsal, Left Lumbar Curve with Displacement of Body to the Right.

Pain.—Painful symptoms are not common in the affection, but when present, such symptoms may be classed as follows:

1. Those due directly to the altered muscular or ligamentous strain.

2. Those due to the abnormal pressure from distorted ribs upon the nerves or ilium, or by vertebræ upon nerves, or to alteration of the size and shape of the thorax, and displacement of viscera.

3. Neurasthenic symptoms from a lack of vitality, superinduced by the limitations as to exercise and activity, consequent on the deformity, and to the impairment of circulation and respiration by the deformity of the chest.

Interruption in the functions of the lungs, heart, liver, stomach, and intestines is occasionally seen in severe cases, shortness of breath and indigestion being frequent symptoms in the severer cases in adult life. In the severest cases in adults the patients are thin, and as a rule lack resistance, being especially prone to pulmonary tuberculosis.

Deformity.—The chief symptom of lateral curvature is the distortion.

The curves of the spinal column vary in degree, situation, and extent. There are, however, common types, which it is convenient to bear in mind in considering the subject of treatment.

Structural and Postural Curves.—Curves will be found to vary not only in their localization and their amount of rotation, but also in their rigidity. This variation is due to the variation in the amount of structural change. For clinical purposes it is convenient to apply

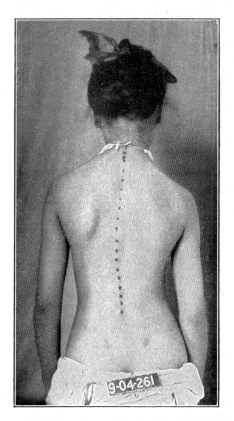

Fig. 195.—Left Total Curve, Showing Elevated Left Shoulder.

the term *structural, fixed,* or *habitual* curves to those with evident changes in the tissues, and *functional* or *postural* to those curves without definite structural changes. The latter are flexible and easily corrected by the patient's effort, by lying down, or by suspension. In such rotation is not a prominent symptom. The terms *primary* and *secondary* curves are also used to define the relative clinical importance or severity of the two curves present.

Lateral curvature either involves the whole spine in one curve, termed by some writers *total scoliosis,* or it is chiefly confined to a region or regions of the spine, when the curvature is called *cervical, dorsal,* or *lumbar scoliosis.* These are defined as right or left, according to the direction of the convexity of the curves.

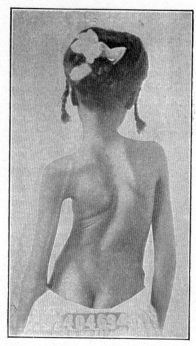

FIG. 196.—Right Dorsal Curve, Showing Elevation of Right Shoulder, Prominent Left Hip, and Rotation of Right Chest Backward.

What is termed *double scoliosis* is met when an upper curve is found in one direction and a lower in the opposite, or *triple scoliosis* when three curves are present.

If one lateral curve occurs in the middle region of the spinal column, one or two other compensating curves, above or below the deformity, are of necessity developed in opposite directions, to preserve the patient's balance, in order that the head be kept erect and in the median line. In some instances one of the compensating curves is of an equal prominence with the so-called primary curve, in which case the spinal column will present the S-shaped curve which is characteristic.

The curves are rarely limited exactly to definite anatomical regions of the spinal column; the upper curve may be so long as to include all of the dorsal and upper lumbar vertebræ. Again, the lower curve may be so long as to invade nearly the whole of the dorsal region, the compensation taking place in the upper part of the cervical region.

Cervical Curvature.—The cervical or cervico-dorsal curves are the least common form of lateral curvature, occurring in about 36 per cent of cases,[1] and are convex to the left more often than to the right.

This form is most commonly accompanied by a long compensatory lower curve. There is elevation of the shoulder on the convex side

[1] Joachimsthal; Hdbch. d. orth. Chir., 1903, iii , 708.

of the lateral curve at the level of the shoulders and the head is tipped to the side of the concavity of the cervical curve.

Dorsal Curvature.—The most common dorsal curve is with the convexity to the right. In these cases the right shoulder will be raised, the right shoulder blade will project backward more prominently than the left, and will be at a higher horizontal level and farther from

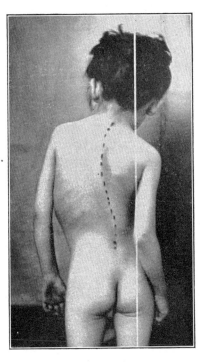

Fig. 197.—Lateral Curvature Due to Empyema of Right Chest. Five months after operation.

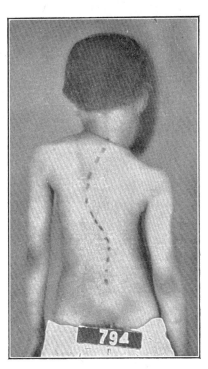

Fig. 198.—Congenital Lateral Curvature Associated with Absence of Ribs.

the median line of the trunk. The back, just below the scapula, will be more rounded backward on the right side and more flattened on the left. In front, in well-marked cases, the breast and front of the chest will be more prominent on the left than on the right side.

In addition to the curve there is displacement of the whole trunk to the right side, as a result of which the right arm, when hanging, will be free from the side, while the left arm, when hanging down, necessarily strikes the hip.

There is also, unavoidably, a change in the outline of the sides of the back. The sides, instead of being symmetrical, as seen from the back, will be different; one side being unnaturally straight, and the other more than normally hollowed.

The normal backward physiological curve in the dorsal region may be diminished so that the upper back is abnormally flat, or it may be increased so that the dorsal region is abnormally bowed. Dorsal curves exist alone in about 20 per cent, and combined with other curves in about 30 per cent, of the cases.

Lumbar Curvature.—Dorso-lumbar or lumbar curvature manifests itself by a prominence of one of the hips; the one on the side of the concavity of the curve appearing in the contour of the trunk higher than on the other side, as the iliac crest is less covered by overlying tissue. It is often termed a " high hip," but incorrectly; measurement showing no difference. In well-marked lumbar curvature there is also a fulness in the back on the convex side, above the crest of the ilium, and a corresponding hollowing on the other. A marked difference in the outlines of the two sides of the back, already mentioned, is seen in this form of curvature. Lumbar curves exist alone in something over 10 per cent of the cases, but are seen most often associated with other curves.

A combination of lumbar and dorsal curves in opposite directions, or compound curves as they have been termed, will present the features of both varieties, the distortion of the most pronounced curve being predominant.

Rotation.—As was explained under the head of pathology, it is impossible for any curvature to take place in the spinal column without being accompanied by rotation, and the prominence of rotation in lateral curvature is, in a general way, a measure of the severity of the case.

Rotation is always toward the convex side of the lateral curve; but in childhood the so-called total scoliosis often shows a general backward prominence of one side (spoken of as reverse rotation, retro-torsion, concave torsion, paradoxical scoliosis, etc.), and the backward projecting shoulder will often be found on the concave rather than the convex side. This occurs only in a flexible spinal curve, where the compensatory curve is not easily recognized or established. It is perhaps the initial stage of the ordinary type of scoliosis, the long curve being afterward divided into two sections.

When school children are examined irrespective of symptoms complained of, many postural curves not brought to the surgeon for examination are seen. Of these, total curves will be found the most common, and of these, the one with the convexity to the left is the most frequent.

VARIETIES OF LATERAL CURVATURE.

Congenital scoliosis and its causes have been already alluded to; acquired scoliosis appears most often in the following forms:

Rhachitic Lateral Curvature.—This form occurs in rhachitic children, but it is not so common a curve as the simple posterior curve

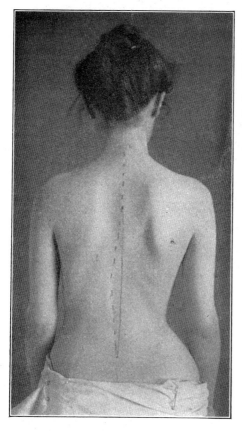

Fig. 199.—Left Lumbo-dorsal Curve.

which appears as a backward prominence in the lumbar region in so many cases of rickets. It is probable that if cases with rickets were more carefully examined, scoliosis would be more frequently observed.

Difference in Length of Legs.—A slight difference in the length of the lower limbs is the rule. But development of lateral curvature directly from this cause is not invariable, because in cases of scoliosis a notable difference in the length of the lower limbs is detected in about the same proportion of cases as in normal children. In children

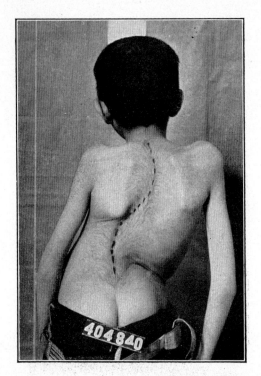

Fig. 200.—Severe Curvature due to Rickets.

with marked inequality in the length of the legs and with diminished resistance in the vertebral column, scoliosis may follow.

Paralytic Lateral Curvature.—In a certain number of cases of paralysis of the muscles of the back lateral curvature of the spine is found. The curvature may be toward the side of the paralyzed muscles or away from them. This form of lateral curvature is most commonly developed after infantile paralysis, but the distortion may be seen after spastic paralysis, progressive muscular hypertrophy, syringomyelia, and similar affections.

Torticollis.—Congenital torticollis, if uncorrected, is always followed by scoliosis. *Inequality of vision* and *hearing* and *congenital* *conditions* causing the head to be held to one side are other possible causes of scoliosis.

Lateral Curvature from Contracture of the Chest.—Lateral curvature may follow empyema. In the purest forms of this type, the contracted side of the chest is on the side of the concavity of the lateral curve.

A curvature is sometimes observed in connection with organic heart disease in children.

Lateral Curvature from Occupation.—Any occupation which necessitates faulty attitudes for long periods daily, favors the development

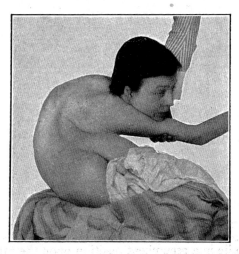

FIG. 201.—Severe Case of Spastic Paralysis in a Patient who had never Walked and who from Childhood had Sat to One Side. The patient is now an adult.

of a spinal curve, but lateral curvatures of severe type due to ordinary occupation are not, as a rule, common, for the reason that laborious occupations are not, in general, entered upon until an age when the spinal column has a sufficient amount of resistance to withstand the superimposed weight without developing great structural change.

Scoliosis seen in school children is in reality generally an occupation deformity, resulting as it does from the constant assumption of faulty attitudes, which produce abnormal pressure and strain upon growing spinal columns lacking in structural resistance.

Alteration in the shape of the vertebræ from disease (Pott's disease, osteomyelitis of the spine, and spondylitis deformans) may cause lateral curvature. It may also occur in sacro-iliac disease as the result of muscular spasm. *Ischias scoliotica,* referred to also as scoliosis neuromuscularis, or neuropathica or ischiatica, is a term which has been applied to lateral curvature in the lower part of the spinal column occurring in connection with sciatica and lumbago.

DIAGNOSIS.

The method of examination of a case of lateral curvature is as follows:

The patient's back should be bared to the level of the trochanters, and the arms should be allowed to hang free. In young children when feasible the whole figure should be unclothed and the position of the lower extremities inspected. The most natural attitude in standing should be noted and also the position of the patient in an attempt to stand in as straight a position as is possible; the tips of the spinous processes are to be marked with a skin pencil, and also the ends of the scapulæ. To determine the central line a string, to which a slight weight is attached, can be used as a plumbline to show a perpendicular. It should be made to hang so as to pass through the cleft of the buttock, and the deviation of the spine from this vertical line can be noted. The distance of the tips of the scapulæ from this central line should be recorded, and also the distances from this line to the points of greatest curvature of the line of the spinous process. The slope of the shoulders, the outlines of the sides of the trunk, and the contour of the back, as well as any lack of symmetry or unilateral fulness, should be carefully recorded. If a side deviation is observed, the patient should be suspended by means of a head sling and also made to lie in a recumbent position upon the face. A marked alteration of the curvature, contour, or outlines following removal of the superincumbent weight is of particular importance. If the curve disappears under these conditions, it is to be classed as chiefly postural. If it does not disappear, it is to be considered structural.

The patient should then bend forward with the knees straight and the arms hanging until the trunk is horizontal. In the normal spine the two sides of the back will be on a level when viewed in this position. Rotation of the ribs or lumbar vertebræ due to structural changes is shown by a greater upward prominence of the side of the back which has rotated backward.

The flexibility of the spine should be tested by causing the patient to stand first with one foot and then the other upon a series of blocks half an inch in thickness, and testing what height can be placed under the patient's foot without preventing her from standing upon both legs with the limbs straight, without flexion at the knee; this tests

the lateral flexibility in the lower part of the spinal column. In testing
the flexibility higher up, the patient should be seated on a stool, and
one hand of an assistant be placed upon her side, above the crest of
the ilium, while the other hand should be placed upon the crest of the
ilium of the opposite side. The patient should then be directed to
bend sideways toward the side of the higher hand, and the amount
of this motion, without tilting of the pelvis, is to be noted.

It is not always necessary to examine the front of the patient's
trunk in the case of older patients. When this is done, the projection

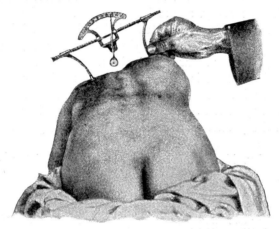

Fig. 202.—Measurement of the Rotation of the Ribs in the Horizontal Position by the Levelling
Trapezium of Schulthess. (Schulthess.)

of the ribs in front, and the difference in the prominence or flatness
of the two breasts, the deviation of the tip of the sternum and of the
umbilicus from the median line are of importance, as indicating the
amount of structural change which has taken place. Asymmetry of
outline is always to be more clearly seen from the front than from
the back of any patient.

The accidental assumption of a faulty attitude does not justify a
diagnosis of lateral curvature but the habitual assumption of such
a position, when the patient stands in the attitude of ease and greatest
comfort, indicates an abnormal condition. The existence of slight
grades of lateral curvature is made more evident by allowing the
patient to stand for a minute before beginning the examination, in
order to obtain the relaxed position due to beginning muscular fatigue.

The amount of structural change is indicated by the amount of
stiffness and by the slight change in the curves and asymmetrical

symptoms as the patient alters the position by standing, lying, bending, twisting, and hanging, and by the extent of the rotation.

Lateral curvature is not infrequently confounded with Pott's disease. In pronounced lateral curvature, the lateral twist and the rotation are essentially different from the curve of Pott's disease, which is chiefly an antero-posterior curve.

Methods of Recording Lateral Curvature.

Of the many methods for recording lateral curvature the simplest, if of sufficient accuracy, are to be preferred.

If the measurements are noted of the distance of fixed points on the spine from a plumb line and these are recorded, the curves can serve as a measure for future comparison.

If a graphic record is desired, a simple method can be employed if the patient with the pelvis secured is placed with the bared back against a transparent sheet of celluloid secured in a fixed position focussed on the portion of the back showing the greatest rotation of the spine.

Photography, if carefully employed, is of assistance.[1] For this purpose the spinous processes should be marked.

The outline of the figure and the line of the marked spines can be traced on a celluloid plate. Accuracy is obtained by the use of fixing the marking pencil in a diopter, easily made by boring two holes in a small wooden block, one oblique holding the pencil and another vertical securing symmetry of the pencil point.

PROGNOSIS.

In the larger number of cases the affection is a self-limited one, occasioning slight deformity, which persists through life, causing no trouble and recognized only by the dressmaker or by some near relative. In other cases, however, the deformity increases, and a pitiable distortion follows, causing a marked deformity, perhaps neuralgic pain, and ill health.

It is impossible to state positively in what instances an increase of the curve will take place and when they can be relied upon to remain stationary. It may, however, be said that when the physical condition during the growing period remains constantly below the proper standard, and when the patient's growth is rapid, an increase of curve is to be apprehended. The decrease or diminution of lateral

[1] Ueber die Messmethoden des Rückens. Hovorka, Wien, 1904.

curvature from simple growth without treatment is not to be expected. Sometimes the disease may remain to a slight extent during early life, developing an increase at a period past middle life. Such cases are dependent upon a loss of general health and upon trophic changes occurring at this period of life.

In determining the prognosis the probable period of growth ahead is to be borne in mind. This can be ascertained by the patient's height, the hereditary tendency toward height as ascertained by the height of the parents and the parents' families. This is of importance, because the completion of growth exerts a powerful influence in arresting progress of the curvature.

In general it may be said that if a patient has gained full height and development in figure, any increase in growth is not often to be expected, and that an increase in curve is not probable after the osseous system has become thoroughly formed and the strength of the spinal column established; except in the severe cases, where there is more tendency to slight increase, even during adult life.

Prognosis under Treatment.—Cases of postural scoliosis should be completely cured by proper treatment. If cases of scoliosis have little structural change, improvement can always be obtained, and in younger children this can be generally made a permanent cure. In cases with marked structural change in the growing years, diminution of the curve is to be expected to follow adequate treatment. In rigid cases an improvement of condition and carriage can be hoped for. The prospects of treatment are, of course, better when it can be carried on during the period of growth.

PREVENTIVE MEASURES.

Certain measures are of importance, not only in preventing scoliosis, but as a preliminary to treatment when scoliosis exists.

Attitude at School.—Correct methods of sitting during school, especially in writing, are of importance, and the matter has received much attention. It is perfectly evident that the continued assumption of a curved and twisted position is a competent cause of scoliosis, and figures show wherever they are taken a constant increase in the proportion of scoliosis among children during school life. For this reason the use of proper school furniture is of great importance and the literature of the subject will be found in the reference.[1]

It is also essential to prevent persistent, faulty attitude at home as well as at school.

[1] Cofton ; American Physical Education Review, December, 1904.

School Hygiene and School Gymnastics.—Proper lighting of schoolrooms and the correct placing of blackboards are essential in favoring proper attitudes. The avoidance of long sitting periods by introducing gymnastic exercises and changes of position is of importance.

Correct Carriage.—Faulty attitudes are frequently assumed in walking and in standing, especially by young children. The inclination to stand upon one leg is usually a habit, but in some cases it may be due to a muscular weakness of one limb or of a knee or ankle. The habit is to be corrected by drill or by muscular exercise, and by encouraging activity with the necessary constant change of position. Incorrect habits in sitting at home are to be remedied by insisting that the children with curvature shall not sit curled up or bent over in reading, but that they shall sit in suitable chairs and hold the book correctly.

Attitude during Sleep.—The most common attitude in sleep is upon the side, but decubitus upon the back is more common than on either single side. The right side is more commonly lain on than the left, but the difference is slight; young children and men not infrequently lie upon the belly, but the attitude is not so often assumed by women or growing girls.

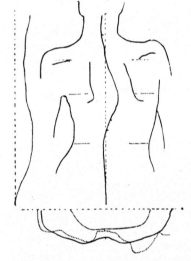

FIG. 203.—A Record Made by the Machine Shown in Fig. 312. At the left is the outline of the upright spine. Below are the contours of the back at three different levels. (Schulthess.)

In ordinary cases the precautions at night which should be observed are that the patient should not be allowed to sleep with many pillows and that the bed should be a firm one. The child should not be allowed to assume a twisted position, but should lie upon the back or the side of the greatest concavity. In threatening cases measures are necessary to preserve a proper position. This can be done by means of bed frames, described under Pott's disease.

Proper Clothing.—T h e modern style of clothing in growing children predisposes to round shoulders, and is a handicap to the treatment of scoliosis.[1] The use of

[1] E. H. Bradford : Trans. Am. Orth. Assn., vol. x., 162.

side garters, which fasten tightly drawn long stockings to waists dragging upon shoulder straps and shoulders, is to be avoided. This can be done by the use of round garters or attaching the garters to properly constructed shoulder straps independent of the waist and designed to draw the shoulders backward and not forward. Heavy petticoats should not be attached to waists with shoulder straps dragging upon the shoulders of growing girls. This can also be avoided by the use of union suits for underwear and light petticoats.

TREATMENT.

Several difficulties are to be met in treating lateral curvature. As the affection is active during the period of growth, treatment, to be efficient, must be carried on for a long time, and is tedious to the surgeon and irksome to the patient. Furthermore, as the disease is one that does not threaten life and is slow and uncertain in its outcome, it is sometimes difficult to enforce the proper treatment for the requisite length of time. Cases will be brought to the surgeon's care presenting varying degrees of deformity and needing different grades of treatment. Cases, however, can be grouped in two classes:

I. Those with slight structural change and curves in the main flexible.

II. Those with structural change showing in curves which are fixed.

I. Treatment of Cases with Slight Structural Change and Curves in the Main Flexible.

Postural Treatment.—The postural treatment consists in the correction of faulty habits, the development of weak muscles, and the retention of proper attitudes. As a raw recruit is taught the position and carriage of the soldier, so children, if faulty habits of attitude are present, are to be drilled into standing and walking in correct attitudes, and the spine is to be made equally flexible in all directions if there is any degree of stiffness present. This method is suited for the simplest cases of beginning curvature. To be thoroughly carried out, it requires that the patient should daily be exercised in walking, standing, and sitting properly for a specified time under the direction of some competent person. The principles of the " setting-up " drill of recruits in all armies are applicable, with modifications, to patients of this class. When resting during the hour of drill the patient should remain recumbent. At other times, such precaution should be taken as will prevent the persistence for any length of time of a faulty attitude. This should not be done (out of the drill time) by constant correction, but by the proper arrangement of the daily routine as to play and school to prevent excessive mental or physical fatigue and a supervision of the chairs when reading and studying. Walking, running, and active games should be encouraged, while reading, except in proper position, should be discouraged.

Gymnastics.—In many early cases of scoliosis the faulty attitudes are clearly the result of muscular weakness. The increase in height

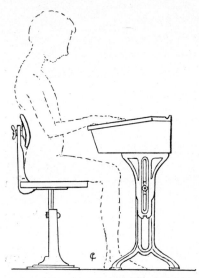

has not been accompanied by a corresponding development in muscle. This condition is frequently met in rapidly growing children, and is one of the common causes of lateral curvature. Here proper gymnastics are indicated, but they should be prescribed and carried out with much care. In the more marked cases the children are unable to bear much exercise without fatigue. Those exercises, therefore, chiefly needed in correcting the deformity should be the only ones prescribed. The usual class-work of a gymnasium is to be avoided, as such cases require the individual attention of a competent person, who will see that no faulty position is taken during the exercises, and each case must be re-

FIG. 204.—Diagram of the Adjustable School Chair Adopted by the Boston Schoolhouse Commission. (F. J. Cotton.)

garded, as far as exercises are concerned, as a separate problem to be worked out individually.

LIGHT GYMNASTICS.—It is not a difficult matter to devise simple and practicable exercises to develop the muscles chiefly at fault.

General developmental exercises for the back, shoulders, and abdomen, when taken with the spine straight and the carriage of the body correct, constitute the best general scheme for the treatment of such cases. Cases will be seen of such feeble muscular strength that it is advisable to begin with those which demand the least muscular effort in maintaining a symmetrical attitude. For these cases exercises with the patient recumbent are desirable.

If the patient has gained sufficient strength, a series of light dumb-bell exercises with bells weighing from one to five pounds can be prescribed, carried on with the patient recumbent, similar to those just mentioned. Care should be taken that they are correctly performed.

After this, follow light symmetrical dumb-bell exercises with the patient standing in a correct position. The work of the patient should be tabulated and carefully graded. This is to be followed by heavier work of the same general type.

Whether light or heavy exercises are used, persistence is necessary for success. It is needless to add that the patient should exercise under careful supervision, rest being prescribed as a part of the daily treatment, the amount of work being regulated each day.

Flexibility Exercises.—In some instances of postural curves abnormal centres of motion of spinal curves and asymmetrical spinal flexibility will be found to exist.

This is to be corrected by exercises to restore normal spinal mobility not designed especially for muscular development, analogous to the measures employed by contortionists to develop abnormal joint flexibility.

These exercises need to be carefully planned for each case, and with checks to prevent motion where free motion in the spinal column already exists, and to develop motion where spinal flexibility is less than normal.

Appliances.—In postural curves, where weak muscles are present, it is sometimes advisable to furnish light appliances to check faulty attitudes, these to be worn at the time in the day when the child shows gradual muscular fatigue and droops into faulty attitudes most readily. These appliances should be light, easily adjustable, and check motion only in the desired direction.

Intermittent Correction.—During this period, not only are the measures for muscular development and the development of normal flexibility required in the treatment of postural and slight structural curves needed, but also more thorough measures.

Flexibility exercises can be given by means of various appliances designed for the purpose, and patients brought daily to institutions or specialists' offices equipped for the purpose can receive the necessary treatment.

But in the majority of cases such treatment is not feasible for as long a period as is needed in the graver cases. Simple forms of appliances, suitable for daily home treatment, are necessary, which can be effectively furnished.

Simple appliances can be made exerting correcting pressure by means of weights, lever pressure, strap pressure—the patient standing suspended, seated, recumbent, or kneeling, and fixed in suitable gas-pipe quadrilateral frames.

The chief difficulty is not in securing simple apparatus but in obtaining suitable home care.

Fixation Appliances.—Recumbency being inapplicable for a long period, and gymnastics being possible only for a limited portion of the day, some form of appliance which checks faulty positions is desirable.

II. TREATMENT OF STRUCTURAL CASES WITH FIXED CURVES.

The treatment of this class of spinal curves demands the exercise of sound judgment, as the proper management of these cases does not consist in the temporary straightening of a curve, which will relapse when the correcting force is removed, nor the constant use of a correcting jacket, which weakens muscular tissues.

Measures should be employed successively in these cases suited to the conditions during the growing years; not for a few months or a year, but until the bones of the spinal column, as well as muscles, are able to bear their load without bending abnormally under the burden.

In some instances it is advisable to disregard the curve temporarily and devote attention to the patient's general condition, with the employment only of such measures as are needed for postural curves.

Where curve correction is needed the most efficient measure is undoubtedly by applying corrective plaster jackets.

Forcible Correction by Means of Plaster Jackets.—In certain cases the curves are too resistant to be altered materially by intermittent correction or gymnastic exercises. In suitable cases attempts can be made to correct the curves by a method of constant pressure, as it has been demonstrated that the shape of bone is altered by constant pressure. For the application of this method, *plaster jackets* should be applied to the patient in as corrected a position as possible. It is evident that this method of correction is adapted to patients during their growing period, though it may be employed occasionally in older cases.

Corrective plaster jackets can be applied with the patient in a standing or sitting position; or recumbent, either lying on the face, back, or side. Correcting force should be used without an anæsthetic.

Suspension or a traction force is of value; but as the affected portion of the spine in lateral curvature is always the most resistant portion, the most economical application of force is by exercising side pressure rather than by pulling each end. Traction force used to straighten the spine by itself will have to be used in large amounts to be effective. If the patient is seated or standing, a head sling may be of assistance, with some suspension force to steady the upper part of the trunk. Traction force may also be used in the recumbent position, though it is rarely effective as a traction force on the resistant curve.

The relative advantages of the different positions of the patient in the application of a corrective jacket are as follows:

With the patient standing or seated it is much easier to apply the bandage on all sides of the patient than when the patient is recumbent, and for this reason is preferable in applying jackets to the neck and shoulders. In the upright position the position of the head relative to the thorax is that usual in locomotion, while in recumbency an alteration in the normal thorax takes place. Recumbently applied jackets are therefore less comfortable to the patients than those applied with the patient upright.

If the patient is seated it is easier to correct lordosis or any torsion of the pelvis than if the patient is standing, but in the seated position the surgeon needs to take especial pains in arranging the seat so as to enable him to apply a jacket which will hold the pelvis firmly.

Much greater correcting pressure can be applied with the patient in a recumbent position, as the superimposed weight is not an influence to be opposed. In recumbency on the face lordosis can be overcome more readily than if the patient lies upon the back. It is less easy, however, to secure a desirable expansion of the chest and arching backward of the spine in the dorsal region in face than in back recumbency. Where there is much rotation to be corrected, the recumbent position is to be preferred. Where side deviation is the more important feature, the upright position is to be considered also.

The simplest method of application of a corrective jacket is for the patient to sit or stand in the centre of a four-upright frame. The head is secured in a head sling with moderate traction. Webbing straps pass from the different uprights and can be made to exert side pressure in different directions as desired. These are included in the jacket, the emerging portions being cut off.

In the recumbent position the patient may be placed with the back supported on a frame with uprights similar to that used in the application of corrective jackets in Pott's disease, except that the pressure points are applied in the back, not upon the transverse processes, but upon the backward prominence of the ribs. Correction of lateral deviation can be furnished by horizontal traction, if necessary, or by side pressure. Felt padding is needed over the portions of the body which

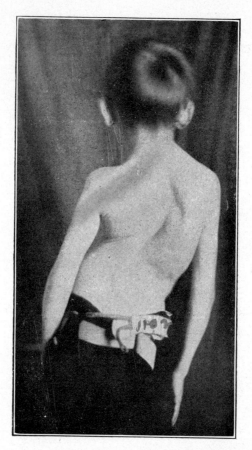

FIG. 205.—Case of Scoliosis Before Treatment.

are but little protected by fatty tissue; the plaster bandages should be applied high up under the drooping shoulder and over the shoulder from behind, across the neck. When the plaster is sufficiently hardened the patient can be lifted, the detachable plates which are thoroughly padded remaining in the jacket.

A simple method of application of a corrective jacket in an inclined or recumbent position is to secure the patient firmly in the centre of the four-upright frame used for applying a jacket in the upright position and inclining the whole frame backward. The correcting straps will need readjustment for proper correcting force when the patient is changed from the upright to the recumbent position.

A useful method in recumbency is to have the patient lie face downward, on two strips of webbing running from end to end on a

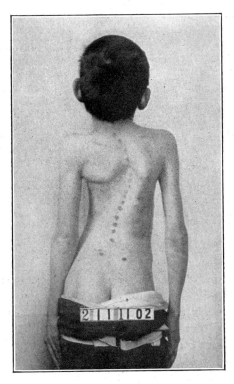

FIG. 205a.—Same Case as Shown in Fig. 205 after Three Years, Treatment by Corrective Plaster Jacket.

horizontally placed oblong gaspipe frame. There are two transverse strips of webbing, one supporting the pelvis and another the shoulders. Side pressure is secured by webbing fastened to the sides of the frame running around the trunk and securing as much side pressure as desired. The patient may lie with the thighs extended or flexed to any desired extent.

In applying corrective jackets, it is to be remembered that there are two elements of the deformity demanding correction—one, the lateral curve, to be corrected by side force; the other, the rotation, to be corrected by a twisting force. Any use of force, to be effective, must be met by counter-points of resistance or the whole spine will be pushed to one side or twisted as a whole.

High dorsal curves are improved by corrective jackets with difficulty, because satisfactory counter-pressure is not easily applied in these curves, if resistant. Lumbar curves are also generally better

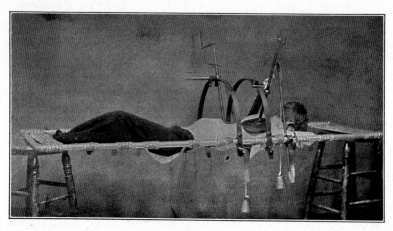

Fig. 206.—Apparatus for the Application of Plaster Jackets during Recumbency on the Face.

treated by other means, because there are no ribs to exert side pressure on this region and direct side force cannot be exerted.

Corrective plaster jackets should embrace the shoulders and, in cases of high dorsal curves, the neck, and should not be removable. In curves in the upper third of the spine a head support adds much to the corrective power of the jacket. Windows can be cut in the jacket over the portion of the trunk where pressure is undesirable, as over the concavity of the thorax. At first the patient will need supervision, but later can go about freely. Jackets should be repeated at short intervals, preferably one, two, or three weeks, and applied as long as further correction can be obtained. This stage of treatment is followed by that of removable jackets and exercises.

The amount of correcting force used is a matter of judgment, as is also the time when corrective pressure treatment should be discontinued. Skill and judgment are needed in the application of braces and removable corsets, after corrective jackets are discontinued. Where the spinal column is not strong enough to carry the superincumbent weight without developing abnormal curves, support is needed, but the constant use of a plaster jacket or stiff, heavy corset for long periods, i.e., a year or more, is not conducive to the development of strength of back. Where such sup-ports are needed during the growing period, the appliance should be light, easily removed, worn without dis-comfort, or disfigurement to the pa-tient, and capable of exerting effect-ive pressure upon the various projecting curves, with no pressure upon the abnormal concavities. Such appliances are not easily made, and should be adapted to the needs of each case. In all mid or upper dorsal curves they should extend above the shoulders. They can be made of celluloid or light stiffened leather, with large windows cut over a region where pressure is to be avoided. Efficient light steel appli-ances can be made, but need much painstaking attention in design and in application. Cases of this class, after the cessation of active correct-ive treatment, need careful direc-tions as to recumbency, exercises— the hours of play, study, etc., and

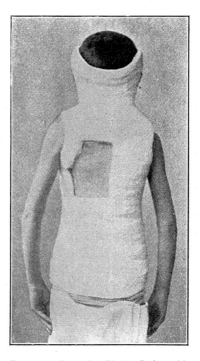

Fig. 207.—Corrective Plaster Jacket with Head-piece Applied for the Correction of Scoliosis. (Wullstein.)

prolonged supervision, with proper record taking and measurement. Resumption of active corrective treatment, or increasing relaxation in gymnastic work, will depend upon the progress of the case.

Treatment by Operation.

Operative attempts consisting of resection of the projecting ribs, performed by Volkmann in 1889 and Hoffa [1] in a few instances, have been made in cases in which the distortion of the ribs resulting from rotation is so severe as to preclude the possibility of correction by other means. The success obtained was not great.

Successful correction of disfiguring rotation by multiple osteotomy of the ribs and the immediate application of correcting plaster jackets is a method which was employed by Hoke, but is rarely applicable.

[1] Zeitsch. f. orth. Chir., 1896, 401.

CHAPTER XII.

OTHER DEFORMITIES OF THE SPINE AND THORAX.

These deformities are either congenital or, in the majority of cases, acquired, dependent on general conditions which in the muscular or osseous system limit the patient's ability to maintain the normal erect attitude.

The physiological normal curves are three, forward in the cervical region, backward in the dorsal, and forward in the lumbar. These curves vary according to the habits, occupation, muscular system, sex, and figure of the individual.

The term *kyphosis* is used to designate an increase in the backward dorsal physiological curve, and the term *lordosis* to describe an increase in the forward physiological curve in the lumbar region.

KYPHOSIS.

An increase of the backward curvature of the spine may be most noticeable in the upper part of the spine, or may practically involve the whole dorsal and lumbar spine. It occurs (1) as a static deformity, which is the commonest form seen, and is known as "round shoulders"; or (2) as the result of an abnormal condition of the bones, or as a result of paralysis.

1. Round Shoulders.

The term round shoulders is generally applied to the stooping attitude which results from the muscular relaxation due to rapid growth, to the assumption of improper attitudes, and to poor general condition. It is generally seen in children and is likely to be observed at any time after the age of three or thereabouts.

Causes.—The affection is to be regarded as a static one connected with improper muscular support. The common causes are as follows:

Improper position at school and at home. Rapid growth, long hours at school, insufficient food, improper arrangement of clothing, and too long an active day, are causes inducing muscular debility and, therefore, favoring round shoulders.

Symptoms.—In round shoulders the dorsal physiological curve is increased, the head is run forward, the shoulders slope forward, the

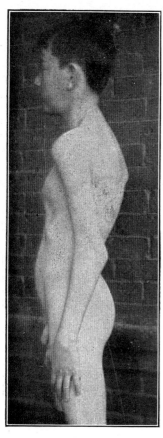

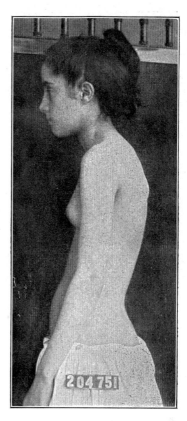

FIG. 208.—Round shoulders. Curve of dorsal and lumbar regions. Marked forward displacement of shoulder.

FIG. 209.—Round shoulders. Kyphosis involves whole spine. (Round back.)

scapulæ are unduly prominent behind and may be noticed through the clothing in severe cases, and the whole shoulder-joint seems to be forward of its normal position; the chest is narrow and flattened, and the expansion deficient. The lumbar spine may present an increased forward curvature, so that the patient stands with an abnormally hollow back (round hollow back), or the lumbar spine may be involved in the backward curve and the lumbar curve diminished or

lost (round back). The patient's trunk swings back and the abdomen
is thrust forward. Some degree of flat-foot is likely to coexist, and
beginning lateral curvature accompanies many of the cases.

With the persistence of the attitude of round shoulders the muscles and ligaments in front of the shoulders become · shortened

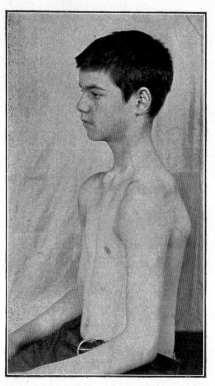
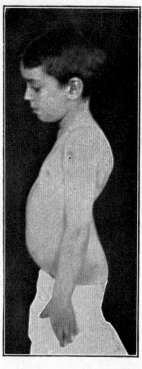

Fig. 210.—Round Shoulders with Forward Displace-   Fig. 210a.—Round Shoulders with
ment of Scapulæ. Back comparatively flat.   Increased Lumbar Lordosis.

and those at the back stretched. If the arms are carried to
a vertical position above the head, it is generally done by arching
the spine forward in the lumbar region, which is made necessary by
the contraction of the muscles connecting the arms and upper chest,
such as the pectoral muscles. Pain may occasionally be present in
nervous children, especially girls.

The attitude may be partially corrected temporarily by the voluntary muscular effort of the patient, but the faulty attitude will be
again assumed almost immediately, as the muscles are unable to maintain the corrected position.

Prognosis.—The prognosis without treatment is not good in pronounced cases, so far as recovery from the deformity is concerned, and it may be carried over into adult life practically unchanged. With proper treatment recovery is to be expected.

Treatment.—In the treatment of round shoulders the patient should be put in the most favorable surroundings possible. Incorrect

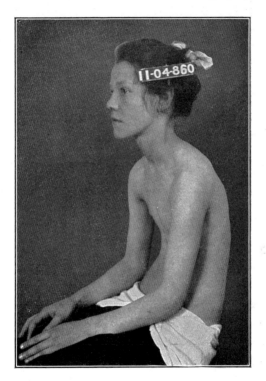

Fig. 211.—Sitting Position in Marked Round Shoulders. The spine is flexible and can be straightened by muscular effort.

attitudes at school and at home should be corrected so far as possible. Errors in vision are to be investigated and remedied if they exist. Undue fatigue and a very long active day are to be avoided.

Round garters should be worn, and the stockings should not be fastened to the waist. The trousers and skirts should, if possible, be supported by a belt, and the waist to which the clothes are ordinarily fastened should be relieved of as much weight as possible.

Gymnastics.—The gymnastic treatment of round shoulders consists in stretching the contracted tissues and in drilling the child in the maintenance of a correct position. The stretching can usually be accomplished by simple measures. Suitable exercises for this purpose are within the range of any good gymnastic teacher and should be done at first daily. In general they should consist of the " setting up

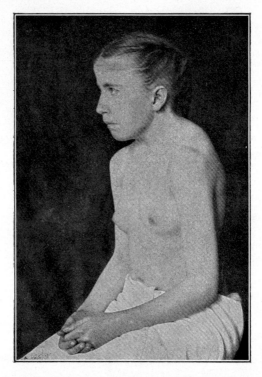

Fig. 212.—Deformity of Shoulders due to the Presence of Cervical Ribs. (Dr. C. F. Painter.)

drill " of the gymnasium and the military recruit, and must be done with force and precision.

The restoration of backward flexibility to the dorsal spine and shoulders before giving corrective work is essential.

The use of a greater degree of force is sometimes necessary to accomplish the desired stretching. This may be accomplished by the application of plaster jackets applied to the spine with the dorsal region hyperextended, and such jackets should include the shoulders, which are pulled backward during the application of the jacket. As soon as flexibility is restored, postural gymnastic work of the type described above should follow.

APPARATUS.—In cases of marked flexible round shoulders, when the children are unable to maintain for any length of time a corrected position, some mechanical assistance to the extensor muscles may be needed. A useful brace consists of a posterior horizontal

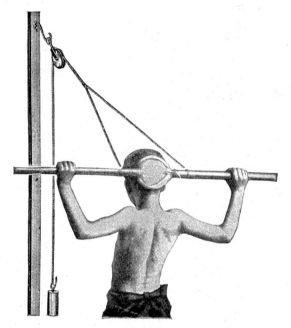

FIG. 213.—Schulthess' Apparatus for Correction of Round Shoulders.   (Schulthess.)

pelvic band, grasping the pelvis at the level of the anterior superior spines. From this run up, at a distance of one inch or less from the spinous processes, two tempered steel uprights, which are turned out on the flat at their upper ends and terminate just below the root of the neck well toward the axillary line, where they are furnished with axillary straps, which run through the arm-pit and fasten to a transverse crossbar on the brace. This brace is furnished with an abdominal band, which runs from the upright around the abdomen, to assist in the maintenance of the correct position.

Treatment by braces should be supplementary to gymnastic treatment, and only used when the latter fails to yield results.

Static Kyphosis from Occupation.—This type of deformity occurs in adults and in children. In adults it is either the result of a condition acquired in childhood carried over into adult life, or it is acquired by some habitual position connected with the occupation of the individual. It is seen in workmen who carry heavy loads upon their shoulders, in tailors who sit cross-legged with the spine bent, cobblers who bend over their work, clerks who sit continually bent over a

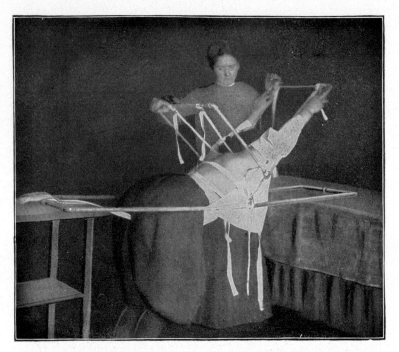

Fig. 214.—Apparatus for Stretching of Round Shoulders.

desk, and in men performing heavy work, such as blacksmiths, who work continually bending over a bench or an anvil. The exaggerated curve of the dorsal spine acquired by children who bend over their desks at school is to be classed in a measure as an occupation curvature.

Kyphosis may also occur in (2) Pott's disease, (3) spondylitis deformans, (4) scoliosis, (5) osteomalacia, (6) rickets, (7) ostitis deformans, (8) paralysis of the back muscles, (9) old age, acromegaly, and secondary osteoarthropathy.

LORDOSIS.

Lordosis is the name applied to the increase of the physiological forward curve in the lumbar region. The amount of this curve, of course, varies in normal individuals from those who have a very flat back in the lumbar region to those who have a very markedly hollow back. The various conditions in which lordosis exists are as follows:

1. Lordosis often exists in connection with the kyphosis of the dorsal spine spoken of in connection with round shoulders as round hollow back.

2. Lordosis also exists in pregnant women and often in persons with large abdomens.

3. Increased lumbar curve may exist as the result of training in professional gymnasts, especially in backward contortionists.

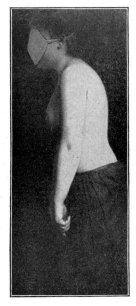 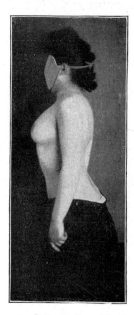

FIG. 215.—Patient with Round Shoulders Before Stretching.

FIG. 216.—Patient One Month Later After Treatment by Stretching.

4. In conditions in which the abdominal or the back muscles are paralyzed, the attitude of lordosis may be the result of an attempt to balance the weight of the upper part of the body without bringing a strain upon the muscles.

5. In Pott's disease of the lumbar region apparent lordosis may be one of the first symptoms to be noticed.

6. In cases of double congenital dislocation of the hip lordosis generally exists.

7. Lordosis exists in many cases of severe rickets.

8. In hip disease, with flexion deformity, lordosis is present.

Contraction of the hip in flexion, for any reason, as in infantile paralysis, causes lordosis.

9. Lordosis may exist in coxa vara and in congenital dislocation of the hip.

10. In spondylolisthesis lordosis is very marked.

Treatment.—The treatment of these curves is necessarily dependent upon the causative conditions and attendant circumstances.

SPONDYLOLISTHESIS.

The name spondylolisthesis refers to a forward subluxation of the body of one of the lower lumbar vertebræ, with the exception of one recorded case in which the upper part of the sacrum was displaced forward.

Pathology.—The essential part of the condition seems to be the slipping forward of one of the lower lumbar vertebral bodies, while the vertebral arches remain practically in place. This implies, of course, an increase in the distance between the body and the spinous process of such a vertebra. The commonest form of the displacement is subluxation of the fifth lumbar vertebra in relation to the sacrum. The displacement may be slight or extreme.

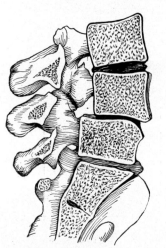

Fig. 217.—Breslau Specimen. Instance of slight forward displacement of the fourth lumbar vertebra. (Neugebauer.)

Etiology.—Spondylolisthesis is recorded as affecting women more frequently than men. It occurs almost always at puberty or in young adult life, and the majority of all cases give the account of a severe traumatism, occurring most often during childhood or near puberty. The deformity may follow immediately upon the accident, or it may develop in after years. In some cases no assignable cause can be found.

Symptoms.—There is a sharp increase in the lower lumbar curve in even the mildest cases, and the spine curves forward sharply from the sacrum, which gives undue backward prominence to the crest of the ilium and the buttocks. The appearance at first glance is the same as that in cases of double congenital dislocation of the hip. Lateral deviation of the spine may be present. With this lordosis

goes a diminution of the obliquity of the pelvis, which causes flexion
of the thighs.   Vaginal examination shows, of course, a prominence

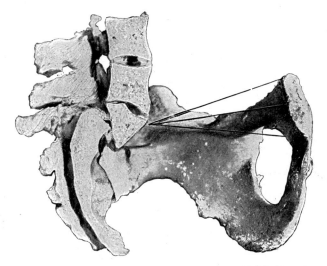

FIG. 218.—Spondylolisthesis due to Vertebral Disease.   (Dr. H. Cushing, Johns Hopkins
Hospital.)

high up on the posterior wall of the pelvis.   The trunk is shortened in
relation to the legs on inspection.   The affection is not one characterized by excessive pain.

Treatment.—The most successful treatment consists in fixation of
the lower spine by a jacket or brace until the fracture, if such has
occurred, has united and the products of the injury have been absorbed; or, if heavy weight-bearing has been the cause, until the
stretched and weakened tissues have resumed as normal a position
as possible.   In cases of great deformity it would seem as if a support
must be permanent.

DEFORMITIES OF THE THORAX.

Pigeon Breast (chicken breast, Hühnerbrust, pectus carinatum or
gallinatum, poitrine en carène, poitrine de pigeon, etc.) is a deformity
more or less common in children, characterized by a prominence of the
sternum and cartilages of the ribs and accompanied by an increase in
the antero-posterior diameter of the chest and a diminution in the
lateral.   The deformity is generally most marked in the median line,
but in many cases the prominence affects chiefly the ribs of one side,
making a unilateral prominence on one side of the sternum.   It is

due to rickets and is associated often with nasal or pharyngeal obstruction in growing children. It is also seen in a marked degree in dorsal Pott's disease, in which it is due to the sinking forward of the upper dorsal spine, carrying with it the ribs. In slight cases the de-

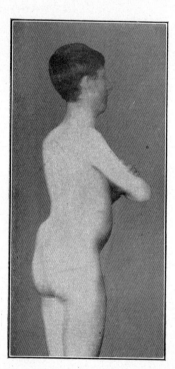 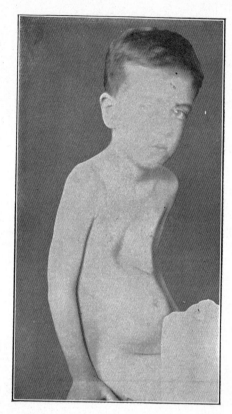

FIG. 219.—Traumatic Spondylolisthesis in a Young Man of Eighteen.

FIG. 220.—Funnel Chest. (J. S. Stone.)

formity is probably outgrown spontaneously, but in the severer cases it may last into adult life.

The treatment consists in children in a combination of gymnastic and respiratory exercises to expand and develop the lateral parts of the chest.

Funnel Chest (funnel breast, Trichterbrust, pectus excavatum, thorax-en-entonnoir) is a name applied to a deformity in which the sternum and costal cartilages are depressed below their normal level. The deformity is as a rule asymmetrical, and in its lighter degrees is not uncommon.   But little is known of the cause of the affection; in many cases it apparently is congenital.   The treatment for this should consist in gymnastic exercises, especially those expanding the chest and developing the muscles, increasing chest expansion; and in the severer cases the temporary use of light braces, checking faulty attitudes.

Congenital Deformities.—Other deformities of the thorax of congenital origin need only to be mentioned.   Among these are absence

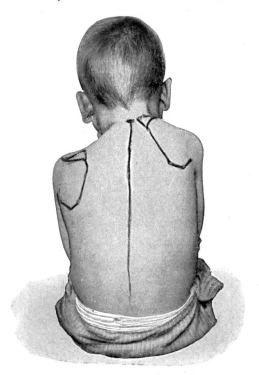

Fig. 221.—Congenital Elevation of the Scapula.

or a defective formation of the ribs, a condition generally associated with lateral curvature of the spine, the presence of cervical ribs, and anomalies or absence of the pectoral and other muscles.   Defective formation or absence of the clavicle has been reported, and malformation of the scapula is sometimes seen.

Congenital Elevation of the Scapula (Sprengel's deformity, angeborene Hochstand des Schulterblattes).—This condition is a somewhat unusual congenital deformity, in which one scapula is raised in its relation to the thorax and clavicle and also to the opposite scapula. The scapula is not only raised, but generally so rotated that its upper angle approaches the spine. Scoliosis exists in connection with it, in the majority of cases, and in some cases torticollis and asymmetry of the face and skull have been noted; the affection is rarely bilateral. One or more of the scapular muscles may be absent and bony anomalies are frequent, and in the majority of cases some congenital defect is present elsewhere in the body. In one class of cases a bridge of bone connects the scapula and the vertebral column; in another class there is a long piece of bone projecting upward from the superior border of the scapula, but not articulating with or attached to the vertebræ. In other cases there is no bony outgrowth and no deficiency of muscles. In some cases the projecting upper border of the scapula is so noticeable in its elevated position that it is mistaken for an exostosis. The symptoms are found in the asymmetry of the shoulders, the secondary changes in the spine, and often an inability to abduct the affected arm to its full extent; but the cases are evidently to be classed with other congenital malformations.

The affection is in all probability due to a congenital survival of the fœtal condition, by which the normal descent of the scapula from the early high position in the early stage is arrested.

In cases seen during childhood extensive division of the shortened muscles holding the scapula in its abnormal position is to be advised, and the removal of any bony bridge or projection, and in resistant cases resection of as much of the upper border of the scapula as may be necessary. Improvement may thus be obtained. In older cases no operative treatment is advisable. The cases can be benefited by persistent gymnastic treatment.

CHAPTER XIII.

TORTICOLLIS.

DEFINITION.

THE name torticollis is given to that distortion of the head which causes it to be held awry, and this condition is either constant or intermittent. The other names by which this affection is known are wryneck, caput obstipum, cou tortu, Schiefhals.

ETIOLOGY.

Torticollis may be (I) congenital or (II) acquired.

I. CONGENITAL TORTICOLLIS.

(*a*) It may exist in connection with other deformities, such as club-foot and similar malformations. In these cases it seems proper to attribute its existence to those intra-uterine conditions causing other deformities. Other intra-uterine conditions to which it may be attributed are:

(*b*) Abnormal pressure of the uterus.

(*c*) Amniotic adhesions.

(*d*) Inflammation of the muscles seems to be proved by the pathological findings in certain cases and must be mentioned.

(*e*) Arrest of the development of the muscles due to an affection of the nerves or nerve centres is a cause often advanced to account for torticollis.

(*f*) Rupture of the sterno-mastoid muscle occurring at birth has been mentioned as a cause of torticollis, and undoubted cases have been observed where torticollis has followed partial rupture of the sterno-mastoid at childbirth. Torticollis, however, has not followed the hæmatomata from rupture of the sterno-mastoid at birth in a number of cases carefully watched by several observers.

(*g*) Imperfections in the atlas and cervical vertebræ have in some reported cases been the cause of congenital torticollis.

251

II. Acquired Torticollis.

As the causes of this form of the affection may be mentioned:
Cicatricial contraction of the skin or deeper tissues, traumatism to
the neck and head, dislocation of the upper cervical vertebræ, inflammation of the muscle ("rheu-
matic" torticollis or acute or
chronic myositis), reflex irritation
of the muscles in caries of the
spine.

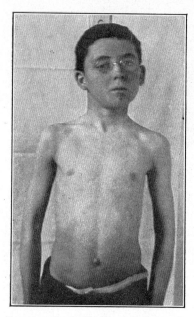

Torticollis may also be seen in
inflammation of the cervical lymph
nodes or with deep cervical abscesses, retropharyngeal abscesses,
inflammations of the ear, parotitis,
adenoid vegetations in the naso-
pharynx, tumors of the neck, and
cerebral lesions. Neuralgia of the
spinal accessory or cervico-brachial
nerves may be accompanied by torticollis. Other causes of acquired
torticollis are:

Difference in the plane or
power of vision of the eyes, lateral
curvature, voluntary habit (physiological torticollis), occupations in
which the overuse of one sterno-

Fig. 222.—Torticollis Showing Contraction
of the Right Sterno-mastoid Muscle.

mastoid muscle is necessary, injury to the nerve centres at the time of
birth, paralysis of the spinal accessory nerve from such causes as
rheumatism or trauma as well as anterior poliomyelitis and the muscular dystrophies.

Spasmodic Torticollis.

In this class are included those cases which arise from nerve irritation. This form may be central and occur in the distribution of the
spinal accessory nerve, or it may be the local manifestation of a more
general nervous irritation and involve several groups of muscles. In
some cases of the spasmodic form, the affection is closely allied to
writers' cramp, spasmodic tic of the face, etc.[1]

[1] Traité des Tort. Spasm. Cruchet, Paris, 1907.

PATHOLOGY.

In some instances of congenital torticollis the contracted muscle appears normal, but more often the muscular substance is replaced by fibrous tissue. This may occur in small patches or the whole muscle may be transformed into a tendinous band. In the majority of

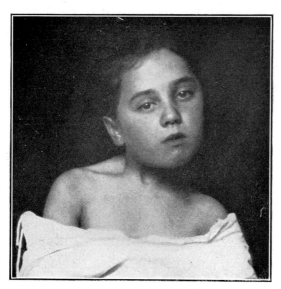

Fig. 223.—Torticollis Due to Contraction of Right Sterno-mastoid Muscle.

cases of fibrous degeneration of the muscle it is adherent to the sheath, and in some instances muscle and sheath are fused in one fibrous band.

The changes described are to be classed as fibrous myositis, and perimyositis has been demonstrated in certain cases. Shortening of the muscle on the affected side may amount to several centimetres.

Secondary changes occur in long-continued torticollis, the most marked of which is asymmetry of the face. It may, on the other hand, be present in birth without the existence of torticollis. This asymmetry diminishes if the deformity is corrected early. Asymmetry of the skull may also be found, as well as a diminished size of the cerebral hemisphere on the affected side. The carotid artery of the affected side has been in certain cases found smaller.

This asymmetry of the face may also occur in acquired torticollis of long standing.

Lateral curvature of the spine will result from long-continued torticollis, and a difference in the length of the clavicles has been noted.

SYMPTOMS.

Congenital Torticollis.—The position held by the head varies necessarily with the muscles affected. When the sterno-cleido-mastoid

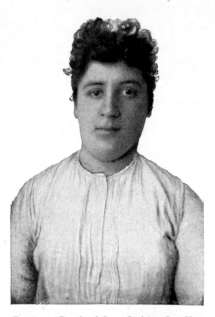

of one side is shortened, the ear of the affected side is brought near to the sternum and the face slightly rotated to the opposite side. If the trapezius or posterior muscles are also affected, the head will also be drawn back, the chin elevated above its normal level, and the features on the side of the spasm drawn below those on the opposite side. In addition to these muscles, the platysma and deep muscles of the neck are sometimes affected, and modify more or less the position of the head. The attitude is sometimes so peculiar as to render it difficult to determine exactly what muscles are affected. On palpation certain muscles will be found to be hard to the touch and others flaccid. Rotation of the head is free up to a certain limit, varying in extent. It is not possible to move the head in a direction against the contraction.

FIG. 224.—Result of Open Incision One Year after Operation in a Girl of Sixteen. Shows also the unequal development of the face.

Acquired Torticollis.—In the acute form the history is that of an acute muscular " rheumatism," an acute glandular inflammation, a traumatism, etc., with sudden onset with a great deal of pain on movement of the head, and the head is held to one side. The acute stage, however, lasts but a short time, and the position assumed by the head is more or less typical and is described above. A chronic form may develop from the acute form.

Spasmodic Torticollis.

The intermittent form of torticollis is not infrequent and occurs mostly in adults. At times the head can be held in a proper position, but locomotion or any excitement or the apprehension of being observed may produce such a contraction of the head that it will be twisted violently to one side and rotated to an extreme limit. A slight pressure of the hand steadying the head will ordinarily correct it, but when the muscular contraction becomes excited, great force is required to hold the head in place in some cases. In certain cases the contraction may be slow and steadily increase to its maximum. In a recumbent position the contraction does not ordinarily take place and usually disappears during sleep. The spasm is sometimes tonic and sometimes clonic, and sometimes pain is excited by the muscular contraction. It is usually confined to the muscles of one side or to associated groups of muscles on the two sides, and may involve the muscles of the back. Slight twitchings of the muscles are sometimes observed for some time previous to an outbreak of the spasmodic condition.

DIAGNOSIS.

There is no difficulty in recognizing the deformity of congenital wry-neck. The head is twisted to one side, the chin being to the right or left of the sterno-clavicular notch, while the face is turned to one side and partly upward. The shoulders are held obliquely to the trunk and twisted, in order to bring the face so far as possible in a vertical line. Certain of the muscles, frequently the sterno-cleido-mastoid, are felt hard on palpation; some rotation of the head is possible, but perfectly free rotation of the head is checked by the contracted muscles.

A diagnosis of the cause and situation of wry-neck is more difficult, as well as an attempt to distinguish it from other affections which give rise to this malformation, a matter which is of great importance. Such affections have been enumerated.

The diagnosis between anterior and posterior torticollis (or torticollis due to contraction of the anterior muscles, chiefly the sterno-cleido-mastoid, and that due to the contraction of the posterior muscles, the trapezius and splenius capitis, etc.), is to be based on palpation chiefly. Palpation also, with a clinical history of paralysis and the evidence of paralysis elsewhere, is sufficient usually to determine the diagnosis of paralytic torticollis.

Torticollis dependent upon enlarged and inflamed glands can usually be recognized by the evidence of glandular enlargement. There is ordinarily little difficulty in recognizing the common acute wry-neck. Its course is acute, the deformity appears suddenly, and it is usually accompanied by pain. Improvement is to be noticed in a comparatively short time.

For the diagnosis of congenital torticollis from that due to Pott's

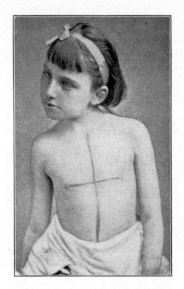 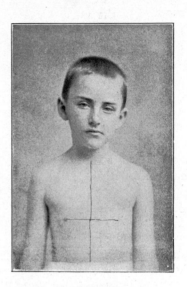

FIG. 225.—Posterior Torticollis Before Forcible Straightening.   FIG. 226.—After Operation.

disease, it may be said that in the latter there is greater rigidity, which involves all the muscles of the neck, and particularly the posterior groups. The pain elicited by attempts to twist the head is greater. When a patient with cervical Pott's disease attempts to lie down or turn over the head is instinctively steadied with the hand, while in true torticollis this is not a symptom.

PROGNOSIS.

Congenital forms of torticollis and the common acquired form (associated with muscular contraction which has become chronic and developed fibrous muscular degeneration) demand surgical intervention. The acute idiopathic wry-neck due to muscular inflammation runs a short course and tends naturally to recovery. Torticollis due to abscess of the cervical glands terminates with the complete discharge of the abscess as a rule.

The deformity is one which is eminently curable by surgical intervention in practically all cases except in the intermittent form, which is dependent upon a general depressed state of the nervous system, in which a cure cannot always be promised even by surgical intervention.

TREATMENT.

In acute torticollis due to the inflammation of the muscles, the treatment is largely the alleviation of the symptoms. This is best

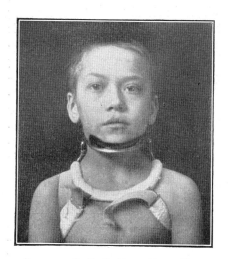

FIG. 227.—Torticollis Brace. Front View.

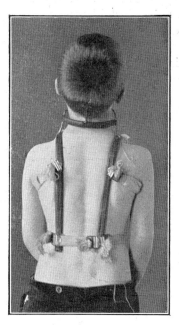

FIG. 228.—Torticollis Brace Applied, Back View.

accomplished by the application of moist heat, rest of the head, and constitutional treatment.

Torticollis due to cervical Pott's disease is treated according to the principles of treatment of that affection. Torticollis due to muscular contraction secondary to cervical abscesses or enlarged glands is corrected by the proper treatment of the local condition. Torticollis due to an affection of the eye should receive proper ocular treatment.

Congenital Torticollis.—The treatment of wry-neck due to permanent muscular contraction is either purely mechanical, or operative, or mechanical and operative.

MECHANICAL TREATMENT.—Mechanical treatment without the aid of operation is usually unsuccessful, except in the lightest cases, in which cases massage and passive manipulation are of value in connection with mechanical treatment; but mechanical treatment is in general to be regarded as of value chiefly in retaining the correction obtained by operative measures.

OPERATIVE TREATMENT.—In the usual form of torticollis the contracted muscle, the sterno-mastoid, is easily divided. Division is made (1) either at the sternal and clavicular insertion, or (2) at its insertion at the mastoid process. Subcutaneous tenotomy is to be rejected as dangerous.

Division at the Sterno-Cleido Insertion.—An incision of the skin is made parallel to the clavicle, laying bare the insertion of the muscle.

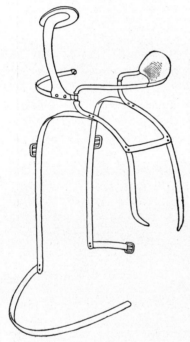

FIG. 229.—Torticollis Brace.

The incision should be sufficiently long to expose the whole attachment, as it is desirable that no undivided fibres remain. It is desirable that the resulting scar should be as low as possible, to accomplish which the skin is drawn upward and divided on the clavicle, after which the skin gapes sufficiently to permit the division of the muscular attachments above the clavicle if the head is retracted, which will also serve to make prominent the contracted muscles. The tissues to be divided are to be carefully freed from all overlying tissue and a director passed under the sternal tendon, care being taken that the director is passed completely under and not through the muscular attachment. It is usually necessary that both the clavicular and sternal attachments of the muscle be divided to prevent any possibility of relapse. With ordinary care there is no danger of dividing the vessels, although they are in close proximity.

Mastoid Division of the Sterno-Cleido-Mastoid Muscle.—A di-

vision of the sterno-mastoid at its origin from the mastoid process
has been advocated on the ground that the incision is away from
the vessels and that the resulting scar is in a less noticeable region.
For this division a skin incision is made behind the ear and the muscle
divided transversely just below the tip of the mastoid process, the
muscle being pulled up by a pointed, curved dissector. The muscular
origin is much thicker than the clavicular insertions and care will be
needed to divide the muscle thoroughly. The writers have been in the
habit of using the clavicular operation with satisfactory results. As
the results are excellent, the technique is simpler, and relapse does not
occur in properly treated cases.

After the operation the neck and chest are covered with sheet
wadding and the head is fixed in an overcorrected position by plaster
bandages applied around the head, shoulders, and thorax at or a day
or so after the operation. It is unnecessary for the patient to remain
in bed longer than a few days, if satisfactory plaster fixation is
furnished. It should be borne in mind that not only correction but
overcorrection is necessary to prevent a relapse, which will follow
to a greater or less degree unless this is done.

After the wound is entirely healed the patient should wear, for
from three to six months, a retaining appliance holding the head
in an overcorrected position. This can be a plaster bandage, a leather
moulded on a plaster form, or a steel appliance. The latter is as follows: A stiff wire collar passes around the neck, furnished with
a plate under the chin, arranged so as to press on the deflected side
of the chin. Pressure is also arranged to be applied to the inclined
side of the head behind the ear. The wire collar is attached to a
ring which rests upon the shoulder, and is furnished with arms which
pass down the back. The asymmetry of the face becomes more noticeable after correction than it was in the deformed position, but in
children disappears gradually if the corrected position is retained.

Posterior Torticollis.—The only efficacious treatment of this form
is that of forcible correction without tenotomy, for the reason that,
as a rule, the muscles are too deep or extensive to be tenotomized.
The writers have divided the outer bands of the anterior scalenus and
trapezius by open incision and can report the feasibility of the procedure. In correcting this deformity the patient should be thoroughly
anæsthetized, and an assistant should hold the shoulders firmly, while
the patient should be so placed that the head projects beyond the end
of the operating-table. The head should be held by the hands of the
surgeon and rotated in all directions, considerable force being used.

The danger of fracturing the spine is in such cases so slight as to be disregarded, and the deformity can be overcorrected. After the operation the head should be fixed, the after-treatment resembling that of the ordinary torticollis.

Spasmodic Torticollis.—This form of wry-neck (known also as intermittent) is resistant to treatment, and in many cases cannot be

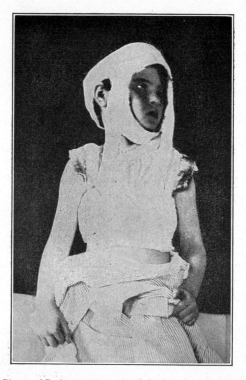

Fig. 230.—Plaster-of-Paris Apparatus Applied after Operation for Torticollis.

relieved by any means known to us at present. The constitutional nature of the affection is an important factor to be considered. The affection may be considered a localized chorea or a disturbance of the proper muscular balance of the muscles holding the head. Of the constitutional treatment nothing need be said, further than that the success of treatment demands the removal of the patient from all depressing influences and the elimination of sources of reflex irritation such as eye strain, etc. The surgical treatment consists of measures of fixation, muscular rest, muscular development, and operative measures.

TREATMENT BY REST AND FIXATION.—Treatment by absolute rest of all muscles sustaining the weight of the head should be tried. This can be furnished by placing the patient in a recumbent position without pillows and fixing the head by sand bags applied at each side of the head. A plaster bandage can be applied or a moulded leather substitute holding the head, shoulders, and trunk firmly, relieving the muscles from any weight-bearing strain. With this the patient is relieved of the restraint of recumbency. Local applications can be made to the muscles with electricity and massage.

TREATMENT BY MUSCULAR TRAINING.—Great benefit may follow carefully directed and graded exercises directed to the cultivation of the groups of muscles which tend to correct the malposition.

TREATMENT BY OPERATIVE MEASURES.—The tedious and unsatisfactory nature of conservative treatment suggests the employment of operative measures. The restoration of muscular balance by myotomy, fasciotomy, and the incidental temporary muscular rest is observed in the surgical treatment of muscular spasm in spastic paralysis, and the same principles can be applied in spasmodic torticollis. The muscles involved are not only the sterno-cleido-mastoid, but the various muscles in the back of the neck. Stretching, division, and excision of portions of the nerves supplying these muscles have been employed.

The nerves to be divided are the spinal accessory from the sternomastoid, and the nerve roots of the deep posterior cervical plexus.

Extensive division of practically all the posterior neck muscles from one sterno-mastoid around to the other has been practised. But the fact remains that relapses after all operations occur, and that both mechanical and operative treatment of the affection are at present discouraging and unsatisfactory.

CHAPTER XIV.

INFANTILE PARALYSIS.

ANTERIOR poliomyelitis, or infantile paralysis, or polio-myelo-encephalitis is an acute infection which attacks chiefly children. It comes on with a sudden onset and deprives certain muscles and often an entire limb of muscular power, and the parts affected undergo rapid atrophy. The paralysis is a purely motor one.

ETIOLOGY.

The disease may occur in epidemics, but is also seemingly sporadic, is apparently contagious, and is a disease affecting chiefly children, and reaching its highest incidence in the late summer. The pathology,

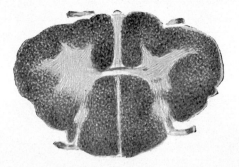

FIG. 231.—Anterior Poliomyelitis. Chronic Stage; Section through Sixth Cervical Segment; Dimunition of Anterior Gray Matter and of Entire Half of Right Side. (Sachs.)

etiology, and symptomatology of the disease are described in medical text-books. In this place will be considered only the surgical aspects of the affection. From this point of view the disease is to be regarded pathologically as a hemorrhagic myelitis, with its chief destruction situated in the cells of the anterior cornua of the cord with the consequent loss of power in the affiliated muscles. These may show parenchymatous or interstitial changes late in the affection. In the severest cases the muscles become mere bundles of interstitial tissue.

SYMPTOMS.

For surgical purposes the clinical history of the disease falls into three stages:

(a) The onset, to which stage belong the acute febrile symptoms and the development of paralysis.

(b) The stage of convalescence, which begins at the time of the full development of the paralysis, and is followed by a brief stationary period, and finally rapid and then slower improvement until a stationary period is reached.

(c) The stage of deformity, in which wasting of the affected limb is present, and static, paralytic, and contraction deformities have supervened.

No arbitrary subdivision of the classes of symptoms can be made, because in reality the stages run into each other.

Infantile paralysis is oftenest ushered in by a mild or severe febrile attack. The elevation of temperature is not excessive, commonly from 100° to 102° F., sometimes even 104°. With this fever are apt to be associated vomiting, convulsions, giddiness, or other cerebral disturbance, sometimes even delirium. The majority of children complain of pain and tenderness in the back and limbs. There is, as a rule, no warning of the attack. The feverish attack at the onset is generally followed by paralysis in from one to four days, although the interval may be longer. In certain cases all feverish and other symptoms are absent at the onset, and the child is suddenly discovered to be paralyzed in one or more limbs.

During the first few days there may be paralysis of the bladder with retention or incontinence of urine.

The paralysis itself very quickly becomes manifest, and having reached its maximum, remains stationary for a short time, when improvement begins. In some cases (probably about 15 per cent) improvement begins immediately after the attack and proceeds to complete recovery. The more common course is for the paralysis to remain nearly stationary for a time varying from two to six weeks, and then to improve, at first rapidly and then more slowly, for three or four months. After six months have passed, further *spontaneous* improvement is unusual.

Vascular changes later become marked, and the temperature of the limb is much lower than that of the other. The limb is generally bluish, with a superficial stagnation of the blood, and when the blood is pressed out of the surface capillaries by the finger it returns slowly.

On account of this vascular sluggishness ulcers may form later on which are slow to heal and very painful. The limb even very early loses its normal appearance, and the flaccid undeveloped look of the foot or hand is most noticeable.

Atrophy of the affected muscles begins to be perceptible very soon after the onset of the paralysis. Muscles seriously affected are toneless

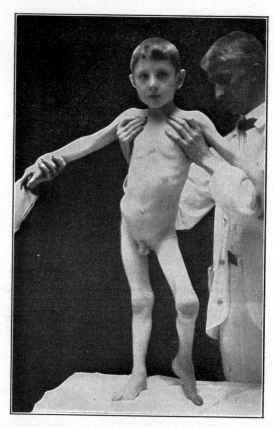

FIG. 232.—Paralysis of the Left Leg, with Talipes Equinus and Contraction of the Fascia at the Anterior and Outer Aspect of the Thigh with Involvement of the Internal Rotators and Abductors of the Leg, Resulting in a Position of Abduction and Eversion.

and flaccid from the first, and in the late stages of wasting scarcely any volume of muscles seems left when the limb is grasped with the hand.

The paralysis is a purely motor one, and although tingling and formication may be present, sensation is very rarely affected. The reflexes are abolished in the affected limb if the paralyzed muscles are those involved in the reflex area.

Often after an attack the paralysis may seem to be general, but the probabilities are that after improving in general, the loss of power will eventually be localized in one limb, and that if one limb originally is paralyzed the likelihood is very great that a certain amount of power will be regained, leaving only certain groups of muscles permanently paralyzed.

The muscles of the back may be paralyzed and the patient be unable to sit erect, or lateral curvature may result—a state of affairs often made worse by allowing the patient to sit erect while the muscles are still weak. The diaphragm is occasionally paralyzed. In those cases of paralysis of the abdominal muscles, the patient leans back to a very marked degree, missing the restraining action of the abdominal muscles. There are, finally, cases of universal paralysis in which death soon takes place from interference with respiration.

Deformities.—The deformities which follow after infantile paralysis are late events in the history of the disease, but develop at times a few weeks after the attack. They are, as a rule, progressive in their character. The deformities fall into two chief classes: (1) deformities due to trophic changes, such as bone shortening, etc.; (2) deformities due to muscular paralysis.

(1) The first class is comparatively unimportant; shortening of the paralyzed arm or leg may take place with atrophy of the bone in every direction. Shortening of the arm is comparatively unimportant in itself, but shortening of the leg may induce lateral curvature of the spine from the necessarily tilted position of the pelvis due to the unequal length of the legs.

(2) The deformities of the second class, which are the result of muscular paralysis, are manifold and form the great bulk of the cases of deformity in anterior poliomyelitis. As a rule they do not appear earlier than two or three months after the onset and more commonly not for many months.

For clinical consideration they fall into two groups: deformities caused by contraction, and deformities due to laxity of the muscles and ligaments.

A word should be said in regard to the reason of the more severe affection of the anterior leg and thigh muscles than of the posterior muscles in nearly all cases. After a paralysis of the leg, the limb lies flaccid and nearly powerless, the toes drop, and, if the sitting posture is assumed, the knees flex and the legs hang heavily down.

As a result of this, the anterior muscles are always pulled upon and slightly stretched, while the posterior ones are lax. If all the muscles are equally affected, this very factor may be enough to make a great difference in the ultimate usefulness of the two groups. Stretched muscles are notoriously at a disadvantage, so far as recovery goes, in any diseased condition, and muscles at rest are much more favorably

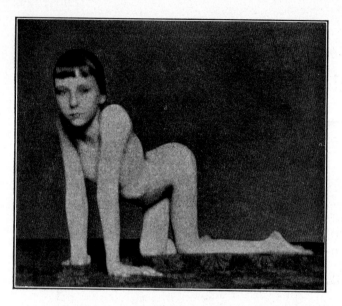

Fig. 233.—Paralysis of the Back Muscles, Causing Saddle-back Deformity.

situated. So that this very point may determine in a measure the relative amount of recovery in the two groups.

Moreover, muscular contraction and consequent deformity occur in cases in which a muscle has been allowed to remain for a long time in a shortened or stretched condition. For this reason it is highly important to support and restrain the affected limb in a normal position (the foot at a right angle to the leg, etc.).

The most important deformities from infantile paralysis which come to the orthopedic surgeon for treatment are those of the lower extremity. Considered in detail, it is best to begin with deformities at the hip-joint and then to pass on to the consideration of knee-joint deformities and distortions of the foot.

Deformities of the Leg.—Paralysis may be complete and a flail-like leg be the result, with wasted muscles and loose, distorted joints, incapable of motion or bearing weight. Such a limb is spoken of as "jambe de Polichinelle."

But more commonly the paralysis is partial rather than complete. The muscles of the thigh commonly affected are the internal and anterior groups. This constitutes a serious combination and renders walking difficult; not only is the leg abducted with a tendency to

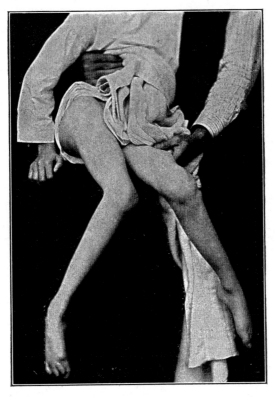

Fig. 234.—Severe Double Paralysis with Marked Knock-knee and Distortion of Feet. This patient was unable to walk.

eversion, but the extensor thigh muscles cannot hold the knee rigid as is necessary in walking, the leg giving way whenever weight is put upon it. The glutei are generally implicated in this paralysis, and the contraction which is likely to result from this paralysis is flexion of the thigh alone or with abduction of the leg, a condition always associated with flexion of the knee.

Flexion deformity at the hip produces in time a most marked

lordosis in the back. When the patient stands with the leg dangling, the weight of it drags upon the pelvis and rotates it on a transverse axis, a compensation which makes it possible for the leg to hang as nearly as possible perpendicularly. This deformity is marked and troublesome.

At the knee, contraction in the flexed position (with often a tendency to subluxation of the tibia backward) is found, and in the more

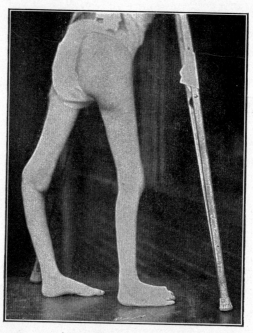

FIG. 235.—Hyperextension of the Left Knee due to Paralysis of the Limb. Varus deformity of the right foot.

severe cases decided knock-knee. In severe cases of this type in which the deformity has been rectified by mechanical or operative means, the tibia may lie in a plane decidedly posterior to that of the femur. The same may be said of the knock-knee which results from the greater prominence of the internal condyle of the femur. The flexion may have been overcome, but still a decided degree of knock-knee may remain in the corrected leg. At other times when laxity rather than contraction predominates, hyperextension of the knee is observed and sometimes lateral mobility also exists.

This hyperextension results in cases in which the anterior muscles are weak and fail to hold the knee extended when walking is attempted. In these cases the patient throws the weight of the body upon the fully extended knee and the strain falls upon the ligaments rather than on the muscles. The posterior ligaments yield in time to this repeated weight and the patient obtains for a time a better bearing. The same deformity is favored by a tendency which these patients have to lean with the hand upon the knee when rising from a chair.

in dorsal flexum. about

Talipes calcaneo-valgus and pure flat-foot are favored by lax ligaments, and the latter may be a progressive deformity, which may increase until a stage is reached in which the inner malleolus almost touches the ground. The bearing of body-weight on a foot, the ligaments and muscles of which are weak, tends to produce flatfoot.

Pure talipes calcaneus seems to be the result of the paralysis of the posterior calf muscles combined with the action of gravity and superincumbent weight, and is commonly associated with what is known as pes cavus.

Deformities of the arms are not common as the result of infantile paralysis. The least infrequent of these results from the paralysis of the deltoid. In addition to the inability to raise the arm from the side, there

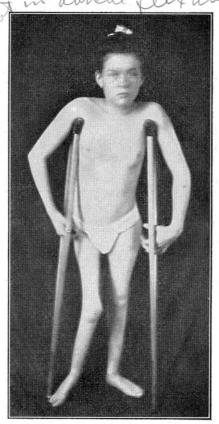

FIG. 236.—Paralysis of Both Legs, severest in right, with knock-knee on that side. This patient was unable to walk without crutches.

are present a flattening of the shoulder and a prominence of the acromion process, and the shoulder presents an angular rather than a rounded outline. The ligaments are loosened, and the arm hangs loosely, so that in some cases a wide gap may be observed between the acromion and the humerus.

The commonest paralysis of the hand is one affecting the adductor muscles of the thumb, as a result of which the thumb is drawn back to a level with the other fingers and the power to oppose it to the other fingers in grasping is thus lost. Paralysis of the erector spinæ muscles results in a permanent arching of the spine and inability to sit erect. Paralysis of the abdominal muscles causes lordosis.

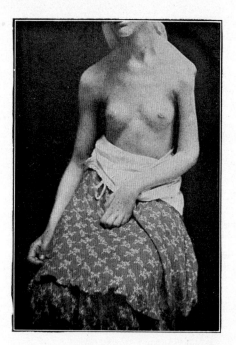

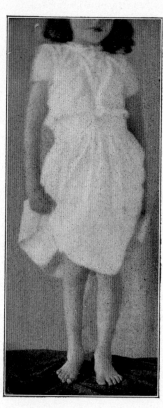

FIG. 237.—Paralysis of the Left Arm Muscles, Deltoid and Serratus Magnus.

FIG. 238.—Moderate Degree of Talipes Valgus, Right Foot.

Lateral curvature of the spine results from infantile paralysis in one of three ways:

(1) From the inequality in the length of the legs due to paralysis of one leg, causing tilting of the pelvis. (2) From the unilateral paralysis of the muscles directly controlling the vertebral column, which might be either a paralysis of the intrinsic spinal muscles or of the erector spinæ group on one side. (3) From faulty

spinal attitudes assumed in consequence of some paralysis elsewhere, as in paralysis of one arm, or of the serratus magnus.

Dislocations from Infantile Paralysis.—Dislocation, complete or partial, belongs to the more uncommon of the complications of infantile paralysis and characterizes severe cases.

Dislocation or subluxation of the hip is the one most commonly met and it takes place either spontaneously or in consequence of weight

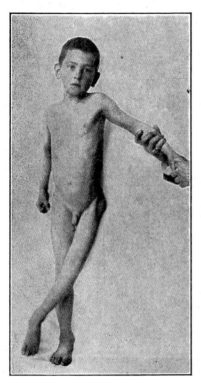 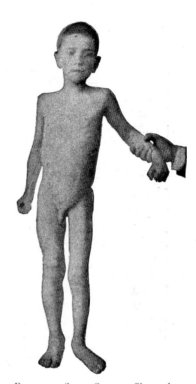

Fig. 239.—Dislocation of Hip, the Result of Infantile Paralysis. In this position the head of the femur (left) is in place, but with abduction it slips out again.

Fig. 240.—Same Case as Shown in Fig. 239, with Hip Dislocated.

being borne upon a limb which is improperly supported by its ligaments. A shortening of one or two inches may be present, as the dislocation is generally on to the dorsum of the ilium; but sometimes it takes the form of a laxity of the joint in all directions, so that the head may be thrown into any position by manipulation of the shaft. Most dislocations of the hip are inconvenient chiefly because of the shortening and insecurity which follow the displacement of the head of the bone, and such legs are sometimes fairly serviceable. Dislocation may, however, occur before any weight is borne upon the affected limb, by the spontaneous action of the muscles, as in a patient eighteen months old, in the experience of one of the writers.

DIAGNOSIS.

In typical cases the diagnosis of infantile paralysis is not difficult. But in other than typical cases the recognition of the disease may be difficult, and it is not possible with our present knowledge to establish a positive diagnosis in the initial stage. At that time the occurrence

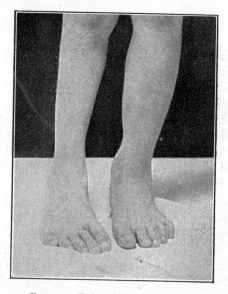

Fig. 241.—Talipes Varus, Right Foot.

of localized pain may be a misleading symptom, and sensitiveness of the affected limbs may suggest rheumatism.

The diagnostic points upon which the practitioner must rely in the stage of established paralysis are the history of the attack, a motor paralysis, rapid muscular wasting, the distribution of the paralysis, and the loss of the tendon reflex. Diagnosis by the determination of the electrical reaction of the muscles requires especial training and skill, although it is distinctive.

Electrical Condition of the Muscles.—Faradic irritability of the affected muscles and nerves begins to diminish within a day or two of the onset of the paralysis, and in muscles severely affected the electric irritability disappears entirely; in the muscles less seriously involved it is merely diminished. The cathodal closing contraction should be normally greater than the anodal closing contraction. When

c. c. c > a c c
here a in aff palw
reverse a c c 7 c c c

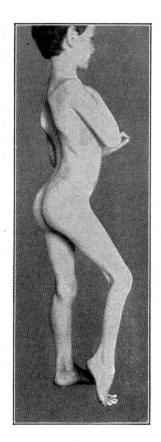

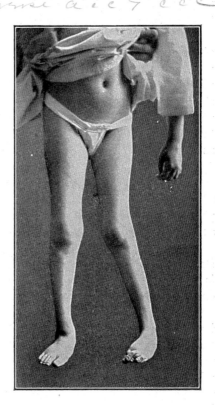

Fig. 242.—Flexion Deformity of the Hip, Knee, and Ankle, due to Contractions.

Fig. 243.—Old Paralysis of Left Leg with Slight Knock-knee and Talipes Varus.

nerves and muscles affected by anterior poliomyelitis are examined, not only a slow wave-like response to electricity instead of a sharp quick jerk is found, but the electrical formula is reversed and *the closure of the positive pole gives the greater contraction.* These qualitative and quantitative changes in reaction to the galvanic current constitute what is known as the " reaction of degeneration," and this affords the most definite ground for the diagnosis of infantile paralysis.

The only affection which may not be distinguished by electrical examination from anterior poliomyelitis is peripheral paralysis caused by interruption in the course of some nerve.

The most available means for the practitioner to adopt in determining which muscles are paralyzed is as follows: The patient is told to dorsally flex the foot, and the examining finger is placed upon the tendons at the front of the ankle to feel which, if any, contract; plantar flexion, adduction, and abduction are each tested in the same way. The activity or inactivity of each muscle can thus be determined. The knee is flexed and extended, with the fingers on the hamstrings and extensor tendons, and the hip is flexed, extended, rotated, and adducted, lying on the back, and abducted lying on the side. Certain muscles will be found to contract feebly and should be classed as " weakened " rather than " paralyzed."

PROGNOSIS.

So far as danger to life is concerned, from 5 to 15 per cent of patients die in the acute attack. If death does occur it is generally at the end of a few days, oftenest from respiratory paralysis.

It is not likely that the paralysis will increase if it has been stationary for twenty-four hours. In cases in which the deformity is only of moderate extent, it is not probable that life will be shortened by it.

When untreated, a case of infantile paralysis will almost invariably improve for one or two months at a rapid rate, then more slowly for two or three months more, and then after a stationary period, contractions, looseness of the joints, and malpositions are likely to begin, which may increase indefinitely. Under treatment the prognosis is much more favorable and the limit of possible improvement extended by many years.

It should be remembered that even in mild cases of infantile paralysis bone shortening may follow. Certain severe cases escape with but little, while a mild case may show, with the wasting of the leg, a shortening of one or two inches in the limb of the affected side, or more in exceptional cases.

A distinct measure of success in the orthopedic treatment of infantile paralysis in the stage of deformity can be expected in a large percentage of cases, exclusive of the hopeless class where a large portion of the body is permanently paralyzed. By thorough surgical care what would be a condition of hopeless affliction can be converted into a slight or endurable disability.

TREATMENT.

The treatment of infantile paralysis varies according to the stage at which treatment is to be undertaken.

The Stage of Onset.—If the fact that paralysis is present, is established during the febrile attack, which is usually the first symptom of

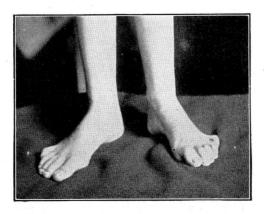

Fig. 244.—Clawed Toes and Pes Cavus following Infantile Paralysis.

the disease, vigorous treatment should be at once begun, to limit, if possible, the destructive process in the cord. Cathartics should be given at once, the patient should be kept quiet and hexamethylenamin administered, although the present evidence is that it acts best as a preventive measure than after the infection has occurred. Its value is probably based on the fact that it sets free formalin in the cerebrospinal fluid. The general condition of the child should in every way be kept as good as possible. The child should be isolated and sputum, urine, and feces disinfected, although there is at present no evidence to show how long the infectious period lasts.

The Stage of Paralysis.—But few cases are seen by the surgeon until the stage of paralysis is present. The question that then presents itself is that the treatment of the paralysis should be such that the ultimate amount of muscular power may be as great as possible. It must be remembered that the tendency of the paralysis is at first very strong toward spontaneous improvement. It is manifest that in the first few weeks treatment should be directed toward producing conditions which shall be as favorable as possible for the spontaneous improvement to attain its maximum.

This stage can be considered to extend from the period of the entire disappearance of the sensitiveness and the contractions of the early irritant stages until the time that all potential power has been regained, or until the deformities require no further attention. Two special demands are important throughout this stage, which are:

1. The prevention of deformity.
2. The regaining of nerve and muscle power.

1. *Prevention of Deformity* —Deformities which occur in the course of recovery from infantile paralysis are those of the limbs and those of the spine, a form of scoliosis. It is especially needful that apparatus be employed in this stage for a twofold object, i.e., first, to prevent the overstretching of the paralyzed muscles during the early stages; and, second, to prevent the permanency of the deformities mentioned.

The need of the early detection of a faulty position of the spine and of early care in the prevention of scoliosis cannot be too strongly stated. On account of the general muscular weakness and of the unequal pull of the trunk muscles, the asymmetrical methods of walking and standing and the faulty superimposed weight, or the one-sided use of the arms in cases of paralysis of the upper extremity, all motions on the part of the patient tend to exaggerate the development of deformity when once under way. For this reason this form of scoliosis presents a most obstinate type for treatment, and as soon as there is any evidence of a beginning deformity of the spine every effort should be directed to check its development.

2. *The Regaining of Nerve and Muscle Power.*—It is possible to gain a return of muscle power after a long period following the onset of disease, even when during the interval there has been no evidence of actual local return of power. It is essential, therefore, that treatment directed to this end be carried out, not only in a most thorough manner, but also over an extended period. The indications during the early convalescent stage are two, viz., for:

(*a*) The stimulation of the motor tracts to prevent all possible degeneration until all possible repair has taken place; and

(*b*) Stimulation and protection of muscles to prevent atrophy and to keep the muscle in condition, that it may respond quickly when nerve impulses are restored.

For stimulation of nerves and muscles the means to be employed are:

1. Muscle training.
2. Physical therapy (including mechanotherapy, hydrotherapy, and massage).
3. Electricity.
4. Baking and different forms of high heat.

1. *Muscle Training.*—Probably no other means at our disposal has a more important place or more extended usefulness, both in the variety of its application and in the length of time that it may be used, than the different methods which may be grouped under this head. It is applicable as soon as any sign of returning power is found, and is best applied through the " assistive form " of exercise, which has the advantage of allowing actual work to the muscle long before power is sufficient to give any practical result in movement. This method is applied in detail as follows:

The part to which the muscle belongs is put through passive movement, with slow rhythm, in the direction that is desired. The patient is then directed to make effort to move the part in the same direction to whatever extent is possible, the assistant supplying the power needed to complete the actual motion. In this way the paralyzed muscle is allowed to contract in the same manner as if it were doing the whole of the work, and has the benefit of the contraction and of the movement during the whole arc of motion. As the muscle becomes stronger, the assistive force supplied becomes less, so that the muscle is allowed to take up more of the work during the whole of the exercise, and receives the maximum amount of exercise possible to a muscle in its condition. In all the other forms of exercise one must be contented with the mere effort of the muscle to make contraction, without allowing contraction through a distinct arc of motion.

Poliomyelitis may weaken certain muscles without paralyzing them; it is desirable to lessen the disability by developing their strength again, and, as far as possible, to secure a return of normal motions of the limb. This can usually be accomplished by systematic exercises carried out regularly once or twice a day. Again, certain muscles may be weakened, not by the disease itself, but by disuse entailed by it, although not in themselves involved in the paralytic attack. For these also it is desirable to use a simple means of exercise.

The aid of an expert is undoubtedly advisable, but the constant daily faithful work of home attendants is more beneficial than occasional treatment at infrequent intervals. It may be mentioned that much more exercise is to be obtained with the patient immersed in a bath, as the weight of the limbs is supported by the water.

2. *Physical Therapy (including Mechanotherapy, Massage, etc.)*.
—Massage, however, should be given a high place in all stages of
this affection after the disappearance of the tenderness. In conjunction with massage, however, it is wise to reiterate the caution that
it is necessary not to rely upon massage alone, but that this means
should be regarded as an adjunct only to the other forms of muscle
and nerve stimulation. Too frequently it is the case that massage

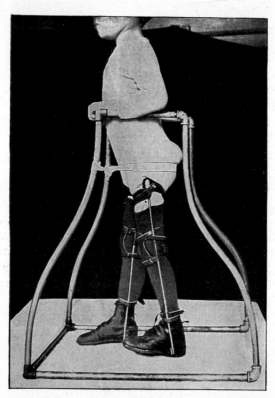

FIG. 245.—Paralyzed Child Strapped in a Walking Frame Wearing Splints to Prevent
Forward Dropping of the Knee. (Boston Med. and Surg. Journal.)

alone is used to the neglect of many of the other means fully as
important.

3. *Electricity*.—The different forms which may be used for this
are the galvanic, faradic, static, and high-frequency currents. In the
early stages galvanism should be used on the nerve trunks and faradism
on the muscles, so long as their irritability for contraction is maintained. When the irritability of contraction to the faradic current is

lost, galvanism should then be used, as having more influence on nutrition. With the returning muscle irritability, faradism should be used. This serves as a distinct exercise to the muscle during its early

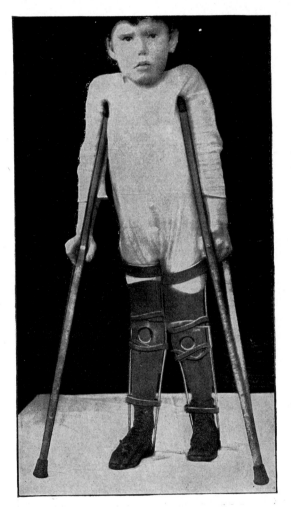

Fig. 246.—Child Walking with Crutches and Splints. (Boston Med. and Surg. Journal.)

stage of weak contraction. High-frequency and static electricity can both be used for their influence on nutrition rather than for their direct action on muscle contraction. It may be stated in this connection that the main dependence for actual results in the use of electricity must be placed upon the galvanic and faradic currents.

4. *Baking and the Other Means of Applying High Degrees of Heat.*—Paralyzed limbs in these cases are almost always cold and the circulation distinctly defective. It is found after the use of baking

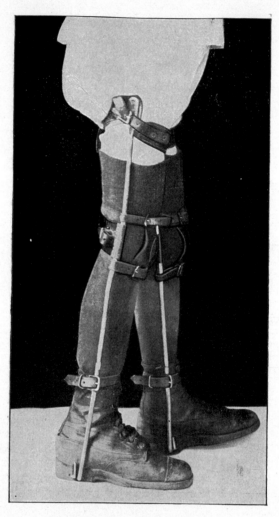

Fig. 247.—Side View of "Caliper" Splint, with Knee Strap and Checks in the Heel to Prevent the Dropping of the Heel or Front of the Foot as may be needed. (Boston Med. and Surg. Journal.)

by electric light and different methods of applying high degrees of heat that the extremities remain warm for a longer time and that the circulation is more active; and that the patient is able to use the very weak muscles better during the time that the limbs remain warm. It is frequently found that after continued use of high degrees of heat this improvement of circulation and the local heat of the limb become more and more permanent, frequently lasting for the larger part of the day or longer.

MECHANICAL TREATMENT.

The objects of mechanical treatment for infantile paralysis are:
1. To correct the deformities of the limb.

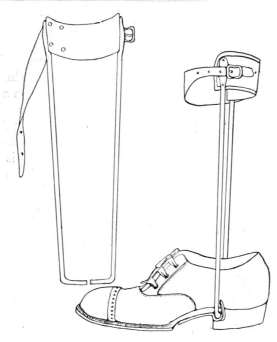

FIG. 248.—Detail of Wire Splint, Showing Adjustment to the Shoe, with Check to Prevent Toe-drop. (Boston Med. and Surg. Journal.)

2. To prevent the development of new deformities.

3. To aid locomotion by furnishing, through the mechanical stops and checks, a substitute for the action of muscles weakened or paralyzed by the disease.

The number of types of appliances which can be devised is great. Those which are simple, light, easily designed, and easily applied are to be preferred. Expensive, heavy, and complicated forms of apparatus are undesirable.

Those which have been for many years used at the Boston Children's Hospital will be referred to here because, in design and construction, they are suited to the practice of any general practitioner who is ready to give personal attention to making, fitting, and adjusting an appliance to prevent the development of deformity in his patient.

Early Stage of Paralysis.—Appliances for this stage should interfere with the circulation as little as possible, since it is desirable to develop the impaired nutrition and circulation, not to impede it. For

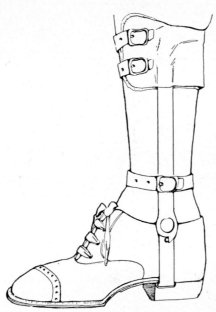

this reason plaster bandages and splints tightly secured by a muslin bandage are less used than formerly.

Toe-drop can easily be prevented while the child is in bed by fixing the limb on a simple posterior wire splint such as one uses for fractures. If this splint be prolonged to reach the upper part of the thigh, and is made stiff enough, contraction of the knee can also be prevented.

Splints for Walking.—These splints are designed for two classes of cases—those in which a flaccid paralysis is present in some of the muscles, and those where, in addition to the paralysis, a con-

FIG. 249.—Apparatus to Prevent Toe-drop Slipping in a Socket at the Heel. An ankle strap secures the leg.

traction and shortening has taken place in muscles which are not paralyzed but have lost their antagonists. In the first class no stiffness or contraction is present, and splints may be needed to prevent (1) toe-drop; (2) dropping of the tarsus to the inner side; (3) dropping of the tarsus to the outer side; (4) walking on the heel; and (5) to hold the knee straight in paralysis of the muscles of the front of the thigh.

Where no stiffness from contraction is present, a simple apparatus can be furnished to prevent toe-drop. It is called a short caliper splint. It consists of two parts, the splint and the socket attached to the boot.

The socket is made of a thin iron plate, made to fit under the

heel and the shank of the child's boot, as far forward as the metatarso-phalangeal joint. The heel of the boot is first removed, and
a deep groove or socket is fashioned in the plate by forging, so that
when it is applied to the boot it will receive at the heel the end of
the upright, as if in a tube. A small spur piece, which is left projecting

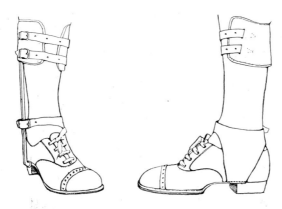

Fig. 250.—Apparatus Similar to Fig. 249, with Ankle Strap to Check Paralytic Valgus. If the upright is applied to the inside with the ankle strap applied to the
outside a varus deformity is checked. (Boston Med. and Surg. Journal.)

outside the boot, is bent up after it is applied, so as to act as a stop,
as shown in the illustration, and the boot heel is reapplied.

At the top the wires are slightly flattened and attached to a thin
metal calf-band fitted to the calf of the leg; at the bottom they are
sharply bent inward at a right angle so as to fit in the socket. The
uprights may follow the shape of the leg, or be left straight. This
brace is held in place by a strap at the top and one around the ankle.

Should the patient, instead of having toe-drop, have paralysis of
the calf muscles, he will walk on his heel. In order to apply the
sole of the boot to the ground, the same splint may be used to advantage if the socket be made so that the stop comes in front of the
upright instead of behind it.

Should the child stand with the foot in the varus or club-foot
position, a stout leather T strap should be added, which is sewed to
the upper of the boot, just in front of the external malleolus; the
horizontal straps buckle into each other and include the inner upright
of the splint.

Should, on the other hand, a pronated or valgus position appear
in weight-bearing, the T strap should be on the opposite side of the

boot below the inner malleolus, and strapped around the outer upright so as to maintain the arch of the foot by preventing the ankle from sagging inward.

Again, if, owing to paralysis of the muscles of the front of the

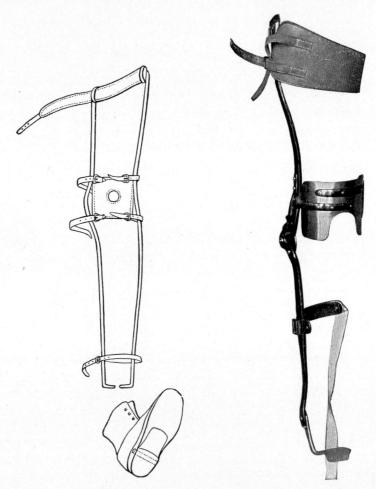

FIG. 251.—Caliper Apparatus for Anterior Poliomyelitis.

FIG. 252.—Supporting Splint for Use in Infantile Paralysis. It prevents flexion of the knee in standing, but is provided with a lock-joint at the knee.

thigh, the quadriceps extensor cruris, the child cannot hold the knee stiff in standing, then the caliper splint should be made to reach the upper third of the thigh and the knee be kept straight by a leather knee cap.

Firmer and more efficient apparatus is the following:

In toe-drop the same end can be accomplished by the application of a walking appliance, described under club-foot as an equino-varus shoe, which should be provided with a right-angle stop at the ankle which will not allow the ankle to be extended to more than a right

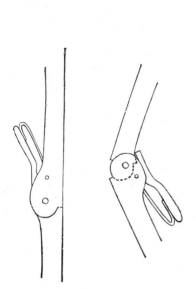

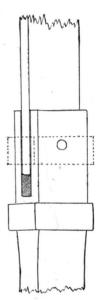

FIG. 253.—Self-locking Spring Catch.   FIG. 254.—Drop Catch.

angle. When in bearing weight upon the leg the ankle assumes a varus position, a varus shoe will correct the tendency to deformity.

If the foot rolls out and is everted into a valgus condition when the body weight is borne upon the leg, an outside shoe is to be applied, in construction like the varus shoe, but which should have a broad leather strap which should pass around the inner malleolus and support it. This apparatus is a difficult one to render quite comfortable to the patient, as much weight must necessarily come upon the strap which supports the inner malleolus. As flat-foot is almost always present in these cases, it is well to arch the steel sole plate of this apparatus so that it serves as a valgus plate as well as a supporting appliance.

If calcaneus is present the apparatus spoken of for equinus is used, with the stop catch reversed to prevent dorsal instead of plantar flexion.

Pes cavus may be treated by inserting a steel sole in the sole of the boot and passing a strap from the sole over the dorsum of the foot. This treatment is made much more efficient if combined with preliminary division of the plantar fascia. Mechanical treatment alone is likely to be unsatisfactory.

It is manifest that the simpler and lighter these appliances are and the less unsightly, the more serviceable they will prove. For

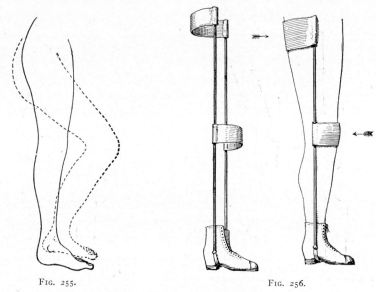

FIG. 255.   FIG. 256.

FIGS. 255 and 256.—Supporting Apparatus in Paralysis of Anterior Thigh Muscles.

this reason they should be carefully fitted and the uprights made to follow the outline of the leg. In very slight cases, in which there is only a slight eversion of the foot with a small degree of valgus, a common valgus plate, such as would be applied for flat-foot, will often answer every purpose in correcting the deformity, and it should be applied as in simple flat-foot.

If the knee tends to drop backward and become hyperextended, it can be remedied by an appliance with a strap passing behind the knee, with an upper band encircling the thigh. In practice this apparatus can often consist of a single outside upright hinged at the knee. It passes to the inside of the leg just below the knee to become attached to a varus shoe. This answers as well as a double upright in many cases.

Other cases, in which the paralysis is more severe, require the two uprights, as they furnish a more definite support. The foot is easily retained to the steel sole plate by straps or a piece of leather lacing over the instep. The fenestrated knee cap is the most comfortable method of holding the knee extended.

Although in walking it is generally necessary to have the knee kept extended by the splint, yet in sitting down it is a great comfort to the patient to be able to flex the knee, and for this reason nearly all splints should be hinged at the knee, especially in the case of older children.

TREATMENT OF CONTRACTIONS.

Equinus Deformity.—In slight degrees, contraction of the short tendo Achillis can be overcome by stretching the muscles with a special splint in walking, if the heel can be held down firmly against a foot plate which extends well forward, while toe-drop is prevented by a stop in the ankle-joint of the upright. At times it is hard to accomplish this because the heel refuses to stay down on the sole-plate, but it may be held there either by a strong ankle strap or by a strip of adhesive plaster attached to the skin of the calf of the leg above and to the lower surface of the sole-plate below. Such an apparatus can be worn inside of the boot, the correcting force being the body weight.

Varus with Slight Contraction.—In paralytic varus deformity a thick leather wedge is pegged to the lower surface of the sole of the boot under the cuboid, so that the foot in walking strikes first on the heel, then on the wedge which projects more than the heel, and forces the foot to turn outward to prevent loss of balance, so that the foot at the end of a step, before leaving the ground, receives the body weight wholly on the abducted front portion.

Valgus with Slight Contraction.—In paralytic valgus deformity, when the contraction of the peronei muscles is slight, the position of the walking foot as it bears on the ground can be improved by supporting the sagging arch, both by an upright and T strap, and by pegging a thick wedge of leather on the lower surface of the sole of the boot, extending forward along the inner side from the heel to the scaphoid, or under the first metatarsal, as the case may require.

Calcaneus.—In cases with slight contraction the position of the walking foot, as it strikes the ground, can be improved by prolonging the heel backwards.

The above-mentioned appliances are only for slight contractions; when firm contractions have developed, they are to be stretched or divided by an operation, under full anæsthesia, either by manual force, tenotomy, or incision, as may be needed; but for a few mild cases the gradual corrections are sufficient which one obtains by plaster bandages or mechanical appliances.

Plaster Bandages.—Gradual correction by the frequently repeated application of plaster bandages is obtained by holding the limb in as corrected a position as possible while the plaster sets, without the aid of an anæsthetic. It is effective in recent contractions in young

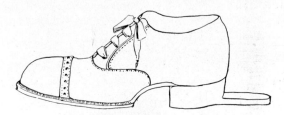

Fig. 257.—Heel Extension to be Used to Check Calcaneus Deformity.
(Boston Med. and Surg. Journal.)

children. The method has to its disadvantage that both muscular atrophy and weakening of undestroyed muscles are favored by the prolonged use of stiff bandages; therefore this method should not be continued during a long period.

The contractions which the surgeon has most frequently to overcome are those of the tendo Achillis, the hamstrings, the tensor vaginæ femoris and fascia adjacent, the psoas and iliacus muscles; also contractions of the tendons and fascia of the foot.

For the correction of contracted ankle, unless the equinus position yields readily to mechanical means, tenotomy of the tendo Achillis, is decidedly preferable.

For a contracted or flexed knee, mechanical measures are better adapted. If the type be mild it can be overcome by the application of a splint resembling Thomas' knee-splint, to which the limb can be bandaged. The corrective pressure is obtained largely from the bandage over the thigh and knee, which should be applied at least twice a day. This apparatus can also be used to walk with. If any form of acquired talipes is combined with the contracted knee, it may be corrected simultaneously in the manner already described.

For contractions of the hip-joint not severe enough to demand operation, two common methods of correction are in use.

1. By encasing in a plaster bandage the limb, with the knee straight, may be utilized to stretch very gradually the contracted muscles and fasciæ of the hip; this may be done either while the child is walking about, or, preferably, while he is in bed, on a bed frame.

Sometimes a separate plaster jacket is required for these recumbent cases, to prevent lordosis of the lumbar spine.

2. A direct pull or traction may be used, such as one would use to correct flexion in hip disease. The patient is then kept on a bed frame with the pelvis fixed (by extreme flexion of the unaffected thigh, if

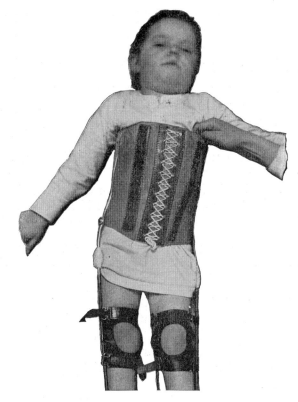

Fig. 258.—Jacket Attached to Caliper Splints Applied to a Case of Paralysis of the Trunk and of Both Legs.

necessary) with the paralyzed leg elevated, and traction is applied in such a position that the line of pull coincides with the new direction of the femur; traction is first made in this direction, and from this position the limb is straightened very gradually day by day.

All contractions at the hip may without doubt be overcome more quickly by the use of the knife, with subsequent fixation, than by mechanical means, but an objection is often encountered in children with extensive paralysis because there remains in the limb so little muscle power that any loss, whether from tenotomy, myotomy, or prolonged use of plaster bandages, is undesirable.

Lateral curvatures from poliomyelitis sometimes require treatment by recumbency to obliterate or diminish the curves, but in most instances plaster corrective jackets are required for the severe types of curvature, and the subsequent use of stiff leather or celluloid corsets is often necessary for a long time to keep the curvature from increasing. (See chapter on Scoliosis.) These can be connected with the leg appliances, if necessary, and will afford assistance in standing. Cases of this sort may be so severe as to require the use of crutches for rapid locomotion.

When the abdominal muscles are affected, waist bands or corsets will serve to correct the malposition of the trunk to a certain extent.

The mechanical treatment of paralysis of the arm is less satisfactory than that of the lower extremity. Apparatus is of little value, and in these cases operative measures offer the best chance of relief. When mechanical measures are undertaken they should consist of protection of the deltoid from all dragging of the weight of the arm, by supporting the latter on a wire support if necessary, which holds it at the level of the shoulder.

OPERATIVE TREATMENT.

The object of operative interference in paralytic affections is twofold:

1st. To correct existing deformity.

2d. To render the paralyzed limb more efficient.

The first division of the subject has been already discussed.

The second will be considered under the subdivisions of (*a*) muscle and tendon transference, (*b*) arthrodesis, (*c*) silk ligaments, (*d*) bone operations.

Muscle and Tendon Transference.

Where certain groups of muscles are paralyzed and the opponents remain strong, a transference of one or more of the strong muscles to perform the function of the weak muscles has been proved to be of benefit. Tendon grafting, that is, the insertion of the tendon of a strong muscle into the tendon of a weak muscle, although temporarily a help, has not, as a rule, been found to be as permanently beneficial as the transference of muscle or tendon with the periosteal insertion of the transferred tendon to a point of bone where a strong attachment can be secured to the periosteum. This gives a proper point for the contraction of the transferred muscle to perform the function lost by the paralytic attack. Where the transferred muscle or tendon is not sufficiently long to furnish a periosteal insertion, the tendon can be elongated by means of silk strands properly prepared. This measure is especially suitable in paralytic affections of the foot, of the knee, and of the shoulder-joint; it has also been used for paralyzed muscles about the hip. Strictly aseptic precautions are necessary. The silk strands should be thoroughly sterilized. Heavy braided silk is sterilized by boiling for an hour in 1-1000 solution of corrosive sublimate; it is then wrapped in sterile towels and handled by aseptic hands or instruments and dried for 24 hours. Then with the same care it is folded or rolled loosely and dropped into boiling paraffin in a closed boiler, in which it is boiled for 30 minutes. The paraffin is then allowed to harden, and when the silk is needed for operation the paraffin is again melted, and from the dish the silk is removed by clean forceps. These silk strands are quilted into the tendon of the muscle to be transferred. The tendon is then divided, and, with the silk strands attached, is passed by means of long forceps through the subcutaneous tissue and brought out through an incision at the point needed for periosteal insertion. The silk strands are then inserted by means of proper needles into the periosteum or bone tissue, the foot being placed in an overcorrected position. In some instances it may be well to supplement tendon transference with silk ligaments.

In quadriceps paralysis of the knee-joint, the hamstrings can be transferred forward and inserted into the patella and into the ligamentum patellæ. In deltoid paralysis, strands of the trapezius have been transferred in such a way. In paralysis of the glutei muscles, the vastus or the rectus femoris have been utilized for transference, and also strands of the erector spinæ. In paralysis of the tibial muscles, the peronei have been transferred, and *vice versa*. In paralysis of the extensor communis of the foot, the flexors have been used, or portions of the tendo Achillis.

For success it is essential that the muscular balance in the paralyzed limb be restored, and for this it is necessary that the transferred muscle pass to its new insertion in the line in which the muscular pull is desired. It is essential that the transferred muscle should not be relaxed and that it should have a firm and an effective attachment.

The operation is done after the limb has been made bloodless by the Esmarch method, and the deformity of varus, valgus, or equinus

must be forcibly corrected with tenotomy and fasciotomy if necessary. The correction of the deformity, if severe, should be preferably
done a few days before the tendon operation. In the more mild cases
the correction can be done at the same sitting
with the operation. A long incision is then
made over the middle of the ankle or the part
of the ankle where the tendons to be operated
on are situated, extending to the dorsum of the
foot. The muscle to be transferred is then
selected and the tendon isolated and cut off as
near its insertion as possible. The end is then
secured by a long, stout, silk suture. The muscular portion is freed above sufficiently to permit a transference of the direction of the
muscle in a nearly straight rather than a
curved course. The desired point of insertion
is then selected, which should be as far forward on the tarsus as is practicable. The tendon itself, or, if it is too short to reach, the
silk attached to the freed tendon is then stitched
securely to the periosteum at the selected point,
the tendon pulled tightly into its new position,
and firmly tied.

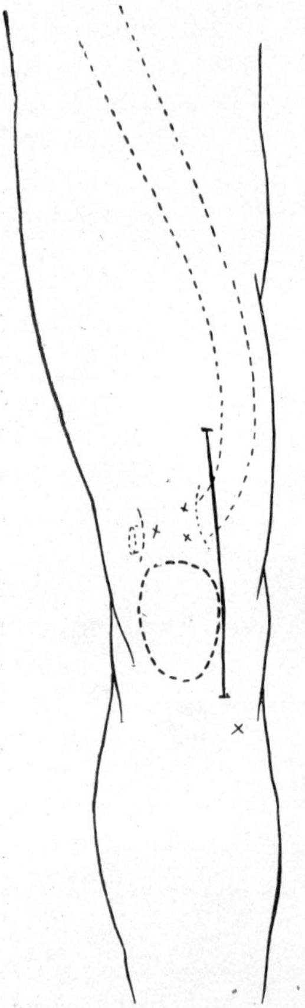

Whether the tibialis anticus or the peroneus
longus, e.g., is selected in a given operation,
depends upon the location of the paralysis and
the muscular pull desired. When the anterior
group of muscles are all paralyzed, as in talipes
equinus, a portion of the tendo Achillis and
one of the peronei can be brought forward to

Fig. 259.—Transplantation of the front of the foot and given an anterior at-
Sartorius to Quadriceps Ten-
don. (Goldthwait.) tachment on the tarsus. In this procedure a
posterior as well as an anterior incision is
needed, and the transferred tendon is passed subcutaneously forward
from the posterior to the anterior incision.

The operative reduction of *calcaneus* or *calcaneo-valgus* is not
permanently accomplished by simple shortening of the tendo Achillis,
because, being paralyzed, the tendon will again stretch and the deformity recur.

If an element of *valgus* exists with the calcaneus, some of the
tendons of the common extensor should be cut and given a periosteal

insertion into the scaphoid or cuneiform. It may also be advisable to change the insertion of one of the peronei muscles to the inner border of the foot.

In *pes cavus* the plantar fascia is to be tenotomized, the foot forcibly stretched, with an osteotomy of the tarsus in extreme cases. Osteotomy of the os calcis is also to be considered in pronounced varus and valgus with distortion of that bone. The proceeding is similar to that in congenital club-foot.

After-Treatment.—After the operation the limb should be protected by sufficient cotton padding and fixed in the desired overcorrected position in a plaster-of-Paris bandage, arranged so as to allow the required inspection after dressing. After six weeks the plaster bandage is to be followed by a retention apparatus, such as has already been described, and the gradually increasing use of the limb allowed, along with massage and passive exercises to develop the transferred muscles to their new work.

Arthrodesis.

If weight is thrown upon a paralyzed lower extremity the knee bends forward and the patient falls. It is evident that if the knee-joint is stiffened in such a way that it cannot bend, the bones will be capable of sustaining the superimposed weight. This can be made possible at the hip, ankle, and mid-tarsal joints. The operation of joint stiffening is known as arthrodesis. The cartilaginous surfaces of the two adjacent bones are removed in the expectation that the bared bone surfaces will unite, forming an ankylosis, and a stiff joint result. Practical experience has shown that this method should not be undertaken in children under ten, as in young children the ends of the bones are largely cartilaginous, and the amount which it is necessary to remove to obtain an ankylosis is considerable; and in addition to this, in children, when a growth of the limb takes place, the limb may grow in a direction of distortion. The operation of arthrodesis can also be applied to the shoulder-joint. In the shoulder-joint the arm should be after operation, during the period of healing, placed in a position somewhat abducted from the body.

Arthrodesis of the hip-joint is less frequently needed, but has been found beneficial in instances where the hip is unstable and subluxated. Arthrodesis at the knee-joint leaves the patient with an awkward limb, which for practical purposes is not as serviceable as one supplied with a suitable prosthetic appliance. In certain instances, however, where it is difficult to furnish a proper apparatus, patients often prefer the inconvenience of a stiff knee to the constant use of an appliance. Arthrodesis of the knee should not be done until the growth has stopped.

In deformities of the foot, where no muscular strength remains and the patients are not young, an arthrodesis between the astragalus and tibia, the os calcis and astragalus, and the midtarsal articulations (the astragalo-scaphoid and calcaneocuboid) is often of benefit; but the use of silk ligaments is to be preferred.

Silk Ligaments.

Limitation of the motion of a joint by means of the insertion of silk strands, properly sterilized, quilted in the periosteum of the bones adjacent to the affected joint, replaces arthrodesis in preventing toe-drop and checking the slighter forms of valgus and varus in children and adolescents. The method is one which requires technical skill and experience.

It has been found that these silk ligaments, properly inserted, remain in the tissues and become in time surrounded by fibrous tissue, which serve the purpose of checks, capable of permanently preventing the development of severe deformity.

If it is desired to prevent toe-drop in a paralyzed ankle, the technique is as follows: The periosteum of the tibia is slit longitudinally 2 or 3 inches above the ankle-joint and silk in size from 14 to 20 is quilted into the everted edges of the periosteum. The two silk strands are then carried down under the annular ligament of the ankle by a flat director with an eye, and brought out through an incision over the desired place of insertion on the tarsus. This may be at the outer or inner side or in the middle line, in the first two instances to correct a tendency toward valgus or varus deformity. At the site of the insertion a pointed heavy curved needle is carried through the bone and by a loop of silkworm gut carried through the eye of this needle; the silk is carried through the bone and knotted firmly, with the strands tight when the foot is in the desired position. The fascia, subcutaneous tissue, and skin are then united over the silk, a plaster-of-Paris bandage is applied over the dressing and worn for 8 to 10 weeks, after which a fixation shoe is desirable to prevent strain on the new ligament for at least 6 months.

The advantage over arthrodesis is that dorsal flexion of the foot is possible while plantar flexion is checked. The application of the technique to other localities does not differ in essentials.

Bone Operations.

Whitman's Operation.—In cases of calcaneus deformity, that is, the paralytic deformity where the weight is borne on the end of the os calcis, the front of the foot not being able to strike the ground, owing to the weakness of the gastrocnemius muscles, a serviceable operation has been devised by Whitman, consisting of the ablation of the astragalus and the slipping of the foot backward, so that the weight is borne upon the middle of the foot instead of its posterior third. A useful foot results, the ultimate functional result being excellent.

Osteotomy may be required to correct severe flexion deformity at the hip, and at the knee to correct the knock-knee and flexion at the same time. At the hip it does not differ from the ordinary Gant operation, and is necessary only in cases in which division of the soft parts is not enough to allow sufficient extension of the thigh on the pelvis.

At the knee a simple transverse division of the femur is made just above the condyles, allowing correction of both flexion and knock-knee at the same time. These operations, of course, have no effect upon the paralysis as such, but merely serve to place the limb in a position suitable for weight-bearing. After operation mechanical support may or may not be necessary.

Excision.—In other cases resection of joints is to be considered on account of the extreme bony deformity which they present, as in severe paralytic knock-knee, in which a stiff knee rather than a movable one is desired. If the latter is preferable an osteotomy rather than excision should be done, as excision leaves a stiff joint. The deformity of knock-knee or flexion at the knee can, of course, be corrected by the plane of the bone section in excision.

Nerve Grafting.—It has been shown experimentally on animals that it is possible to divide and transplant a motor nerve so that its efferent impulses are transferred from its own peripheral distribution to that of the nerve into whose distal part it is transferred. This has been applied to the treatment of infantile paralysis, a healthy nerve, or a portion of one, being divided and sewed to the cut peripheral end of a paralyzed nerve. Varying degrees of success have attended this procedure, but the percentage of practical failures is still so great that the method cannot be regarded as having passed beyond the experimental stage.

CHAPTER XV.

SPASTIC AND OTHER PARALYSES.

SPASTIC PARALYSIS.

THE condition is known under the following names: Spastic paralysis, cerebral paralysis, and Little's disease.

Motor disturbances in children which are due to cerebral lesions are manifested clinically in one of three ways: (1) As a single hemiplegia; (2) as a diplegia; (3) as a paraplegia. Contractures, choreiform movements, mental impairment, aphasia, epilepsy, incoordination, etc., may be the accompaniments of any one of these forms.

The condition is rarely congenital and most frequently acquired.

CONGENITAL SPASTIC PARALYSIS.

It is usually not recognized at birth, as it consists of a lack of muscular co-ordination common in infancy, which persists in certain muscles during life. The origin of it is to be found in cerebral defects, intra-uterine cerebral hemorrhage, and lack of development of the brain.

NON-CONGENITAL SPASTIC PARALYSIS.

Symptoms.—The condition may follow cerebro-meningitis in an acute attack with cerebral disturbances, or as a result from chronic hydrocephalus. The onset may resemble very closely that of infantile spinal paralysis; it often begins with an illness of some sort. Frequently paralysis develops in the course of an infectious disease, sometimes after a slight feverish attack, sometimes after a fall or a slight blow on the head. Commonly the onset is marked by convulsions. Delirium or screaming spells may accompany the onset.

When the paralysis is noticed, it is found to be most often hemiplegic in distribution. Monoplegia is rare. The face is paralyzed in a moderate proportion of all cases, and the arm is generally affected

more severely than the leg and recovers more slowly. The facial
paralysis ordinarily is not complete and disappears first of all the
paralyses. Strabismus is common; the reflexes of the affected side
are much increased from the first. As in the hemiplegia of adults,
rigidity of the affected muscles comes on in about seventy-five
per cent of all cases at a varying time after the onset of the
paralysis. The rigidity, when present, is increased by any attempt
to use the limb; it is excited by passive manipulation and it disappears

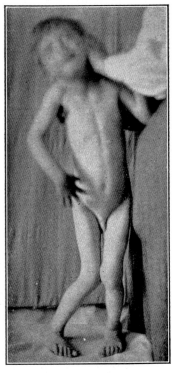

Fig. 260.—Case of Right Hemiplegia
Attempting to Walk.

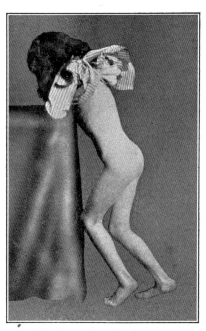

Fig. 261.—Attitude in Attempted Walking,
Spastic Paraplegia.

during sleep and usually under an anæsthetic. Post-hemiplegic movements follow in a certain proportion of cases.

Mental enfeeblement, varying from complete idiocy to simple back-
wardness, develops in a large proportion of all cases. The mental
disability may be manifested in the milder cases by an excessive irritability and a disposition to do mischief and perhaps to destroy play-
things wantonly. Furious outbursts of temper are not uncommon.

The mind may, however, remain perfectly clear in spite of a severe hemiplegia, and no sign of mental deterioration may be present in the early or the late history of the disease. Such children as escape mental deterioration in childhood may develop psychoses later in life.

Epileptic attacks appear in one-quarter to one-half of all cases reported. Ordinarily they come on in two or three years after the paralysis, but they may be delayed, and ten or even thirty years may elapse sometimes; on the other hand, they may begin within a few weeks of the onset.

To the later history of the affection belong the atrophy and contractions of the limbs. In hemiplegia the affected side rarely recovers

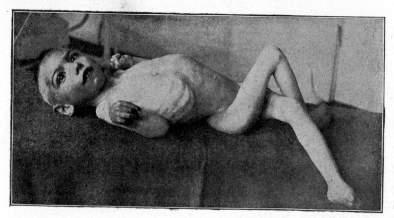

Fig. 262.—Severe Infantile Spastic Paralysis.

entirely, and often the growth of the bones may be retarded. The muscular atrophy, as a rule, is not so great as in infantile spinal paralysis.

The permanent contractions that come on are most noticeable in the arms, legs, and feet. The arm is held close to the side, the elbow is flexed strongly and firmly, the hand is flexed, and the fingers are drawn into the palm, usually embracing the thumb. The humerus is rotated inward, and outward rotation is resisted by muscular contraction. Supination and extension of the fingers are resisted.

The leg in bad cases is adducted and flexed at the hip, the hamstring muscles of the knee are contracted, and flexion of the knee results, while the foot is in a position of talipes equino-varus or simple equinus. In very mild cases only the finer movements of the hand may be lost, and the leg movements may be impaired only enough to cause a limp.

Post-Paralytic Disorders of Movement.—In certain cases of hemiplegia, single and double, a disturbance of motion occurs at a later

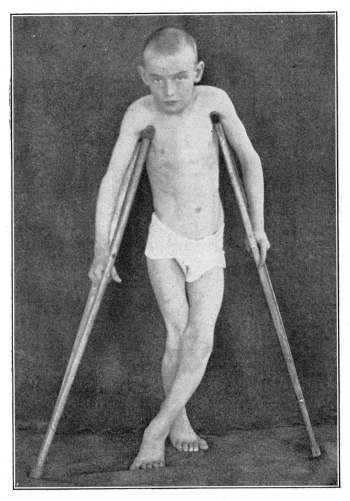

FIG. 263.—Severe Spastic Paralysis with Cross-legged Progression on Attempted Walking.

stage, which is spoken of under many different names, such as athetosis and chorea spastica.

Spastic Condition of the Muscles.—At times the tonic spasm of the muscles becomes the most prominent feature of the case, and there is a persistent stiffness and constant spasm of the muscles of the legs and sometimes of the arms; the legs are rigid, and the feet are extended, and when an attempt is made to walk the child stands on tiptoe, and often the spasm of the adductor muscles is so great that the legs are crossed. The walk is almost characteristic—a clinging gait, in which the feet are scraped along the floor with much effort and straining at every step, if indeed the spasm is not so great that walking at all is out of the question.

In the severest cases the children have strabismus, a stupid, idiotic

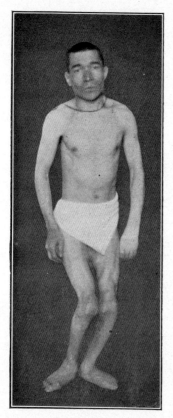

FIG. 264.—Spastic Paraplegia in an Adult.

face, the saliva drips from the mouth, and the teeth decay very early. In the more severe cases it is often impossible to demonstrate the increased tendon reflexes either at the knee or at the ankle on account of the great stiffness of the legs, because the muscles are continually at their maximum of contraction. In the milder cases exaggerated reflexes are almost constant. The electrical reaction in these and in the hemiplegic cases is unchanged.

Pathology.—The pathological condition is much the same in hemiplegia, diplegia, and paraplegia. These conditions in general are due to embolism or hemorrhage, and the resulting retardation of growth of the affected portion of the brain, together with the secondary changes in the spinal cord. Autopsies made later in the disease show wasting and sclerosis of a greater or less part of the brain and the condition known as porencephalus. Porencephalus occurs as a loss of substance in the form of cavities or cysts.

The pathology of the condition is a lesion of the motor tract of the brain with consequent atrophy and retarded development of the affected portion, and descending degeneration of the pyramidal tracts and lateral columns of the cord.

Diagnosis.—Spastic paraplegia is characterized by tonic contraction of the muscles which yields to steady resistance, except in the advanced stages where fibrous changes have taken place. The galvanic reaction is normal. At times the muscular rigidity is so excessive that the exaggerated knee-jerk and ankle clonus cannot be obtained. In estimating the child's mental condition, very little weight can be attached to the parents' account of the patient's capacity.

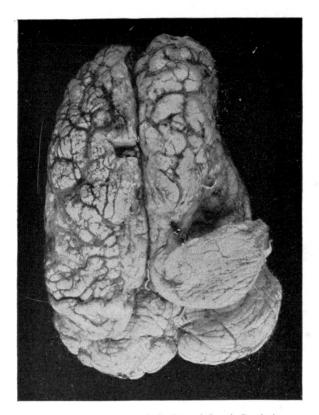

Fig. 265.—Diseased Brain in Case of Spastic Paralysis.

Prognosis.—The prognosis in these cases should be most guarded, and is dependent upon the extent of the central lesion, not always easily recognized. When marked mental impairment is present little benefit can be expected from surgical treatment. The spastic muscular condition is to be regarded as a difficulty in addition to the mental condition which especially needs treatment. When no mental impairment is present much benefit can be expected from suitable surgical treatment.

Treatment.—In spastic paralysis the treatment will be considered under the following heads: (1) Muscle training and exercise; (2)

operative lengthening of muscles, tendons, and fasciæ; (3) tendon transference; (4) alcohol injections; (5) division of the posterior

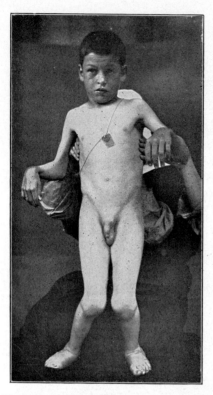

nerve roots. In spastic paralysis it is at times possible to accomplish much by muscular *training* and developing *exercises*. The muscles which are most strongly contracted are the thigh adductors and the calf muscles. Such a patient should be given exercises calculated to develop the abductor muscles and the dorsal flexors of the foot, which by increased power will in a measure counterbalance the muscles which are too powerful. In walking the patient should be cautioned to go very slowly, to lift each foot well off of the ground, and to turn out the toes with much care. In connection with massage and rubbing, this method of treatment is capable of accomplishing much in the milder cases.

The disappearance of the aphasia is aided by systematic training, and it always proves more tractable than in the adult.

FIG. 266.—Spastic Paralysis before Operation.

Apparatus is of little advantage in cerebral paralysis except in retaining the limbs in proper position after operation. Post-hemiplegic movements are at times relieved by placing the member at rest for some weeks or months under restraint, and contractions of the wrist may be stretched by means of a palmar splint hyperextending the wrist.

OPERATIVE TREATMENT.—*Tenotomy, Myotomy, Fasciotomy, Tenotomy* (complete division and plastic tenotomy).—Clinical evidence has proved that tenotomy, especially of the tendo Achillis, in this class is of great benefit in suitable cases, not only in improved walking, but sometimes in improvement of the general condition and diminution of the general irritability, from the benefit of increased activity. If tenotomy of the tendo Achillis is done in cases of marked talipes equinus the contraction ceases, and though the strength of the muscle is not lost in a number of cases which have been watched by the writers for several years, there is little tendency to a reappearance

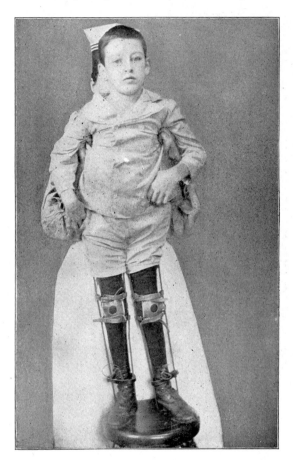

FIG. 267.—Spastic Paralysis after Operation.

of the equinus deformity. Plastic lengthening of the tendo Achillis by dividing halfway through the tendon on opposite sides at different levels and then pulling the two halves of the tendon by each other is in the writers' opinion to be preferred to complete division of the tendon on account of the danger of overcorrection sometimes seen.

Division of the hamstring tendons by open incision should be done when they are sufficiently contracted to prevent the full extension of the knee. This operation is preferable to subcutaneous tenotomy because it offers a better chance to divide contracted tissues other than tendons. In the severer cases with adductor spasm division of the adductor tendons is also of benefit.

Myotomy and Fasciotomy.—In resistant and severe cases not only must the tendons be divided, but contracted bands of fasciæ must be

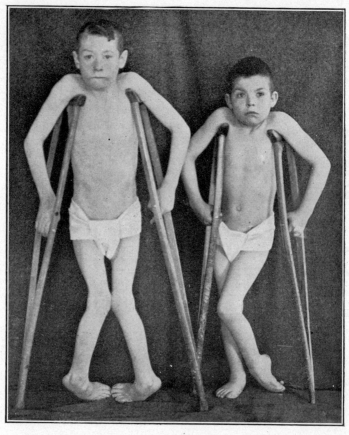

FIG. 268.—Two Cases of Severe Spastic Paralysis of Different Types.

cut. The removal of portions of the contracted muscles is advisable in the most marked cases in order permanently to weaken such muscles, e.g., in extreme adduction of the legs the resection of the adductor muscles may be of permanent value and in marked inversion of the feet it is desirable to remove a strip of the tensor vaginæ femoris.[1]

[1] Gibney : Am. Journ. Orth. Surgery, ii., 1.

After the operation the limb is to be fixed in an overcorrected position by means of plaster-of-Paris bandages or retentive appliances for several weeks. This is to be followed by muscle training, gradually increasing exercises, with limbs held by ambulatory retention appliance (similar, as a rule, to what are to be used in infantile paralysis) until the proper muscular balance has been established, when appliances are to be discarded.

It is to be remembered that the affection is not strictly a paralysis, but a disability from imperfect muscular co-ordination, increased by muscular contraction in certain muscles. The treatment consists in not only restoring the muscular balance, but in muscle training to re-establish the proper muscular co-ordination. Care is necessary during the process of muscle training with apparatus not to overstretch the divided tendons.

Tendon transference has been recommended in this affection, especially of the hamstrings forward, to reinforce the lengthened extensor curis by a procedure similar to what is employed in poliomyelitis. The procedure should be reserved for the more severe cases, as it necessarily results in a loss of muscle balance.

Arm and Hand.—Tendon transference, however, is of great advantage in the spastic contraction of the forearm. The pronator radii teres may be converted into a supinator,[1] and the carpal flexors may be converted into carpal extensors. In the first operation an incision, two or three inches long, is made in the middle of the front of the forearm. The upper and lower borders of the pronator are cleared and the tendon with its periosteal attachment is freed from the radius. The tendon is then passed through the interosseous

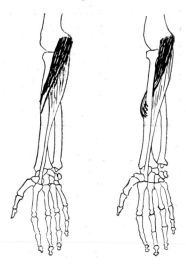

Fig. 269.—Transplantation of the Pronator Radii Teres in Spastic Paralysis of the Arm.

membrane close to the radius and the tendon reinserted on the outer side of the radius, if possible at the site of its former insertion; if not, at a new roughened place on the radius.

In the other operation[2] the flexor carpi ulnaris is divided just

[1] A. H. Tubby : Brit. Med. Journ., September 7, 1901.

[2] Robert Jones : Tubby and Jones, " Surgery of Paralysis," London, 1903, p. 225.

above the annular ligament and inserted into the tendon of the extensor ulnaris, and the flexor carpi radialis divided at the same level and attached to the radial extensor.

Alcohol Injection.—On the ground that the muscular irritability is constantly increased by active irritative impulses arising from the cortical motor cells it has been possible to secure the temporary isolation of muscular groups by the injection of certain nerve trunks with alcohol (70-80%), thus resting and apparently much benefiting the affected muscles. The nerve is exposed by dissection. For adductor spasm one exposes and injects the obturator nerve; for overaction of the hamstrings the branches of the sciatic supplying these muscles; for the gastrocnemius the internal popliteal nerve; and for the anterior tibial group, the anterior tibial nerve.[1]

Division of the Posterior Nerve Roots.—The operation of division of the posterior nerve roots has been advocated and performed on the theory that the cessation of afferent impulses will give a period of rest to the irritated centres. A laminectomy is done and several of the lower posterior nerve roots supplying the legs divided on each side. Although successful cases have been reported, the mortality is high, and the operation cannot be regarded as having passed the experimental stage.[2]

There are certain motor disturbances affecting children which come under the notice of the orthopedic surgeon so frequently that a brief mention of their characteristics deserves a place here. These affections are:

I. Pseudo-hypertrophic muscular paralysis. Progressive muscular atrophy.

II. Hereditary locomotor ataxia, obstetrical paralysis.

PSEUDO-HYPERTROPHIC MUSCULAR PARALYSIS.

Pseudo-hypertrophic muscular paralysis is an affection of the muscular system characterized by a diminution or loss of the functional energy of certain muscles and an abnormal increase in their size, which, together with diminution in the size of other muscles, is pathognomonic. Modern classification places the affection among the progressive muscular atrophies.

The *etiology* of the affection is not known. The disease develops usually during childhood, and affects males more commonly than fe-

[1] Allison and Schwab: Am. Journ. Orth. Surg , viii., 1, 95.
[2] Förster and Tietze: Mitt. aus d. Grenzgeb. der Med. u. Chir. xx., 3, 493.

males. The disease is more apt to occur in family groups than in isolated cases.

The *pathological* condition consists in the overgrowth of the connective tissue in the muscles and the wasting of the muscular substance proper, while a deposit of fat takes place to a greater or less extent. No constant or characteristic pathological condition is found in the spinal cord.

The first *symptoms* to attract attention to the child's condition are muscular feebleness and peculiarity of gait. Such children tire very easily in walking and they have especial difficulty in going up and down stairs. They fall often and in rising from the ground they adopt a procedure which is one of the most characteristic features of the disease. Inasmuch as on account of muscular weakness they cannot straighten the back or extend the knees without assistance, they rise from the ground by climbing upon the thighs, which they extend by pushing them down with the hands, using the muscles of the arms to accomplish what the leg and back muscles cannot do.

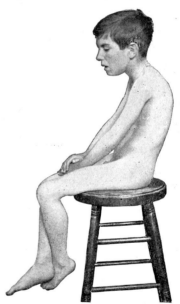

In walking these children throw the centre of gravity of the body well over each leg in turn as it supports the bodyweight, and the result is a waddle more or less marked. They may stand with marked lordosis of the lumbar spine, even in moderately advanced cases, chiefly due to a weakness of the lumbar muscles. The lordosis disappears when the patient sits down and a bowing backward of the whole vertebral column takes its place. In kneeling on the hands and knees at times there may be noticed a characteristic saddle-shaped depression of the back, which is due to the weakness of the erector spinæ muscles. The enlargement of

FIG. 270.—Kyphosis in Pseudo-hypertrophic Paralysis.

the muscles is usually most marked in the calves of the legs. The affected muscles are hard and resistant to the touch.

Atrophy of some of the muscles of the upper extremity is apt to be present. The scapular muscles, the serrati, the latissimus dorsi, and the pectoralis major are often wasted.

Talipes equinus and flexion of the knees and hips may occur from muscular contraction. Lateral curvature of the spine may follow, and at other times a permanent flexion of the spine occurs from weakness of the erector spinæ muscles, and the child sits bowed forward. The late stage of the affection is characterized by a helplessness more or less complete.

Neither the reflexes nor the electrical reactions are modified in any degree until the muscles have reached a marked stage of atrophy. Then they are diminished in proportion to the muscular wasting, and finally they are lost. Very often the skin over the affected limb is mottled and subject to vascular changes, indicating some vasomotor disturbance.

The *prognosis* is as unfavorable as possible. Recovery is all but unknown, and arrest of the disease is rare. The course of the disease is essentially chronic.

Treatment is practically without benefit, and there is no reason to believe that drugs have any effect in retarding its progress. Electricity, massage, and gymnastics are sometimes of benefit in connection with other treatment. Tenotomy is of use as soon as the heels are drawn up. Often walking may become impossible, chiefly on that account, and division of the tendo Achillis on both sides may restore for a time the power of walking; also tenotomy of the hamstring tendons at the knee may be indicated in severe cases.

PROGRESSIVE MUSCULAR ATROPHY.

Progressive muscular atrophy is an affection characterized by a wasting of the voluntary muscles, and a consequent diminution in their power, which pursues a chronic course and attacks successively individual muscles and groups of muscles.

In muscular atrophy as it occurs in children, the only cause assignable is a congenital tendency, often inherited. Males are more often affected than females, and the time of onset of the disease is most variable.

Progressive muscular atrophy has, since the days of Aran and Duchenne, been subdivided into different types.

1. In the Aran-Duchenne type the atrophy begins oftenest in the small muscles of the hand, spreads to the forearm, and perhaps the shoulders and back. It may begin in the muscles of the thighs. The atrophied muscles show fibrillary contractions, and the reaction of degeneration is present. The affection has a pathology and is of spinal origin.

2. The hereditary form is of the same general type as the preceding. It is very unusual and may occur in more than one member of a family.

3. The peroneal form or leg type of progressive muscular atrophy affects in most cases the lower extremities. The extensor muscles of the toes are first affected, then the small muscles of the feet, and finally the entire leg. Talipes equinus or equino-varus is a common result. Sensory changes are generally present. The reflexes in the lower extremities may be diminished or lost if the disease is sufficiently advanced. The electrical reactions, as a rule, are altered both quantitatively and qualitatively. Cases of club-foot occurring in this type may be successfully operated on.

The changes in the muscles consist in atrophy of the fibres, a loss of transverse striation, and a proliferation of the nuclei. Degenerations of the nerves are present, but changes of importance in the spinal cord have not been established.

4. Erb's type. The juvenile form of progressive muscular atrophy is very rare and is characterized by progressive wasting of certain groups of muscles. These are the muscles of the shoulder girdle, the upper arm, the pelvic girdle, the thigh, and the back. The forearm and leg muscles remain, for a long time at least, intact. There are no fibrillary contractions, no reaction of degeneration, and no sensory disturbances.

5. The Landouzy-Dejerine type or the facio-scapulo-humeral variety occurs at times in children. The muscles of the face are first affected and the atrophy spreads to the shoulder and arm muscles. In exceptional cases this type may begin in the arms or legs. The reaction of degeneration and fibrillary twitching are never present.

The medical *treatment* of all these affections is hopeless. When muscular contractions occur tendons should be cut and deformities rectified. Rest to the atrophied muscles, massage, and electricity are useful.

HEREDITARY ATAXIA.

Hereditary ataxia, known also as family ataxia and Friedreich's disease, deserves mention as a serious motor disorder which is sometimes met in children. It is dependent upon a family predisposition, but is not often directly inherited, but more commonly appears in several members of one generation. The cases are rare.

Aside from the influence of a congenital tendency the cause of the disease is as yet unknown. The disease develops most often early in life.

In examining sections of the cord in these cases, changes are found similar to the lesion of locomotor ataxia.

The *symptoms* resemble very closely those of locomotor ataxia. The patient notices a feeling of weakness and uncertainty in walking, and soon it becomes apparent to others that the motions of the legs are not properly co-ordinated. The feet are placed wide apart in standing, and in walking the gait is practically that of locomotor ataxia. The movements of the hands become irregular and inco-ordinate, and a jerky irregularity develops in the movements of the head and neck, so much so that it may assume the aspect of an irregular tremor. Speech may also be impaired. The knee-jerk disappears, but the plantar reflex remains. Sensation is affected in varying degrees in different cases, and trophic disturbances of the skin are not present. As a rule the sphincter muscles are not affected. Nystagmus is often present and the Argyll-Robertson pupil is absent.

Deformities are apt to come on in the later stages of the disease, lateral curvature may be present, talipes equinus or equino-varus, and permanent flexion of the knee are likely to occur. The disease is essentially progressive, and the prognosis is bad in proportion to the rapidity of progress.

The *treatment* should be similar to that in common use in locomotor ataxia. Deformities should be corrected by tenotomy, etc., as they occur.

Among similar affections is *the cerebellar type of hereditary ataxia* described by Marie, differing chiefly in having exaggerated reflexes and ocular symptoms in addition to those described above.

OBSTETRICAL PARALYSIS.

Obstetrical paralysis of the shoulder is an affection which is fairly common and most often results in a disabled arm. It occurs generally after difficult labors when traction is made upon the head in head presentations, or upon the trunk when the head is delivered last. It may occur, however, after normal labors.

The injury appears to be due to injury to the two upper roots of the brachial plexus, the muscles chiefly involved being the biceps, deltoid, and supinators of the forearm.

The condition is made manifest immediately after birth by an inability to use one arm; it hangs powerless at the side, with the palm turned backward, and often the fingers are flexed tightly. If the arm is lifted from the side it falls lifelessly back into place, and although movement of the fingers is generally present, it is impossible to

use the arm to any extent on account of the paralysis of the sh
muscles.

If the arm is allowed to remain hanging in this position d ...
growth the adaptive changes resulting simulate very closely congenital
dislocation of the shoulder.

Three types are recognized, the upper arm, lower ar   d entire
arm types.

The *prognosis* in the severer cases is not good as to recovery.

Treatment.—For the treatment of the newborn the ai n should
be kept in a sling at an angle from the side, checking the w idency
to adduction of the limb. An axillary pad or splint should be used,
accompanied by measures to stimulate the circulation—massage, gentle
passive exercises. If the arm and hand are affected the tendency to
pronation is to be checked.

In older cases of confirmed contraction the arm should be treated
on the same principles that are of use for the contractions of cerebral
paralysis elsewhere; viz., myotomy and fixation for a time in an overcorrected position, followed by muscle training.

Resection of the affected nerves and the surrounding cicatrix in
the cervical plexus has been employed, but the method of myotomy,
overcorrection, and muscle training has, as a rule, given better functional results.

Ischæmic Paralysis.—Also known as Volkmann's paralysis, as first
described by him, is a condition of disability of the forearm following
fracture at the elbow and the pressure of retaining splints; sometimes
also the prolonged use of an Esmarch tourniquet.

The affection consists of a myositis, due to a temporary ischæmia,
resulting in the severe cases in a fibrous degeneration of the muscles,
the nerves being compressed by cicatricial contraction.

Sensory and motor paralysis results with flexion and contraction
of the wrist and fingers, with disturbances of the circulation in the
hand and atrophy.

The treatment consists, in the milder early cases, in measures to
stimulate the circulation; but in the severe cases operative interference is necessary. This consists in correcting the contractions by
myotomy and fasciotomy, by freeing by dissection the median nerve
if compressed by contracted tissue. In the more obstinate cases improved function has been obtained by shortening the bones of the
forearm, removing a section of bone, and in this way relieving the
tension of the muscles.

CHAPTER XVI.

FUNCTIONAL AFFECTIONS OF THE JOINTS.

UNILATERAL ASYMMETRY.

FUNCTIONAL AFFECTIONS OF THE JOINTS.

FUNCTIONAL or neuromimetic or hysterical are names applied to a class of joint affections where there is no evidence of organic disease, yet where active disability exists.

Etiology and Occurrence.—At present one recognizes, however, certain cases largely in emotional women and children where excessive pain and symptoms exist without demonstrable organic lesions, and again in the same class of patients, pain and symptoms of a severe character accompanying organic lesions of a slight grade. Trauma and an antecedent organic lesion, such as a synovitis, are the commonest exciting causes, but the affection occasionally arises apparently without assignable cause.

Symptoms.—The symptoms are generally much the same as those of an organic lesion of the same joint. Pain, lameness, muscular irritability, and spasm, the slight atrophy of disuse and malpositions are the accompaniments of the affection. But the subjective signs are out of proportion to the objective, and are fluctuating and inconsistent with each other. Muscular spasm, for example, relaxes when the patient's attention is diverted, and the pain and lameness are not only variable but are out of all proportion to any demonstrable organic cause.

The stigmata of hysteria may or may not be present when an organic lesion exists or has existed; the subjective symptoms are out of proportion to the cause, and in many cases are to be classed as "habit pains." The cases of mixed organic and functional character are the most difficult to handle. The purest type of hysterical joint affection is seen in girls just at or before puberty, where symptoms of excessive pain, lameness, and malposition exist in the hip, knee, or ankle, e.g., without demonstrable organic cause.

Diagnosis.—The diagnosis is a dangerous one to make, and should be formulated only after the most painstaking and thorough examination, eliminating all organic causes. The lines on which it should proceed have been indicated above.

Prognosis.—The prognosis in recent cases is favorable, and in cases of longer standing is less favorable in those where the duration has been long and in those where the neurasthenic or hysterical condition is marked.

Treatment.—The treatment consists first in the general improvement of the patient's mental and physical condition, and generally removal from home conditions is necessary for the re-education of the patient, in which the treatment largely consists. The surgeon must be sure of his diagnosis, because no success will follow a treatment formulated to cover either a functional or organic lesion, and temporizing is fatal to a successful issue.

The second part of the treatment consists in correcting malpositions if they exist by traction, manipulation under ether, or by apparatus, and then beginning with the progressive use of the affected joint without regard to the increase of pain caused. This course is pursued until the normal use of the joint is regained. Massage, exercises, and similar measures to restore the circulation and muscles of the affected joint are of use. The prolonged use of apparatus, crutches, etc., is undesirable. In cases of long standing tenotomy may be required to correct malpositions.

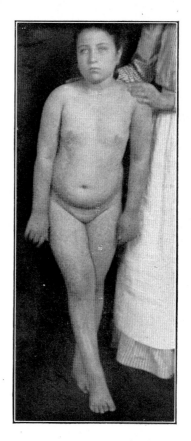

Fig. 271.—Attitude in Walking in a Case of Hysterical Affection of the Joints of the Leg in a Girl of Thirteen.

Functional affections of the especial joints are sufficiently well covered by the general description; but the spine requires separate mention, both as to symptoms and treatment.

FUNCTIONAL AFFECTIONS OF THE SPINE.

This condition is described under the names of irritable spine, spinal irritation, neuromimesis of the spine, hysterical spine, weakness of the spine.

Etiology and Occurrence.—The affection occurs frequently, is uncommon in children, and affects adolescent and young adult women more often than men or than older persons. Patients affected by it are generally of less than the average physique and resistance, and are most often of the emotional, neurasthenic, or excitable temperament.

The condition frequently follows trauma, either severe or slight, overuse or overstrain of the back muscles, or it may occur apparently spontaneously.

Symptoms.—The symptoms are irritability, pain, and sensitiveness in the spine, generally aggravated by standing, walking, forward bending, and sometimes by sitting. The pain and irritability frequently extend into the buttock and thighs. The lower part of the back is more frequently affected than the upper, and pain and tenderness in one or both sacro-iliac joints is a frequent symptom. It may be accompanied by hyperæsthesia of the skin, and muscular irritability and spasm are frequently found in the erector spinæ muscles.

The condition varies from a degree where there is occasional moderate backache after exertion through all grades to a condition where the patient is bedridden and helpless, an instance of the " spinal invalid." This spinal affection, although not strictly organic, yet seems to have a definite mechanical basis. In the erect standing position the weight of the body is held from falling forward by the posterior muscles, which for this purpose are all stronger than the anterior, e.g., the gastrocnemius is far larger than all the anterior muscles combined. Under conditions of general muscular laxity and other disturbances, which we do not now understand, the strain thrown upon the posterior muscles of the back and thighs is increased, and undue overstrain, pain, tenderness and irritability develop in the muscles, fasciæ and joints of the lower back, pelvis, buttocks, and thighs. Hence the lumbar and sacral pains, the pain and tenderness in the sacro-iliac joints and thighs (so often classed as sciatica), and the less frequent pain in the dorsal spine and back of the neck. On inspection such patients most often show a " slumped " relaxed position of the spine, with rounded dorsal and flattened lumbar region. On the other hand, others stand with a slight lateral curve, in which case the pain is most often unilateral and on the convex side of the body, but as a rule of the same general character as that described. Certain cases are associated with static troubles in the feet or intra-pelvic disease or malposition.

A preceding trauma may or may not be found in the history, as for example the post-operative backache following the stretching of the lumbar muscles in certain operations; the traumatic cases, as a rule, present more stiffness of the spine, and have already been spoken of under spinal sprains.

Diagnosis.—The diagnosis of the condition consists in the elimination of organic spinal disease, such as tuberculosis and arthritis deformans of the spine. If intrapelvic disease or malposition exists it is a competent cause of the symptoms described. After the careful elimination of all these factors a functional disorder may be assumed to exist, presumably largely of mechanical origin.

Prognosis.—The condition is notoriously resistant to treatment, and the outlook is least favorable in cases of long standing, associated with marked neurasthenia, especially if no obvious mechanical defect exists. It is most favorable in recent cases, with a demonstrably bad standing position and absence of marked neurasthenia. Under these conditions in patients of average resistance a cure should be generally effected.

Treatment.—The treatment should be directed to the cause of the condition, namely, the backstrain. The back muscles being irritable and overstrained, should first be rested in the severest cases by recumbency for part or all of the time, with the hollow of the back supported. In the standing position a jacket, brace, or corset should be worn at first, when the muscles are irritable and weak, to splint the back and relieve the overstrained muscles. A tight pelvic band is generally comfortable, probably acting as an annular ligament to the glutei and pelvic femoral muscles. Exercises to cultivate a correct standing position are the real means of cure, and should be begun very gently, with the aim of inducing a correct standing position; and massage is of value, given in moderation and not too early. If a short leg exists in connection with lateral deviation it should be corrected by increased thickness of the sole. The general condition should of course receive attention.

UNILATERAL ASYMMETRY.

Apart from pathological conditions causing asymmetry in corresponding bones on the two sides, difference in the length of corresponding bones in healthy individuals is apparently the rule, perfect symmetry being exceptional. In the arms this difference is of no importance, but in the bones of the leg leads to slight obliquity of the pelvis and consequent curving of the spine to one side in the standing position. It has been shown by observation that in healthy boys something more than half show a difference in the length of the legs of from ⅛ inch to 1½ inches.[1] The conventional measurement from the anterior superior pelvic spine to the malleolus is unreliable, because of the uncertainty of the bony landmarks, because of the variations in the positions of the anterior superior spines in the pelvis, and because it does not take into account pelvic asymmetry. So far as the spine is concerned, the equal length of the legs can be ascertained by building up the short leg by a series of pamphlets placed under the foot until the spine is in the middle line of the body. Inferences drawn from other methods are likely to be misleading.

Long continued pain in the back and hip, generally unilateral, may be due to the shortness of one leg, and is relieved by its correction.

Hypertrophy of one member, or part of one member, of very marked degree may occur as the result of dilatation of the blood vessels (angioma), from disease of the lymphatics (multiple plexiform fibroma), and as the result of congenital anomalies.

[1] Morton : Phila. Med. Times, July 10, 1886.

CHAPTER XVII.

CONGENITAL DISLOCATIONS.

CONGENITAL DISLOCATION OF THE HIP.

CONGENITAL dislocation of the hip is neither a common affection nor one of very great rarity. Among 6,969 orthopedic patients applying at the out-patient department of the Children's Hospital, there were 152 cases of congenital dislocation of one or both hips.

The affection is much more common in girls than in boys; girls present 88 per cent of the cases of the deformity. No satisfactory

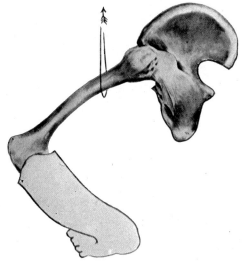

FIG. 272.—Congenital Dislocation of the Hip in Full-term Fœtus. (Warren Museum.)

explanation has been advanced to account for this preponderance in girls.

Etiology.—The etiology of the affection is not known. True congenital dislocation without doubt is an affection of uterine life, congenital dislocations having been found in the fœtus. It would seem also that it is not an arrest of development like harelip, but, like congenital club-foot, rather a perversion of it, a malposition of bones

317

with the resulting structural changes of the soft parts. Violence at birth alone is not considered the cause of true congenital dislocation.

In a few instances there appears to be an hereditary influence, and in other cases two children of the same family have been afflicted with the affection. This is, however, not the rule.

Pathology.—The changes in the anatomical structures seen in congenital dislocation are found in the capsule, in the muscles, and in

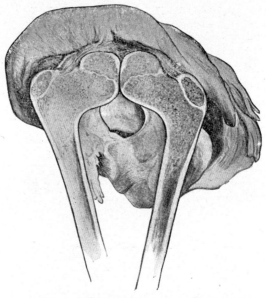

Fig. 273.—Congenital Dislocation, Child of Ten. Femur sawn and sides reflected, showing dislocated position of the femoral head, the capsular pouch, the capsular hymen in front of the acetabulum, the acetabular cavity, and capsular constriction at the mouth. (Warren Museum.)

the bones. The changes in the capsule are such as would naturally follow a prenatal dislocation before the joint structures were formed. Normally the capsule passes from the rim of the acetabulum to the neck of the femur, the head being placed well in the socket and held firmly by the cotyloid ligament. In congenital dislocation, when the head lies out of the socket and above the acetabulum, the capsule is stretched. Furthermore, the weight of the body, as soon as the individual walks, rests not on the head of the femur placed under the acetabulum, but falls upon the capsule, which stretches like a strap from the acetabulum to the trochanter, and this capsule necessarily becomes thickened. As it is stretched across the acetabulum it becomes adherent at the rim and to a portion of the ilium, so that the acetabulum seems obliterated, being covered by thick, strong, fibrous tissue, reaching from rim to rim. This portion of the capsule is entirely shut off by adhesion from that which surrounds the head, save for a small opening at the upper portion of the rim. This opening may be, and usually is, in older cases, smaller than the head, and

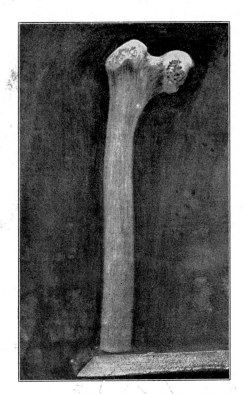

Fig. 274.—Femur in Congenital Dislocation, Showing Alteration in Angle of Neck.

not easily stretched, as the tissues lose their elasticity owing to the fibrous bands which form from the use of the capsule as a weight-bearing structure.

In the infantile cases the capsule is loose and there is a lack of development of the cartilaginous prolongations of the rim of the acetabulum and of the cotyloid ligament.

The muscles are changed in consequence of the altered position of the head. Some of the muscles are shortened, others are lengthened. The muscles which are shortened are the adductor group, the psoas and iliacus, and the muscles reaching from the tuberosity of the ischium to the leg, i.e., the hamstring muscles. The alteration in the bone consists of a flattening or alteration of the shape of the

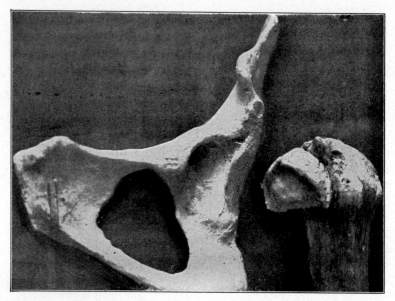

Fig. 275.—Old Congenital Dislocation of Hip with Alteration of Neck of Femur to Shape of Acetabulum. (Warren Museum.)

head, a twist of the neck (the consequence of malposition of the head), and in the shape of the acetabulum, which is sometimes triangular in shape and shallow.

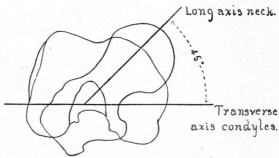

Fig. 276.—Twist of Neck in Congenitally Dislocated Femur, Looking from Above Downward.

If the point of suspension is directly over the proper place for the acetabulum, the patient's pelvis is hung in a comparatively normal plane, but if much behind it, the pelvis is tilted and severe lordosis results, the latter being the more common condition.

Symptoms.—The deformity often attracts no attention until the child learns to walk. Then, in double cases, it is noticed to stand ordinarily with its back very much arched and to waddle most

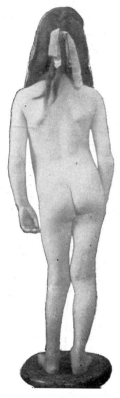

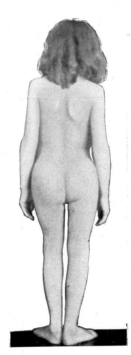

FIG. 277.—Unilateral Dislocation of the Hip. (Fiske Prize Fund Essay.)

FIG. 278.—Prominence of Trochanters in Double Congenital Dislocation of the Hip. (Fiske Prize Fund Essay.)

markedly when walking is well begun. This is characteristic and very marked. When the dislocation is only unilateral, the gait becomes an exaggerated limp; in stepping on the leg the child leans to the affected side, and the leg seems to have grown shorter. In double dislocation in young children, the prominence of the trochanters is not marked enough to attract attention; in older persons, however, the prominence of the trochanters is most noticeable. There is no complaint of pain by children suffering from this affection.

Diagnosis.—The diagnosis is not difficult in children who are old enough to walk. The limp is characteristic. There is shortening of the limb. On palpation the trochanter is high, and the head, except in large, plump children, can be felt above and behind its normal place.

On pulling the leg with gentle force the trochanter will be felt in younger cases drawn down, if the other hand is placed upon it, and to slip back when the leg is released, and a measurement will

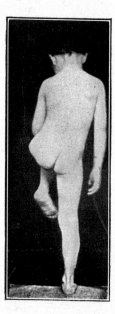

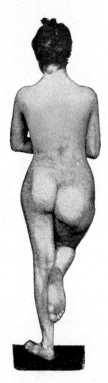

FIG. 279.—Coxa Vara, Showing Elevation of Pelvis when Patient Stands on Affected Limb.

FIG. 280.—Congenital Dislocation, Showing Dropping of Pelvis when Patient Stands on the Affected Limb.

show that the leg has been lengthened temporarily by the traction force.

The muscles, although not normally developed, are not paralyzed, and the children are healthy. In unilateral dislocation the leg of the affected side is slightly smaller than the other.

In larger children and adults the conformation and outline of the hips are so distinctive that the diagnosis may be made almost at a glance; but in young children palpation or a skiagraphic examination is often necessary.

Trendelenburg has called attention to an important diagnostic symptom. When a normal child stands upon either limb and flexes

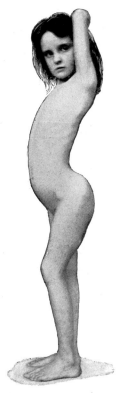

FIG. 281.—Lordosis in Double Congenital Dislocation of the Hip. (Fiske Prize Fund Essay.)

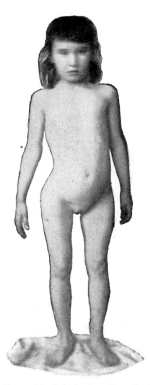

FIG. 282.—Broadening the Perineum in Double Congenital Dislocation of the Hip. (Fiske Prize Fund Essay.)

the other at the knee and thigh, the opposite buttock will be seen not to drop. In the case of congenital dislocation of the hip, however, the opposite buttock will be found to drop to a noticeable degree if the patient takes this attitude. This is to be explained by the fact that in congenital dislocation of the hip, owing to the fact that the head of the femur is not in the socket, the muscles from the great trochanter and the pelvis (which serve to keep the pelvis level) when supported on one side have no purchase and are therefore inefficient.

A skiagraphic picture is of great value in diagnosis, and if accurate is conclusive.

Coxa vara, or the distortion of the neck of the femur, which shortens the limb and raises the trochanter above Nélaton's line, may be confounded with congenital dislocation. The mistake can be avoided if the fact is borne in mind that in coxa vara the head is in its normal socket, while in congenital dislocation the head is to be felt outside of the acetabulum.

Prognosis.—The disability caused by this affection in childhood is slight, but the limp is noticeable, and, in double congenital dislocation,

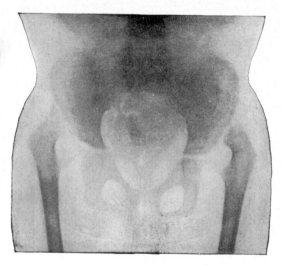

FIG. 283.—Double Congenital Dislocation Unreduced.

may be distressing. In single dislocation the defect in adults may entail only an inability to engage in active occupation, accompanied by occasional attacks of severe muscular pain, with muscular cramps. These attacks subside under rest, but if the patient becomes heavier or feeble they may necessitate the use of crutches and cause severe disability. Muscular patients suffer less than those with feeble muscles. In double dislocation the trouble is increased.

Treatment.—In a few instances of congenital dislocation of the hip seen in infants under one year of age, a spontaneous recovery has been observed, but in other cases operative treatment is needed.

In a majority of cases manipulative reduction under an anæsthetic is the method to be employed.

MANIPULATIVE REDUCTION.

There are several manipulative methods employed, all based upon the plan of stretching the contracted soft parts, muscles, capsule and ligaments, so that the head can be forced successfully through the

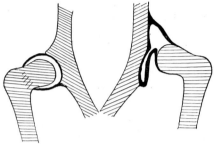

FIG. 284.—Diagram of Section of Capsule in Normal and in Congenitally Dislocated Hip.

distorted capsule into the socket. The following method will be found serviceable:

Complete anæsthesia is necessary. The child's ankle is grasped firmly and a strong pull exerted, counter-pull being furnished by an

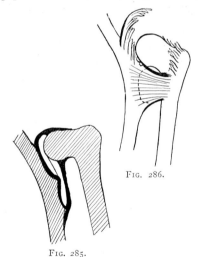

FIG. 286.

FIG. 285.

FIGS. 285 and 286.—Diagram Showing Difficulties in Reduction. 1, In the capsule covering the acetabulum; 2, in the shortened capsule between the acetabular rim and the lesser trochanter.

assistant who presses upon the perineum. The limb should be rotated forcibly to both the outer and inner side, and then forcibly abducted both with the knee flexed and straight.

It is essential that the adductor group of muscles should be over-stretched. After the limb has been brought to nearly a right angle with the axis of the trunk, the knee being straight, it should be again brought in a line of the axis of the trunk and then forced upward with the knee straight, until the thorax is almost touched by the front

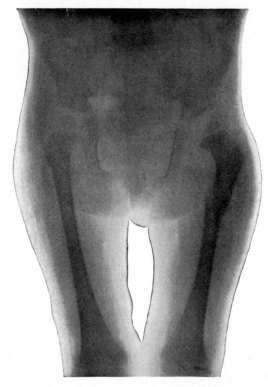

FIG. 287.—Congenital Dislocation. Reduction by incision. Osteotomy of shaft to correct twist of neck.

of the thigh, thus stretching the hamstring muscles. The child should then be turned upon its face and forcible hyperextension used, both with the leg abducted and straight. The child is then placed upon its back and reduction attempted, the surgeon holding the patient's limb just below the knee, which is flexed and abducted strongly with one hand, the other hand being placed upon the pelvis, the palm pressing on the crest of the ilium and the thumb passing behind and beneath the trochanter.

The child is then placed upon its back and an attempt at reduction made. If the tissues have been sufficiently stretched by the above-mentioned manœuvres, the reduction can be made with the exercise

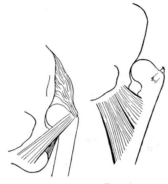

FIG. 288.   FIG. 289.

FIGS. 288 and 289.—Diagram Showing Pelvi-trochanteric and Pelvic Muscles in Congenital Dislocation of Hip.

of a little skill. The surgeon holds the patient's limb just below the knee with the hand, abducts the limb strongly, flexing it at the knee. The other hand is placed upon the pelvis, the palm of the hand

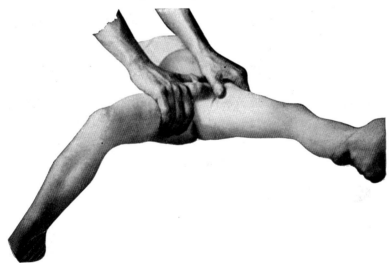

FIG. 290.—Manipulative Reduction in Congenital Dislocation of the Hip. Traction and reduction.

resting on the anterior spine, and the thumb being placed under the trochanter, while an assistant steadies the pelvis by pressing upon the opposite side. The patient's knee is moved outward and toward the plane of the operating table, while the trochanter is pressed upward and slightly forward. In successful cases the head will be felt to slip into the acetabulum with a sudden movement characteristic of the reduction of a dislocation.

It is often necessary to give slight rotary motion to the limb and

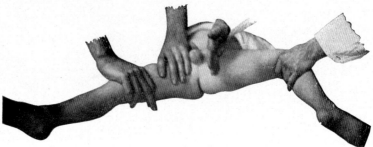

FIG. 291.—Manipulative Reduction. Forced abduction stretching the adductors with blows upon the adductor attachment.

slight manipulation is often necessary. The surgeon should by manipulation determine the size and depth of the acetabulum, and the firmness with which it is held in the acetabulum is also to be noted.

In the more resistant cases a padded, wedge-shaped block placed

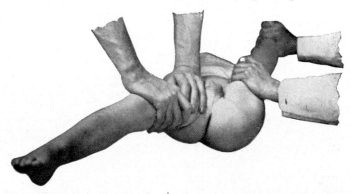

FIG. 292.—Manipulative Reduction. Forced flexion with leg straight at knee.

behind the trochanter will be of assistance, serving to push the trochanter and head of the femur forward, while the patient's knee is pressed downward. When the head of the femur is well in the acetabulum it can be felt on careful palpation, lying under the point of intersection of a line following the femoral artery, with a line crossing the pelvis at a level with the top of the symphysis pubis. A tightening of the hamstrings will usually be observed after reduction of the hip. After the reduction has been made, the limb should be

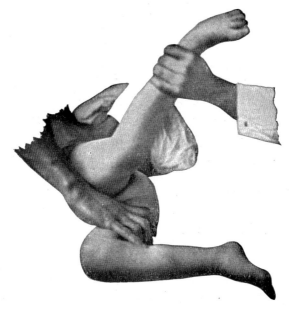

FIG. 293.—Manipulative Reduction. Hyperextension.

carefully brought into a straight position, i.e., parallel with the long axis of the trunk. If dislocation occurs during this manipulation

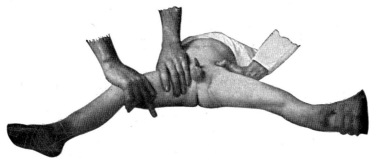

FIG. 294.—Manipulative Reduction. Head of femur pressed into acetabulum by manipulation after all contracted tissues are relaxed by overstretching.

the tissues must be stretched still further and the head again placed in the acetabulum.

Reduction with the Aid of Mechanical Force.

In the younger cases little difficulty will be encountered in stretching the shortened muscles by the use of manipulation as described, but in older cases much force is necessary, which involves danger of fracture of the femur or pelvis, both of which accidents have occurred in manipulative reduction. A difficulty encountered where manual force is employed is in holding the pelvis. This is essential to the accurate employment of force, and the accurate employment of force is of the greatest importance if much force is to be used.

It is for this reason that mechanical aids have been advised in the reduction of congenitally dislocated hips.[1]

The appliance at present employed by the writers will be found to be of service.

Traction is furnished by means of a movable traction rod playing upon a socket placed near the hip-joint. Traction is furnished by a screw force pulling upon a leather anklet bound on the patient's ankle. A counter force is furnished by uprights pressing on the perineum to prevent the riding upward of the trochanter. As the limb is abducted steel pegs are placed upright above the trochanter and close to the pelvis, inserted in a steel plate on which the patient lies. On these and on the perineal uprights steel plates are placed, preventing movement of the ilium and symphysis pubis. The pelvis is firmly held. A steel lever rod, with its end inserted in a hole in the steel plate held by the surgeon, can be made to press on the trochanter and femoral neck and serve to exert force downward and inward on the head and neck or to lift it over the acetabulum ridge. While the limb is strongly pulled and abducted by this means the head can often be forced safely through the capsular constriction in resistant cases where manual manipulation fails.

Reduction by Open Incision.

In the more resistant older cases, where manipulative reduction has failed, reduction by incision can be employed with success. This procedure is one which requires the exercise of skill. Traction is first applied to pull the head as near to its proper place as possible. It

[1] One of the most efficient of apparatus for the purpose is an appliance devised by Mr. Ralph W. Bartlett, of Boston. For a full description of this excellent apparatus the reader is referred to the former edition of the authors' Treatise on Orthopedic Surgery, and to the Journal of Med. Research, December, 1903.

is then cut down upon, with as little injury to the muscles as possible, the capsule is opened, and capsular constriction divided by means of a herniotome and stretched. All ligamentous and fibrous bands which are obstacles to reduction are cut, the head reduced, and the capsule stretched firmly around the neck. The operation should be

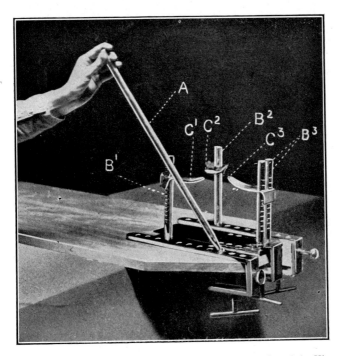

FIG. 295.—Apparatus for Reduction of Congenital Dislocation of the Hip.

done under the strictest asepsis and the limb secured by a plaster bandage in an abducted position.

After the reduction the redundant capsule can be closed, with a wick for drainage, or packed, according to the judgment of the surgeon. When absolute confidence can be placed in thorough asepsis, closing the wound in this way at the time of operation saves for the patient a long period of wound-healing. The limb should be fixed by means of a plaster-of-Paris spica reaching from the thorax down to the foot, holding the limb in a strongly abducted position. The position of the limb should be that of strong abduction.

Accidents.—The method of reduction of congenital femoral dislocation by manipulation is not without danger and requires the exercise of considerable judgment. Fracture of the femoral head, fracture of the pelvis, death from shock, rupture of the femoral artery, and temporary and permanent paralyses have all followed the in-

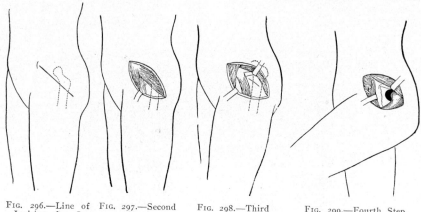

FIG. 296.—Line of Incision for Operative Reduction.   FIG. 297.—Second Step.   FIG. 298.—Third Step.   FIG. 299.—Fourth Step.

judicious use of force in correcting this deformity. These accidents can be avoided if the method is limited to the less severe cases.

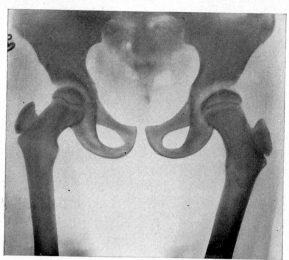

FIG. 300.—Result of Reduction in Congenital Dislocation of the Hip.

From the experience at the Boston Children's Hospital it would appear that the danger of injury in forcible reduction is diminished by the employment of the mechanical appliance mentioned. Great care and judgment, however, are necessary in the use of this as of all powerful aids.

AFTER-TREATMENT.—After the hip has been placed in the acetabulum, it is necessary that it should be held in the socket until the capsular tissues are sufficiently strong to prevent a relapse.

The child, while still under the anæsthetic, is placed upon a pelvic

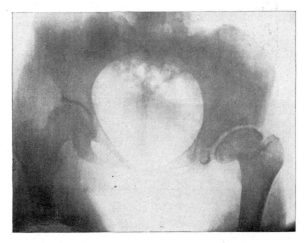

FIG. 301.—Skiagram Taken Seven Years after Reduction of a Dislocated Right Hip, at the Age of Twelve Years.

support and a firm plaster bandage applied to the thigh and pelvis, protected by stockinet, felt, and cotton.

Surgeons vary in their recommendations as to the best position in after-treatment. This must necessarily vary in different cases according to varying conditions. The writers ordinarily prefer to place the limb with the patella pointing forward and the leg (the knee being bent) pointing backward, the thigh being strongly abducted and flexed. For the first two weeks the plaster bandage should pass around the hip not operated upon to give greater fixation. This can later be removed and more motion of the affected limb permitted. The child can then walk about with crutches.

The length of time during which it is necessary that the plaster bandage should be worn varies, with each case, from two to six months, with a change of plasters as may be required for cleanliness and examination of the hip. After the time has passed when plaster fixation is no longer necessary, daily exercise should be given, directed to increasing the motion at the hip-joint. It is necessary to stimulate the muscles which are not being used, and to stretch by gradual exercise the muscles which may remain contracted. The patient should be given both passive and active exercises. In the passive exercises the manipulator should place one hand upon the pelvis with slight pressure above the trochanter, and with the other move the femur in the

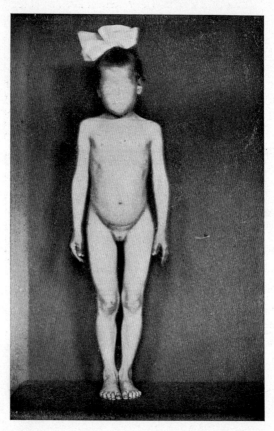

Fig. 302.—Six and One-half Years Old. Congenital dislocation of left hip. One year after reduction by operative mechanical stretching and manipulation.

direction of flexion and adduction, the patient being recumbent. Movement should also be made to straighten the limb at the knee and turn the foot inward, bringing the limb gradually in the direction parallel with the other. Similar active exercises can be undertaken and conducted with care daily.

Relapse may follow where the capsular tissue fails to hold with sufficient firmness in the acetabulum the femoral head after reduction.

This takes place when a cotyloid ligament is not developed, and when the muscles are not sufficiently strong to keep the femoral head in place, or when tissues, contracted in the flexed and strongly abducted

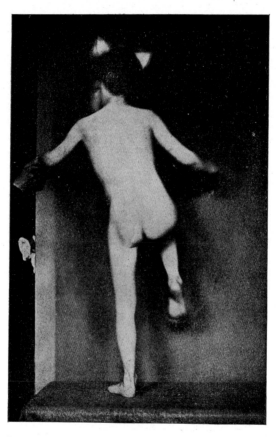

FIG. 303.—Showing Strength of Reduced Hip by the Trendelenburg Test.   Motion and gait of reduced hip normal.

position of after-treatment, prevent the placing of the limb in the normal position without causing displacement.

Care in after-treatment may prevent relapses in many instances of this class. Careful examination of the cases during after-treatment by manipulation and with the skiagraph, the use of gymnastics, and massage will be of advantage in restoring the muscles to their normal condition.

Relapses result also from abnormality in the shape of the femoral head and in the shape of the acetabulum. It is impossible by manipulative reduction to place securely a distorted femoral head into an equally distorted and smaller acetabulum. Permanent reduction is also made difficult by the twist of the femur, which gives an abnormal direction to the femoral neck and consequent abnormal muscular rela-

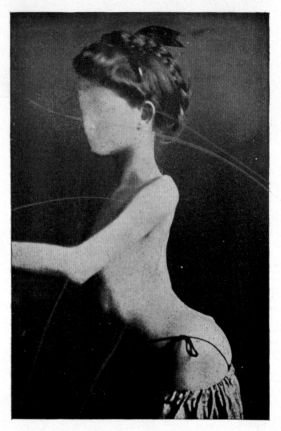

FIG. 304.—Untreated Case of Double Congenital Dislocation.   Unable to walk without crutches.

tion. The importance of the femoral twist in causing relapse after congenital dislocation has been exaggerated. It has been found by the investigation of Mikulicz and also by Soutter that a femoral twist may exist to a considerable extent without causing noticeable disability. When a femoral twist of ninety degrees is present, it is impossible for the patient to walk normally with the femoral head in the socket. Under these circumstances an osteotomy of the femur is necessary.

OSTEOTOMY.—When osteotomy is necessary it can be performed by the use of an osteotome, dividing the femur beneath the lesser trochanter by a linear osteotomy.

PROGNOSIS AFTER TREATMENT.—The results obtained in the treatment of congenital dislocation of the hip show a gratifying

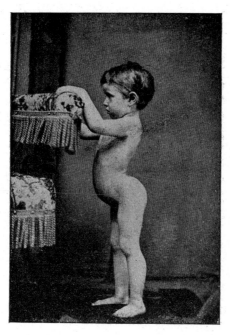

FIG. 305.—Double Congenital Dislocation of Hip. Child aged four. Untreated.

increase in the percentage of permanent cures as the knowledge of the pathological conditions of the deformity has been more thoroughly understood and as technical skill has increased. Permanent cures (i.e., successful anatomical replacements, with re-establishment of motion) can be expected in 80 to 90 per cent of cases suitable for operation (i.e., between 2 and 10 years of age). In some of the younger children and in the double cases a second reduction is sometimes needed, when the head is not held firmly in the socket after the first operation.

SUMMARY.

Surgeons will vary somewhat in their choice of methods of operation, according to their experience and success with the methods of reduction by forcible manipulation or by open incision, but these facts may be said to be generally accepted:

As a rule no attempt at reduction is advisable under two years of age, as the tissues are not sufficiently developed to prevent relapse.

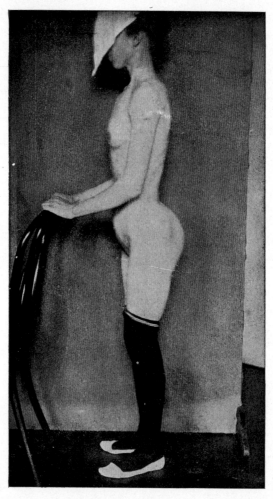

FIG. 306.—Same Patient, Age Twenty-eight. Untreated case. Patient able to walk actively with little limp.

In the early cases, from two to five years of age, reduction is easily accomplished by forcible manipulation.

In older cases, from five to ten, except in children with weak muscles, although reduction by forcible manipulaticn is often not difficult, reduction is much easier after mechanical stretching, and in some cases reduction is impossible without such aid.

In resistant cases, where there is reason to believe alteration of the shape of the head and acetabulum or a firm and narrow hourglass contraction of the capsule exist, reduction by open incision after a thorough stretching of the muscular tissues is advisable.

In cases of doubt as to which method to employ, the surgeon can regard it as a safe rule to follow to attempt reduction first by forcible manipulation, employing open incision if relapse follows.

The length of time needed in after-treatment must be determined by the condition found after reduction, and must be left to individual judgment in each case.

Double cases are to be regarded as more than twice as difficult as single. Attempts at reduction by forcible manipulation should be made on both hips at the same time, but if open incision is employed, as a rule two separate operations are necessary.

KNEE.

Congenital dislocation of the knee is seen with greater frequency than that of some of the other joints.[1] It occurs most often in the form of hyperextension of the leg on the thigh, which has been considered by some writers a displacement rather than a true dislocation forward. In some cases the lower epiphysis of the femur is bent forward on the shaft.[2] It is in any event a congenital affection of importance when it occurs. It is frequently double, and the displacement may be directly forward or forward and to one side. The leg forms a right angle with the thigh, the apex of the angle being backward, and the condyles of the femur can be felt in the popliteal space; the patella is often small and occasionally absent, and lateral mobility may be present. The affection is also known as genu recurvatum. Modifications in the shape of the bone, ligaments, and cartilages in the knee-joint, even to the point of ankylosis, have been recorded in some of these cases. The deformity may be associated with malformation of other parts, and the cause can be given no more clearly than that of other congenital deformities.

Forward displacement of the leg at the knee is to be treated by manipulation in the direction of correction and the application of a

---

[1] Drehman : Zeitsch. f. orth. Chir., vii , 22 (98 cases).

[2] Delanglade : Rev. d'Orthopédie, May, 1903.

repeated plaster bandage to the knee to force the limb into a corrected position.

PATELLA.

Dislocation of the patella is among the more common of the congenital dislocations; many cases reported as congenital have, however, been doubted.

The type most frequently seen is outward dislocation existing with some degree of knock-knee. It may be displaced inward or upward, in the latter case being associated with lengthening of the patella

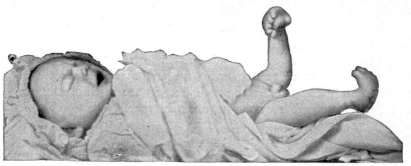

FIG. 307.—Congenital Dislocation of the Knee. (Genu recurvatum with club-foot.)

tendon. There may be, in connection with the dislocation outward, absence or flattening of the outer condyle of the femur.

The disability may be slight or there may be marked impairment of the extension power of the leg on the thigh. Treatment by operation would be similar to that described in speaking of slipping patella.

CONGENITAL ABSENCE OF THE PATELLA.[1]—The patella may be absent or tardy in its development. If it is absent the knee appears broad and flat and there may be marked impairment of the function of the knee. In other cases the knee is useful. It may coexist with other malformations of the knee, especially genu recurvatum. It is often bilateral and is frequently associated with club-foot and similar deformities.

The treatment consists in the use of apparatus to support the defective joint, and massage and muscle training to the extensor muscles.

SHOULDER.

True congenital dislocation of this joint is rare, and many cases reported as congenital have proved on investigation to be dislocations

[1] A. Thorndike : Orth. Trans., vol. xi.

due to paralysis or due to injury to the shoulder at birth, resulting most often in a separation of the epiphysis. The dislocation found is the subspinous, but other varieties have been recorded, such as the subcoracoid and subacromial. Double dislocation of the shoulder has been described and in some cases has been associated with other malformations. The glenoid cavity is likely to be malformed, as in a case reported by Smith, where there was hardly a trace of the normal glenoid cavity. In other cases it is approximately normal. The limitation of function is similar to that in traumatic dislocations. Cases of dislocation of the shoulder-joint in young infants have been reduced with or without incision, with improvement in the usefulness of the arm; cases of true congenital dislocation, however, improved by operation are few. Cases were operated on by Phelps by doing what was practically an arthrodesis through a posterior incision, and the redundant capsule was removed. The chances of successful replacement would be greater in cases with a normal glenoid cavity and in cases undertaken early in life. In later childhood the prospect is less good.

In addition to the operative reduction, reduction by manipulation is to be considered, following the lines indicated in the operation for congenital dislocation of the hip. After replacement the arm should be held by a plaster bandage for some months in a position of abduction and outward rotation.

ELBOW.

Congenital dislocations of the elbow are very rare and of comparatively little practical importance. The reported cases do not conform to any one type, following a wide range of variation.

In connection with congenital dislocation of the elbow may be mentioned a deviation from the normal line of the arm occasionally seen. If the arm of the adult hangs at the side with the palm of the hand directed forward, the line of the forearm should form with the line of the arm an angle of about 169 degrees with a variation of 10 degrees in either direction. The outward deviation of the forearm is a few degrees greater in women than in men. *Cubitus valgus* is the name applied to the condition in which the forearm is displaced too far to the radial side; *cubitus varus*, the condition in which it is displaced to the ulnar side. Trauma is the most frequent cause of the marked varieties. They are also associated with rickets and the element of inheritance apparently plays a part. In case either deformity should be severe enough to require operative treatment, an osteotomy may be done similar to the Macewen operation for knock-knee.

WRIST.

Pure congenital dislocation of the wrist is extremely rare. The ordinary form in which it is seen is in connection with club-hand.

SPONTANEOUS SUBLUXATION OF THE WRIST.—A displacement of the wrist has been described by Madelung, in which the hand is displaced to the palmar side of the forearm and probably to either the radial or the ulnar side laterally, generally to the former. In such cases the lower border of the radius and that of the ulna are prominent at the dorsum of the wrist, and the bones are somewhat separated from each other. The wrist is much increased in thickness and the function of the hand is impaired. Active and passive dorsal flexion are affected and some pain may be present, especially in dorsal flexion. The hand can be replaced only in the lighter grades of the affection. There is excessive mobility of the intercarpal joint and there may be slight forward bending of the lower extremity of the radius.

Aside from the pain which may be present, the symptoms are weakness and sensations of discomfort about the wrist. The causes of the affection are given as relaxation of the ligaments, stretching of the muscles by hard work, irregularity of growth at the lower end of the radius, and possibly a malposition lasting over from rickets. The treatment is at first hyperextension of the joint by means of bandages and splints, the use of massage and similar measures, and osteotomy in cases with bony deformity sufficient to require it.

CHAPTER XVIII.

TALIPES, CONGENITAL AND ACQUIRED (CLUB-FOOT).

THE name talipes signifies a deformity of the foot, and, although it was originally used to indicate a form of talipes now known as equino-varus or club-foot, the present use of this word is as a prefix to the descriptive adjective designating the variety of the deformity which exists.

TALIPES EQUINO-VARUS (CLUB-FOOT).

The term club-foot is popularly applied to a deformity characterized by an inversion, torsion, and depression of the front part of the foot with an elevation of the heel.

In walking on a foot thus deformed, the weight of the body is borne, not by the sole of the foot, but by the outer side, and in extreme cases by a portion of the dorsum of the foot also.

The deformity is either congenital or acquired.

Frequency.—Club-foot is by no means an uncommon distortion. In 6,969 orthopedic patients applying at the out-patient department of the Children's Hospital, Boston, there were 488 cases of club-foot. Congenital club-foot is by far the most frequent of the congenital deformities of the foot.

Pathological Anatomy.—The deformity is a displacement inward of the anterior part of the foot. The scaphoid bone will be found articulating with the side of the head of the astragalus rather than with the anterior surface. The articulation is also more toward the under side of the astragalus, the head of which is thus partially uncovered.

The cuneiform bones, being intimately connected with the scaphoid, follow the displacement of the latter, and the same is true of the metatarsal bones and the phalanges, so that the long axis of the front of the foot forms a right angle, or even an acute angle, with the axis of the leg. The cuboid is necessarily displaced to the inner side and does not articulate with the front of the os calcis, the facet of which also inclines obliquely to the inner side.

In fully developed cases, and in older children or adults, there is a more marked and important alteration in the shape of the bones.

The os calcis, by the elevation of the tuberosity, is drawn from a horizontal into a position approaching the vertical. It is also more or less rotated on its vertical axis, so that its anterior extremity is directed outward and the posterior extremity inward, and thus the anterior articulating facet is oblique to the axis of the bone. The

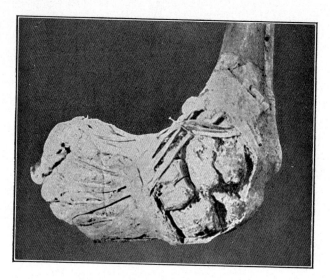

Fig. 308.—Dissection of Club-foot.

cuboid bone maintains its connection with the os calcis, but follows the inward direction of the anterior extremity of the foot.

The different tendons assume an abnormal direction and in general are carried farther to the inside than is normal; this is especially true of the tibialis anticus, the common extensor of the toes, and the long extensor of the great toe. Synovial bursæ may form on the outer edge and back of the foot, which may become inflamed and suppurate; corns and callosities are also formed on the skin, from the pressure of walking. No change has been found in the nerves or the spinal cord in cases of club-foot.

In extreme cases there may be slight alteration in the shape of the femur and a laxity at the knee-joint; the tibia has also been found altered. The muscles are never found paralyzed in congenital club-foot, but the contracted muscles seem more developed than the lengthened muscles. The muscles of the leg atrophy from disuse, and the leg is much smaller and the foot shorter than normal.

Etiology.—In regard to the etiology of congenital club-foot, various theories have been advanced in explanation of the deformity.

A popular idea is that the distortion is due to maternal impressions, but no conclusive evidence in regard to this has been obtained.

Heredity, on the part of both the father and mother, has been

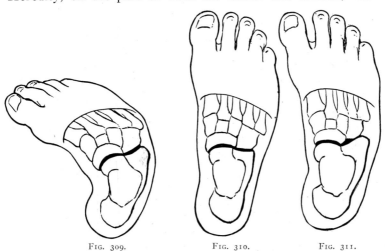

FIG. 309.   FIG. 310.   FIG. 311.

FIG. 309.—Diagram Indicating Mid-tarsal Articulation in Club-foot and the alteration in the positions of the scaphoid and cuboid in their relation to the astragalus and os calcis—with alteration in the shape of front of os calcis.
FIG. 310.—Diagram of a Normal Foot.
FIG. 311.—Diagram of a Club-foot Partially Corrected, Leaving the Projection of Front of Os Calcis Unchanged, and the Consequent Imperfect Reduction of the Cuboid. A relapse necessarily follows.

established without doubt in a certain number of cases, but in a very large majority no trace of similar deformity in ancestors can be found.

Symptoms.—Club-foot gives rise to great inconvenience in walking. In uncorrected cases, however, the amount of skill and agility patients acquire in locomotion is surprising, even though the deformity remains unchanged. Bursæ and callosities form over the unprotected portions of the foot, and may inflame and cause much discomfort, limiting the amount of the patient's activity.

Diagnosis.—There is no difficulty in recognizing the deformity of club-foot. The history of the case establishes a diagnosis between the congenital and non-congenital forms of club-foot. The paralytic form can also be recognized by the evidence of paralysis of the muscles on the anterior and external surface of the leg.

Prognosis.—In regard to the prognosis of the deformity, it may be said that the distortion does not correct itself, and, if left uncorrected, remains the most obstinate of malformations. The deformity is one which is essentially curable through surgical intervention.

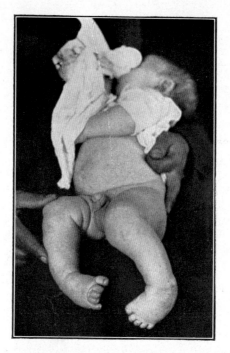

FIG. 312.—Double Congenital Club-foot.

In infantile cases the time required for correction is relatively short, but retentive appliances are needed for a longer time. It may be said in general that the older the cases and the larger the foot the more difficult the correction, but the less the danger of relapse after correction.

In regard to the permanence of the cure and the danger of relapse, it may be said that if perfect correction is attained relapse is exceptional, if moderate care is used in the employment for a sufficient time of retentive appliance.

But it must be borne in mind, especially in the case of young children, not only that the correction must be complete, but that efficient appliances for keeping the proper position of the foot in walking (retentive or walking appliances to be described) must be worn until the gait and attitude are perfect. In club-foot half-cures are practically no cures. Relapsed cases are invariably resistant and difficult to correct.

Treatment.—The object of treatment is the correction of the distortion and the retention of the foot in a corrected position until any

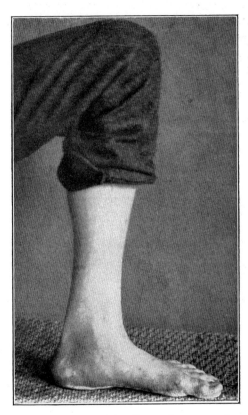

Fig. 313.—Congenital Club-foot. Cured club. Twenty-four years after correction in infancy by tenotomy, manual force and retention, walking appliance worn for two years. Patient able to walk without limp or discomfort twenty miles a day.

return of the deformity is impossible, the tendency to relapse being very strong.

The treatment should be purely mechanical, or both operative and mechanical.

The treatment of club-foot, therefore, requires:

1. A rectification of the misplaced bones and a lengthening of shortened and contracted tissues.

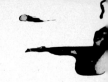

2. A retention in a normal position until the abnormal facet of the astragalus and the other tissues become, under the pressure of new position, normal.

At the present time few procedures in surgery are as precise in their indications and as certain in their results as the methods for the correcting of club-foot.

The correction of club-foot should be divided into two steps, whether the treatment is mechanical or operative.

1st. Correction of the varus deformity.

2d. Correction of the equinus deformity.

In other words, the front of the foot should be twisted out and afterward be raised. This will be found of practical importance, as the foot is more easily twisted before than after the equinus deformity is overcome.

Operative treatment in some form is the method to be selected in cases of congenital club-foot, except in young infants and in older children when some contra-indication to operation exists.

The mechanical procedures for correcting club-foot are as follows:

Manual manipulation.

Plaster-of-Paris bandages.

Apparatus.

The operative procedures which are to be considered in treating club-foot are:

Tenotomy.

Division of the ligaments.

Open incision.

Forcible correction and osteotomy.

MECHANICAL CORRECTION.

Manual.—The simplest method of correction is by the use of the hands, and in the case of a new-born infant with club-feet the mother may be directed to manipulate the foot, and having rectified the deformity by gentle force several times daily, to hold it as straight as possible for a minute or two each time. This process continued daily over a period of months is in intelligent hands capable in the less resistant cases of restoring the foot to its normal mobility and position, after which retention treatment should be begun. The method, however, is too tedious and uncertain to be relied upon.

Plaster-of-Paris Bandages.—Another method in correcting club-foot is by repeated fixation in a plaster-of-Paris bandage, the foot

being held as nearly in a corrected or in an overcorrected position
as possible at each application of the bandage until the bandage
hardens. The application of a plaster-of-Paris bandage must be made
with care and skill to prove efficient.

The foot should be wound with sheet wadding, pads should be
temporarily placed between the toes, and the foot should be held over-

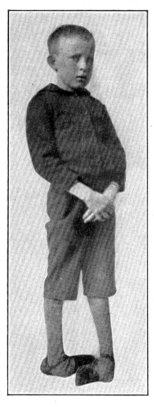

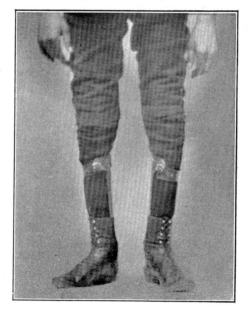

FIG. 314.—Congenital Double Club-   FIG. 315.—Double Club-foot. Two months after correc-
foot Walking Before Operation.   tion by forcible manipulation, wearing walking reten-
                                              tive appliances. Same case as Fig. 314.

corrected, with the knee flexed, from the first during the application
of the bandage by an assistant, who shifts the fingers from place to
place to keep out of the way of the bandage, yet who maintains the
overcorrection.

The circulation of the toes must be carefully watched after the
application of such a bandage.

The bandage should reach above the knee, where the limb should be bent to prevent the plaster bandage (which should be renewed every two or three weeks) from rolling around the limb, and to prevent the child from kicking it off. In the case of small children

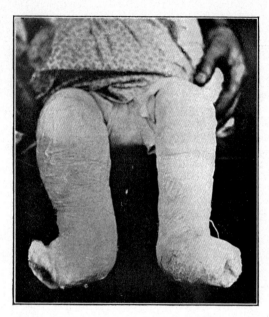

Fig. 316.—Double Club-foot in Plaster Bandages After Operative Correction.

with plump legs, and in resistant cases, it will, however, be found difficult to prevent the heel from being drawn away from the bandage, and stretching of the tendo Achillis will by this method be tedious.

This method has the disadvantage of being tedious, except in young children; but it has many advantages in being a practical method, readily applied, and not leaving details of application to the patient's parents. It is evident that correction in this way, if persistently applied, is possible, but, except in very young children, it is advisable to perform tenotomy first. If the Chinese can produce an extreme deformity by bandaging the children's feet, the same method could be employed for the correction of deformity. It is especially adapted to the deformity in infants under 4 months of age. The plaster bandage can be protected from softening by urine by painting it when dry with jap-a-lac paint.

Apparatus.—Mechanical correction (without tenotomy) by means of appliances has been successfully employed in very young cases.

The method, however, requires much persistence on the part of the surgeon if a perfect cure is expected, and is not to be advised.

Although treatment by apparatus is not sufficiently effective to cure any but the mildest forms of congenital club-foot in young children, it is often enough to bring about a cure in acquired club-foot of moderate severity. The form of apparatus is the same whether used as a corrective or as a retentive appliance, and will be described here. The object of such apparatus is to retain the tarsal bones in proper

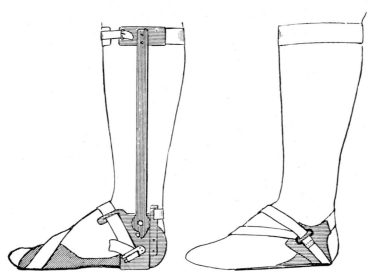

Fig. 317.—Splint for Club-feet, Inner and Outer Views.

position until the muscles and ligaments have adapted themselves to the normal position, and until articular facets have been formed in the proper direction, or the astragalus and os calcis have assumed, under altered pressure, a relatively normal shape.

The corrected foot tends to relapse in two directions—inversion and elevation of the heel. If this is unchecked and walking is done in improper attitudes, hurtful pressure and strain fall upon the bones and ligaments of the foot, and relapse takes place. This should not occur if proper retention and walking with a proper attitude of the foot are cared for.

As these appliances are to be worn a long time, they should be light, readily adjusted by the nurse, not unsightly, and in no way limiting locomotion, walking, or running. The best are worn within the shoe.

It is to be remembered that in all appliances it is necessary that the pressure preventing a faulty position of the foot should be applied precisely, pressing the front of the foot and the inner tip of the heel outward, the front of the foot, especially the outer edge including the cuboid, upward, and the back sole (i.e., the end of the os calcis) downward.

Inward pressure should be exerted upon the outer edge of the front of the os calcis and astragalus, and not upon the cuboid, as is too

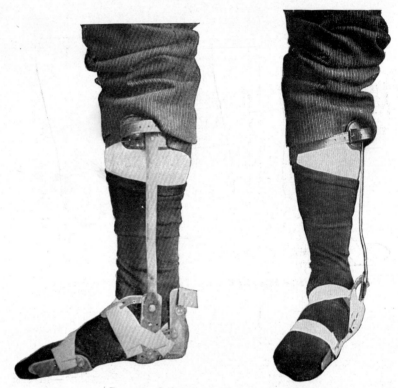

FIG. 318.—Splints for Equino-varus Applied.

commonly done in inefficient apparatus. As the latter bone is in front of the mediotarsal joint, inward pressure upon it not only fails to correct the deformity but tends to increase it. This explains the occurrence of many relapses, faulty apparatus being not only useless but injurious.

The apparatus, which is a modification of Taylor's varus shoe, consists of a sole plate small enough to fit in a shoe secured to a

jointed upright furnished with a stop to prevent the plate from dropping into the equinus position. The foot is secured to the plate by
means of straps.

The appliance can be worn inside of a shoe, opened like a bicycle
shoe well down to the toes.

OPERATIVE TREATMENT.—A combination of operative and mechanical methods of treatment is at present the most common mode of
treating club-foot at all ages, apparatus being used after overcorrec-

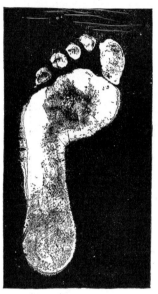
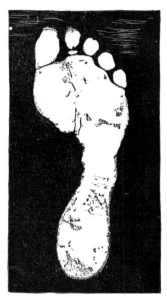

FIG. 319.   FIG. 320.

FIG. 319.—Imprint of Foot of a Child Sixteen Years Old. Treated when one year old for congenital club-foot.
FIG. 320.—Imprint of Normal Foot.

tion has been obtained as a means of retention until the normal
muscular balance has been restored. The operative interference most
frequently resorted to is tenotomy and subcutaneous division of the
fasciæ or ligaments.

Tenotomy.—The structures to be divided are, of course, those
which hold the foot in its deformed position. The tendons may be
divided by entering the tenotome under the skin and cutting the
tendon from without inward, or by passing the tenotome under the
tendon and cutting outward. The advantage of the former is that
there is no danger of making a large skin incision by a slip of the
tenotome. There is, however, danger of incomplete cutting of the

tendon.   The tendon which is most frequently divided in equino-
varus is the tendo Achillis.

Section of the Tendo Achillis.—The patient should lie upon his
face or side and an assistant should hold the foot; the surgeon enters
the knife parallel to the border of the tendon, passing the tenotome

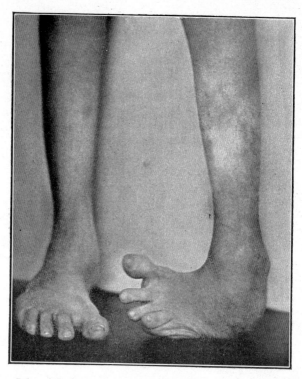

FIG. 321.—Relapsed Resistant Congenital Club-foot in a Boy of Eight.   Front view.

flatwise between the tendon and the skin.   This having been done,
the blade of the knife is turned toward the posterior surface of the
tendon and the assistant raises the end of the foot so as to stretch
the tendo Achillis slightly.   The left index finger presses on the skin
over the back of the tenotome, and in this way the sensation of the
cutting of the tendon can be felt.

The only precaution necessary is to be assured that the tendon is
completely divided.   When the operation is done, the extravasated
blood is squeezed out of the opening and a small amount of aseptic
gauze is placed over the wound.   The operation should be done
aseptically and an aseptic dressing applied.

In older cases, especially in paralytic equinus, the tendon can be half divided at two levels, one on the anterior and the other on the posterior part, and the rest of the tendon torn by manipulative force. A lapping flap may thus be secured, facilitating more rapid development of a strong tendon.

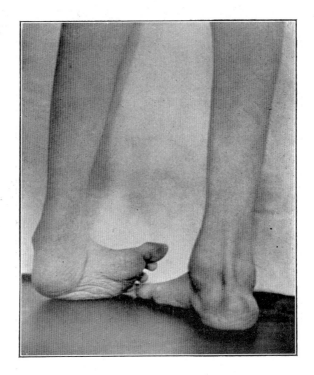

Fig. 322.—Relapsed Resistant Congenital Club-foot in a Boy of Eight.   Rear view.

The insertions of the tendons of the tibialis anticus and posticus muscles can be divided, and at the same time the shortened ligaments on the inner and under side of the articulation between the astragalus and scaphoid by a free use of the tenotome inserted at the inner side of the astragalo-scaphoid articulation.   If the point and edge of the tendon is kept close to the bone there is little danger of serious injury to the artery.

Division of the Plantar Fascia.—It is often necessary to divide also the plantar fascia, preferably before division of the tendo Achillis, as the latter acts as a means of support for stretching the foot when the plantar fascia is divided. The plantar fascia is divided in the same way that the tendons are incised. The most prominent portion of the fascia is the point of election for subcutaneous incision. The fascia, it must be borne in mind, is not a narrow band, but a broad ligament needing a long subcutaneous incision. The tenotome should be inserted on the inner side of the sole nearly halfway between the os calcis and the ball of the foot, but nearer to the os calcis. The

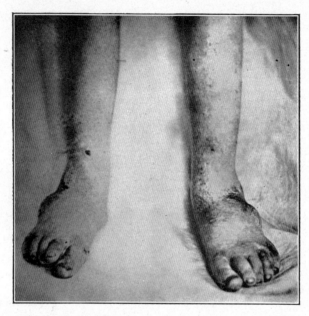

Fig. 323.—Same Case. Three weeks after forcible correction, immediately after removal of plaster retention bandages.

tenotome is to be pushed subcutaneously nearly across the sole, the edge of the knife turned toward the fascia, and the knife drawn across the fascia, which will be felt to give way as it is divided; an assistant should make upward pressure upon the ball of the foot, in order to put the fascia on the stretch. As the artery lies deeply, there is no danger of injuring it, if ordinary care is used.

The tenotomes used should be strong at the neck, and the cutting edge should not be too long, as the skin is necessarily divided if they are too long; infantile cases require a much smaller instrument. The blunt-pointed tenotome is but little used now, and the sharp-pointed ones are used for all subcutaneous work.

Tenotomes as furnished by instrument-makers are ordinarily much too large, and though serviceable in myotomy, are better for tenotomy in children if smaller.

The Repair of Divided Tendons.—When a tendon is divided, the cut ends are separated to a variable extent, depending upon the retraction of the muscle to which it belongs; but a strong tendon results by natural repair if the sheath has not been extensively injured by the tenotomy.

The calcaneo-cuboid ligament should also be divided in severe cases. The tenotome should be inserted a short distance behind the

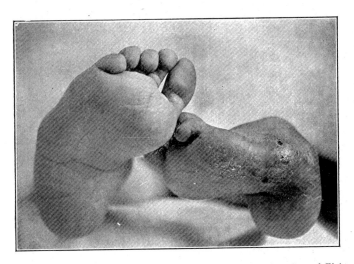

Fig. 324.—Soles of Relapsed Resistant Congenital Club-foot in a Boy of Eight.

head of the fifth metatarsal bone, near the articulation of the os calcis and cuboid, which can be felt on palpation. The sharp-pointed tenotome should be inserted to the bone, and then by careful motion the whole ligament should be divided.

In case the correction has not been perfect, as sometimes happens with more resistant feet, a second operative correction is necessary.

When the plaster bandages are removed the retention appliance, described above, is to be used so long as there is any tendency to an incorrect position.

The permanence of the correction depends on the establishment of an accurate balance of the antagonism of muscles and other soft parts when the foot is in normal position. The after-treatment by retention must be persisted in until the child is able, without special effort, to walk with the foot in a natural position; otherwise a relapse will occur.

The use of retention apparatus will be necessary for some time

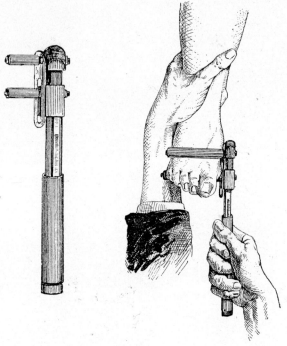

FIG. 325.—Thomas Club-foot Wrench, Modified.   (Hoffa.)

and should be discontinued gradually.   The parent may aid in the treatment by daily manipulating the feet into the overcorrected position.

OPERATIVE CORRECTION.

In cases too resistant to be corrected by the means described the following radical measures may be employed:

1st. Open incision.

2d. The use of extreme force.

3d. Tarsal osteotomy.

OPEN INCISION.—The chief difficulty is in obstinate cases to stretch the contracted tissue on the concave side of the distortion. Phelps' open incision on the inner and plantar surface is of use in these cases.

The advantage of open incision in club-foot is the facility of complete and thorough division of all the soft tissues to the bone. The method by which this is done is as follows: The skin is divided along the inner side of the foot, from the tip of the malleolus well

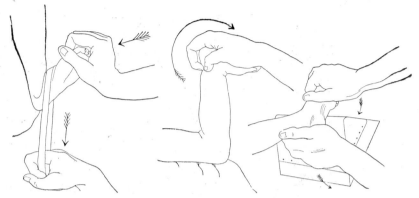

FIG. 326.—Manipulative Correction of Club-foot.   (After Lorenz.)

down on the inner edge of the first metatarsal bone. After the skin is incised, the other tissues are cut with care, using a director if necessary. The insertion of the tibialis tendon is found and cut across. The artery can be spared by careful dissection, but if necessary it can

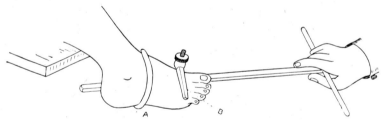

FIG. 327.—Lever Correction Apparatus Applied.

be divided and tied. The plantar fascia on the sole of the foot should be divided by the use of a tenotome, or long, thin knife. A cross incision toward the sole of the foot from the middle of the long incision is sometimes necessary, but it is desirable to avoid this if possible. A triangular incision with its apex upward toward the ankle, instead of the cross-cut of the skin and fascia, is equally efficient and diminishes the gap after correcting the foot.

FORCIBLE MANIPULATION.—Even if tenotomy and thorough open incision are done, a certain amount of resistance remains from the interosseous ligament connecting the tarsal bones. Considerable force is often necessary to bring the foot into an overcorrected position. This can be done either by manual force or by the aid of mechanical force. Several wrenches for this purpose have been devised; that of

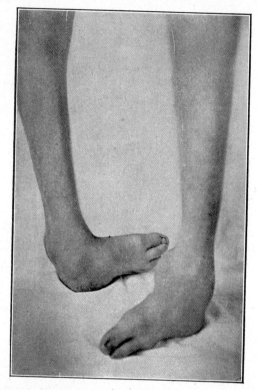

FIG. 328.—Double Congenital Club-foot Before Operation.

Thomas is the simplest and is sufficiently efficient when no bone obstruction exists. The foot is then brought into as normal a position as possible, thorough aseptic dressings are applied, and the foot is then fixed in a plaster-of-Paris bandage reaching above the knee and holding the well-padded and aseptically dressed foot in an overcorrected position. If the dressing is provided with efficient protectors and sufficient dressings, no change in the bandage need be made for a fortnight or longer. If necessary, however, a window can be cut in the plaster over the wound and the dressings changed. After the plaster-of-Paris is discarded the retention shoe is to be worn.

In applying the bandages, it is of course important that the foot should be held in an overcorrected position until the plaster becomes hard, as no further correction can take place under the bandage. In the majority of cases perfect correction or overcorrection is possible, and the foot can be held in proper position for the application of the fixation bandage without much force.

OSTEOTOMY.—When but a slight amount of osseous distortion is present forcible correction aided by tenotomy or open incision will

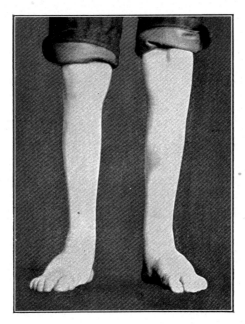

FIG. 329.—Same Case Six Weeks After Operation by Forcible Correction.

be sufficient to overcome the deformity, but in the more resistant cases changes in the shape of the tarsal bones forming the mediotarsal joint prevent perfect cure, and operation upon the bones is necessary.

Astragaloid Osteotomy.—An examination of the anatomy of resistant club-foot shows that the facet of the astragalus in the astragaloscaphoid articulation is on the side instead of in front. There is also some obliquity of the neck of the astragalus. If this obstruction of the bone can be corrected and the front of the foot brought into place, there would be less tendency to relapse.

It is essential, in every inveterate case of club-foot, that if the foot is to be unfolded, the shortened tissues in the arch of the foot and in the inner side of the foot must be stretched, torn, or divided. This can be done safely by means of tenotomy, forcible stretching, or open incision; but the deformity of the astragalus still remains. In many cases of younger children, even if somewhat resistant, if the deformity is rectified and the foot held a sufficient time in the proper position, and a proper walking shoe used for a year, a new facet of the astragalus will be formed and a cure effected. In a few cases this is not the case, and in such instances osteotomy of the neck of the astragalus suggests itself as a suitable operation.

The procedure will not be found a difficult one. Tenotomy or open incision and division of the fascia and ligaments should be done, and the foot stretched and manipulated into as nearly normal a position as possible. An incision through the skin is made from the tip of the malleolus to the inner side of the head of the first metatarsal, which will be found in severe cases close to the malleolus. The incision is close to and nearly parallel to the tibialis anticus tendon, and in the direction of the metatarsal. The incision should be made to the bone and the foot straightened, as the metacarpal bone is separated from the malleolus. The scaphoid will be seen before the astragalus is encountered, if the deformity is great, and it will be first within the reach of the knife in all cases. If the foot is still further stretched, the scaphoid begins to uncover the side of the astragalus, and the neck of the astragalus is seen; a small osteotome is entered and placed upon the neck of the astragalus, to the proximal side of the scaphoid articulation, and the neck of the astragalus divided or nearly divided. The foot is then forcibly straightened, and the neck of the astragalus unchiselled is fractured. The result is similar to that in Macewen's operation for knock-knee, and the distortion at the neck of the astragalus is removed. It is manifest that the line of section of the bone at the neck of the astragalus should be transverse to the axis of the bone, and at such a plane that when the equinus deformity is corrected the resulting gap at the section should not be greater than necessary. The foot should be fixed in an overcorrected position. A wedge-shaped resection of the neck of the astragalus through a skin incision in the outer and upper surface of the foot has been performed, but linear osteotomy would seem to be preferable.

Osteotomy of the Head of the Os Calcis.—The relation of the cuboid to the os calcis is frequently masked, lying deeper than that of the scaphoid and astragalus, and it may in treatment be but partially corrected. The distortion of the os calcis at its anterior aspect, if not corrected, increases, and forms an obstacle to the complete restoration of the cuboid to the normal position, although the rest of the deformity may have been corrected.

When the cuboid is cartilaginous and the ligaments are well stretched, the defect at the anterior portion of the os calcis can be overcome by forcibly correcting the foot and retaining it in the corrected position by means of a plaster-of-Paris bandage, care being taken, however, that the cuboid be restored to place, and in time it

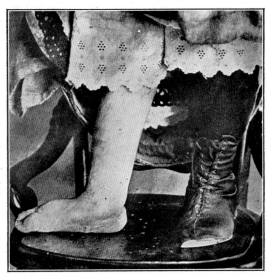

Fig. 330.—Case of Bad Relapsed Congenital Club-foot in a Woman of Thirty-four, Corrected by Force with the use of a Wrench. Photograph taken three months after correction, showing cicatrix of the tear of the skin caused by correction.

will be found that the cartilaginous abnormality in the shape of the os calcis is gradually changed under corrected pressure.

When distortion of the head of the os calcis is great, no amount of mechanical treatment can overcome the obstacle, if it is of bone and if the ligaments are strong, binding the bones in a distorted position. It is manifest under these circumstances that the rational treatment is a removal, not of the astragalus or cuboid, but of a part of the projecting portion of the head of the os calcis.

After complete stretching or division by tenotomy, force, or open incision of the contracted tissues on the inner and under side of the foot, tendons, ligaments, and fasciæ, if it is found that the front of the foot cannot be brought to a perfectly corrected or overcorrected position, an incision should be made on the outer side of the foot, passing from behind the external malleolus forward and downward. The incision should be a curved one, and the chief convexity should be at the forward portion of the os calcis. This incision should reach to the bone and should expose the peroneal tendons. These can either be drawn to the side or divided to be stitched later. The upper portion of the incision should reach behind the external malleolus, and should extend far enough up to allow sufficient retraction of the flap to give room for the osteotomy. After the bone has been reached, and the periosteum divided and pushed aside, an osteotome should be inserted far enough back to remove a sufficient amount of bone. The direction of the insertion of the osteotome should be such as to allow the placing of the cuboid, after the bone has been removed, in a normal position. This step of the operation requires some nicety and judgment, as it is of importance that the front plane of the bone, after the wedge has been removed, should be in the direction of the normal facet of the front of the os calcis. A wedge-shaped portion of bone should be removed from the anterior and outer part of the os calcis, and the cartilaginous ends saved in order to allow a proper amount of motion between the cuboid and the os calcis after recovery. The wedge-shaped portion of bone that should be removed should be ample and enough to allow the replacement of the front of the foot in a normal or overcorrected position and the restoration of the proper direction of the os calcis.

The wound should be carefully washed out to remove any fragments of bone that may have been left, and subsequently stitched; the tendon of the peroneus longus, if divided, being stitched. The foot should then be dressed with proper dressings and fixed in an overcorrected position by plaster bandages according to the ordinary rules in osteotomy.

Whether or not this operation should be done in connection with an osteotomy of the neck of the astragalus, and with an open incision, is a matter of judgment.

Imperfect results are due to neglect of thorough asepsis, failure to remove a sufficient amount of bone, failure to remove it in such a direction as to cure the deformity, and lack of care in placing the foot in an overcorrected position after operation.

While the plaster is hardening the cuboid is pressed upward and outward, and the front of the foot pressed outward and upward, counter-pressure being applied on the astragalus on the outer and upper side, and the os calcis twisted into its normal position.

Treatment can be carried out with a plaster-of-Paris bandage until the foot is thoroughly healed, and also until locomotion has been re-established. After this the use of the club-foot shoe is advisable for at least some months.

RELAPSES.—No error is greater than a common one, namely, that tenotomy alone is sufficient to correct club-foot. In fact, tenotomy is only the beginning of a course of treatment. If the foot is rectified and held in place for a month, it is supposed by some surgeons that a cure has been effected. But such is by no means the case.

Moreover, it must always be borne in mind that relapses will *invariably occur* unless the distortion is overcorrected, and little reliance can be placed on the curative effect of time. Efforts at correction should be continued until the foot can be easily abducted beyond the median line, and while slightly abducted, can be flexed so that the dorsum of the foot shall form less than a right angle with the leg, the sole of the foot being flat, and there being no twist in the front of the foot. After this the correction appliance can be gradually omitted while manipulation of the foot is still carried on, and the case should be kept under observation.

Relapses occur in a certain number of cases simply from the carelessness of the parents, who are not aware of the necessity of retaining the corrected foot in the proper position for a long time. In such cases a second operation is advisable.

Relapses in older children are due to incomplete correction, either from a lack of thoroughness or from the existence of an unusual amount of distortion of the astragalus or os calcis not suspected, and demanding osteotomy, or from too early removal of the fixation or retention appliance.

In some instances of resistant club-foot it is found difficult, in correcting the foot, completely to overcorrect the equinus deformity, and to enable the foot to be brought to within a right angle with the leg. If this is not done, inconvenience is felt by the patient in taking a long step, and the foot is turned in to facilitate this. The smaller the foot the greater this danger. If this is not corrected, it may, in some instances, seriously interfere with the excellence of the result.

It should always be borne in mind that a distortion in the neck of the astragalus or in the head of the os calcis exists, even in infantile club-foot, and that the feet are not permanently corrected until the alteration of the facets into a normal position has taken place. This is independent of bringing the foot into a normal position, and demands fixation in an overcorrected position for some time. In some cases this is more needed than in others, probably because the alterations of the facets of the astragalus are in some instances slight.

Too great overcorrection of the deformity and the development of a splay-foot have sometimes resulted from overzealous treatment. This danger is, however, not great; and instances are rare, and are to be overcome by the treatment for a valgus foot.

Inversion of the foot, after cure of the club-foot, may in a few instances be observed from imperfect strength of the outward rotatory muscles at the hip. This, however, causes but little disfigurement, the inversion usually being slight, and correcting itself by the normal development of the muscles. A marked toeing-in of the foot in running persists a long time in some instances in which the foot is entirely corrected and the walking is normal. It disappears with the increase of muscular strength. In such cases the ordinary Taylor shoe should be carried up to the hip by means of an upright on the outside of the leg and a posterior arm carried back from the level of the trochanter, as in the knock-knee splint. By tightening this, eversion is secured.

A relaxed state of the knee-joint causing inversion of the tibia is not uncommon in infantile club-foot; it usually corrects itself in the development of the child after correction of the foot. In rare instances, however, it may persist, requiring the longer use of a walking appliance.

The muscles retarded in club-feet by disuse need development before a complete cure is effected. Ordinarily the muscles develop of themselves after complete correction, if the limbs are actively used. In some cases the development is slow and massage and electricity are advisable.

In addition to retentive appliances, in cases of imperfect muscular balance, shoes (worn over the appliance, if necessary) with a high sole wedge under the cuboid are sometimes needed. This corrects at each step, as the weight comes upon the sole, the dropping of the cuboid.

The most common form of acquired talipes equino-varus is that following infantile paralysis.

The correction of paralytic club-foot is to be conducted on the same principles as that of the congenital type. Correction is, however, much less difficult, as osseous changes are present only in the old severe and neglected cases.

Tenotomy of the contracted muscles can be done as in congenital cases, though overcorrection after tenotomy is to be avoided. Immediate correction and fixation in a corrected position are to be used after tenotomy as in the congenital form.

In paralytic equino-varus, tendon transference, referred to under infantile paralysis, is of importance, and arthrodesis in older cases.

TALIPES EQUINUS.

(Pes equinus, Horse heel, Pied bot equin, Pferdefuss, and Spitzfuss.)

Talipes equinus is the name given to a condition in which the foot is held in a position of plantar flexion and cannot be dorsally flexed to the normal extent (twenty degrees beyond a right angle).

Varieties.—Talipes equinus may be congenital or acquired. Congenital equinus is an uncommon deformity, constituting about five per cent of all cases of equinus.

In the acquired forms all degrees of deformity are met, from the slight condition in which the foot cannot be flexed dorsally beyond a right angle with the leg, to one in which the foot and leg form practically a straight line.

Etiology.—The causes of acquired talipes equinus are as follows: Infantile paralysis of the anterior muscles of the leg. Cerebral (spastic) paralysis. Shortening of the leg after joint disease or fracture may lead to an adaptive talipes equinus which serves to make the legs of equal length for walking.

Talipes equinus may be a symptom or result of disease of the ankle-joint. Long confinement to bed may cause talipes equinus, which is merely the result of the long-continued plantar flexion of the foot.

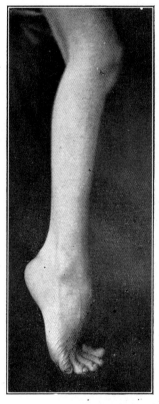

FIG. 331.—Talipes Equinus of Marked Degree. This represents the weight-bearing position.

Fractures may result in talipes equinus either from injury to the ankle-joint or from fixation during repair in a plantar-flexed position.

The contraction caused by posterior cicatrices or the loss of power due to division or injury of the anterior muscles and tendons of the leg.

Symptoms.—The deformity in its slighter degrees is not particularly disabling. In its severer grades it is the cause of a severe limp and at times of much discomfort.

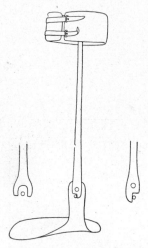

The detection of talipes equinus is a simple matter. The normal foot should be capable of flexion about twenty degrees beyond a right angle, and any cause which restricts this flexion is a degree of talipes equinus.

Treatment.—The division of the tendo Achillis will relieve the deformity in all cases except those in which bony deformity exists at the ankle, as in the cases following fracture and tuberculosis of the ankle-joint. In such cases or in extremely severe instances of deformity from other causes, osteotomy of the tarsus may rarely be required for rectification.

FIG. 332.—Apparatus for Talipes Equinus, with Stop Catch. On the Right of the Picture is a Detail Drawing of the Stop for Talipes Calcaneus, on the Left a Catch Allowing Slight Motion.

The deformity should be at once corrected after tenotomy and a plaster-of-Paris bandage applied. If a retention appliance is required after operation, a modification of the club-foot shoe, with the ankle-joint arranged to stop extension at a right angle, will be found to be effective and simple.

TALIPES CALCANEUS.

Talipes calcaneus is the name applied to a condition in which the foot is held in a position of dorsal flexion.

Varieties.—The deformity may be congenital or acquired.

It is a comparatively rare congenital deformity, the form ordinarily seen being a paralytic calcaneus, often combined with a valgus deformity.

Symptoms.—The patient walks upon the heel and the gait is inelastic, because the spring of the foot is absent and the patient walks bearing the whole weight on the os calcis.

Treatment.—In congenital cases the foot should be daily manipulated by the parents into a position of plantar flexion. As soon as the anterior muscles are stretched, it is advisable to put the foot up in a position of plantar flexion, to bring about adaptive shortening of the posterior muscles. In the severer cases the application of a series of corrective plaster bandages holding the foot in plantar flexion may be necessary. Tenotomy of the anterior tendons is rarely required. When the foot can be plantar-flexed to the normal amount, a reten-

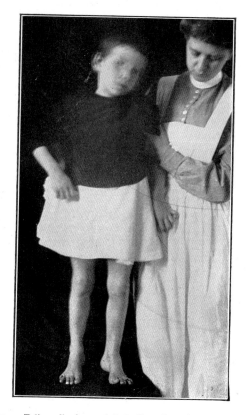

Fig. 333.—Talipes Equinus of Left Foot Resulting from Paralysis.

tion shoe preventing dorsal flexion may be applied, but in slight cases this is not necessary. The foot can be supported in a splint with an upright jointed at the ankle, but with a stop preventing extension of the foot upward, or by prolonging backward the heel of the shoe. The paralytic form is discussed under Infantile Paralysis.

TALIPES VALGUS.

Talipes valgus is the name given to a condition which is not in all cases to be clearly differentiated from what has been described as flat-foot. Talipes valgus may be congenital or acquired. As a *con-*

genital deformity it is one of the less common of the congenital deformities of the foot.

Acquired Talipes Valgus.—The most common cause of acquired talipes valgus, not of the purely static variety, is anterior poliomyelitis. It also occurs following inflammation of the ankle-joint, and in cer-

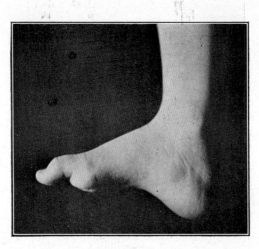

Fig. 334.—Talipes Calcaneus.

tain cases of spasm of the peroneal muscles. Treatment, if the congenital form, consists in repeated correction by plaster bandages, aided in the severer cases by midtarsal osteotomy. In the paralytic cases, after correction of the deformity, muscle transference or arthrodesis or the use of a retention shoe is needed.

TALIPES VARUS.

Talipes varus is the name given to a condition in which the front of the foot is turned inward.

Treatment.—In the congenital form the treatment is practically the same as that of equino-varus, except that it is not necessary to cut the tendo Achillis. In the acquired form retentive apparatus is useful, preventing inversion of the foot.

TALIPES CAVUS.

Talipes cavus (hollow foot) is the name given to a condition in which the arch of the foot is increased and the anterior part of the foot is approximated to the heel. It is not necessarily associated with any other deformity, but may occur in connection with talipes equinus, calcaneus, or varus. It is rarely congenital in its severe forms, but a markedly high arch to the foot may be an inherited peculiarity sometimes sufficiently marked to justify classing it as pathological. In

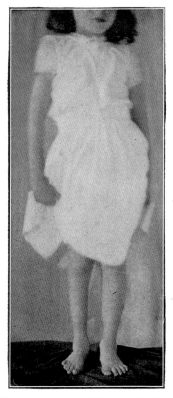

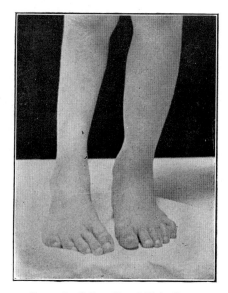

Fig. 335.—Moderate Degree of Talipes Valgus, Right Foot.

Fig. 336.—Talipes Varus, Right Foot.

the acquired form it exists in most cases as the result of anterior polio-myelitis, and is also to be classed as a shoe deformity. The patho-logical changes show nothing besides the effects of a continued mal-position of the bones. The deformity varies more or less in degree. The most marked form is to be found in the foot of the Chinese lady of high rank, in which the heel and front of the foot are approxi-mated by bandaging in early youth, and a degree of pes cavus is in-duced which does not exist except under these highly artificial condi-tions. From this extreme grade all degrees of the affection are seen,

the slightest being an increased elevation of the arch not accompanied
by symptoms, in which the foot rests upon the ground in standing,
touching only on the heel and ball of the foot. It is less disabling
than pes calcaneus, and is frequently associated with the other deformities mentioned. The two types commonly seen are, first, those

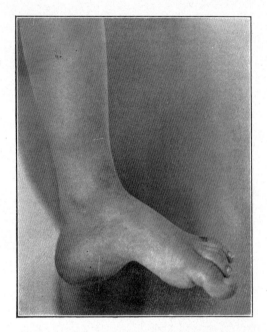

Fig. 337.—Pes Cavus with an Element of Calcaneus.

resulting from anterior poliomyelitis, in which a paralysis more or
less extensive has involved the foot and leg. In a second form, generally milder in grade, it apparently develops as a shoe deformity in
middle childhood, and appears to be the result of wearing too short
a shoe or of a shoe narrower than the front of the foot; the front
of the foot being held back by the front of the boot, the tendency in
weight-bearing is to approximate the heel and the toe, and in this way
to approximate the front of the foot to the heel. In the slightest
grade it apparently forms one of the varieties of the condition described as *contracted foot*. The plantar fascia is contracted and bands
may be felt under the skin. The symptoms in the slighter varieties
are those of a sprain of the arch of the foot and the muscles of the
leg, owing to insecure balance of the foot in standing. Corns and

callosities may develop in the front of the foot; the elasticity of the gait is impaired.

The treatment of the slighter forms consists in the use of a boot with sufficient room in the upper. If any element of equinus coexist, the tendo Achillis should be lengthened by stretching or tenotomy. Operation is required in the severer cases. The plantar fascia is thoroughly divided by a subcutaneous tenotomy, and the foot is forced

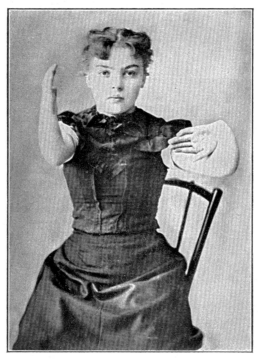

FIG. 338. - Club-hand due to Congenital Absence of Radius. (Sayre.)

into shape by means of an osteoclast, after which the foot is put up in a plaster bandage, which should flatten the arch of the foot as much as possible. When walking is begun, which should be as early as possible after operation, the steel sole plate and strap described above should be adjusted to the shoe.

PES PLANUS.

This consists of an abnormality at the metatarso cuneiform articulation, chiefly of the first metatarsus.

It is frequently seen in babies and is not uncommon in the old and feeble, with weakened plantar muscles. It is of little pathological significance, except when combined with a valgus deformity constituting plano-valgus, or flat-foot, referred to elsewhere.

CLUB-HAND.

In German the distortion is known as Klumphand, and in French as main bote.

Congenital club-hand is a rare condition, analogous to congenital club-foot. The name is applied to a deviation of the hand, at the wrist, from the line of the forearm; this deviation is almost always in the direction of flexion.

It may occur without malformation of bones, but more commonly they are deformed, or the radius may be wanting wholly or in part. The carpus may be normal, or incompletely developed, or almost entirely wanting. When the radius is deficient, the lower end of the ulna is enlarged to articulate with the carpus.

The **diagnosis** is evident, and any pathological process which is accompanied by this malposition is classified as club-hand.

In early childhood correction should be attempted by repeated plaster bandages.

When operation is attempted in older cases it should consist in bone plastic attempts to supplement an absent radius by splitting the ulna and inserting the carpus between the split fragments.

Treatment.—In the mildest cases, particularly if the bony structure is normal, treatment should consist of manipulation to stretch the contracted tissues and retention in the correct position by means of a splint.

CHAPTER XIX.

FLAT-FOOT.

Definition.—The term " flat-foot " is applied to a faulty condition of the foot impairing its weight-bearing strength. It may be defined technically as a static pes plano-valgus.

The human foot normally changes in shape as the superimposed body weight is shifted in the different static conditions incident to human action. Man as a hunter and fighter needs not only swiftness of foot but firm play and agility in his footing while using his arms and hands in combat. This is secured by a function of the tarsus, peculiar to man, whereby a side play of the midtarsus is possible while the heel and front of the foot are firmly planted upon the ground. When the body weight is supported equally on both feet, the weight falls through the astragalus on the end of the os calcis and the heads of the metatarsals; but if the load is shifted to either side, the midtarsus moves with it, the limb rotating at the midtarsal articulation and at the hip-joint. The normal check to too great outward twist is in the locking of the midtarsal bones as the weight falls on the outer edge of the foot, giving a firm base of support, but for inward rotation the check lies in ligaments and muscles.

When the front of the foot is turned out too far or too constantly while the midtarsus is twisted in, a condition of

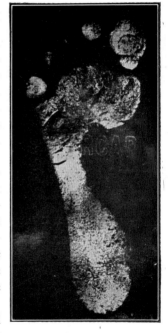

Fig. 339.—Print of Arab Foot.

chronic strain follows which may lead to ligament irritation, too great inward play of the midtarsus, or abnormal position of the tarsal bones; in short, to pes plano-valgus or flat-foot.

375

Up to a certain limit this movement occurs in normal feet, but beyond this what must be regarded as a pathological condition is reached, attended by symptoms of pain and disability, and is the first step in the formation of flat-foot.

The deformity, strictly speaking, is not a flattening of the foot, but consists of an exaggerated midtarsal drop and twist, occurring

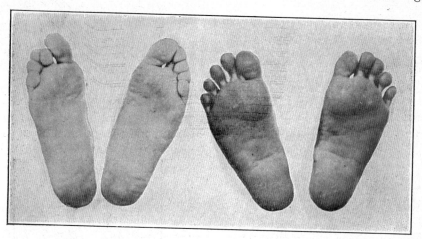

FIG. 340.—Casts of Civilized and of Savage Feet.

normally within limits. The movement is a combination of inward rolling and dropping to the inside of the middle of the foot. The individual stands with the front of the foot turned out to give a wider base of support. The internal malleoli are unduly prominent, corresponding to the well-known knee deformity. This may be termed a knock-ankle deformity.

PATHOLOGICAL ANATOMY.

Alterations in the shape of the bones are noted in severe cases, the external malleolus being at times somewhat flattened and rounded, but the chief distortion in the bones occurs in the astragalus, os calcis, scaphoid, and cuboid. In extreme cases the astragalus has dropped from above to the inside of the os calcis, the latter being rolled to the inside with a deviation of its forward end to the inside. The front of the foot is turned outward, the scaphoid and cuboid being practically dislocated. At the outer side the cuboid may be displaced upward. Changes in the direction of the metatarsus and of the phalanges are found and exostoses are at times developed.

There is a loss of the normal play of the bones in the tarsal articulations from loss of elasticity of the ligaments, and changes in the shape of the bones result from abnormal pressure. The muscles are changed in their strength, the tibialis being weakened and the peronei contracted. The plantar ligaments are stretched and displaced, and those bearing strain are thickened.

Varieties.—As has been already mentioned, talipes valgus resembles flat-foot, and they are

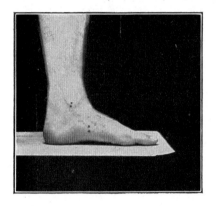

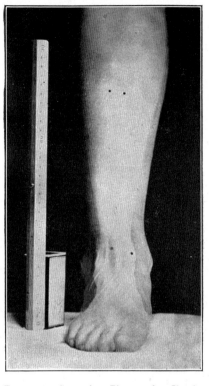

FIG. 341.—Composite Photograph, Showing Excursion of Malleolus and Arch with and without Weight-bearing. (Dane.)

FIG. 342.—Composite Photograph, Showing Lateral Excursion of Lower Leg and Foot with and without Weight-bearing. (Dane.)

often classed together. For clinical reasons it is more convenient to consider the subjects separately. The same is also true of congenital valgus, sometimes called congenital flat-foot.

Causation.—In general terms it may be said that the deformity is caused by a disproportion between the weight to be borne and the muscular power which bears it. Footwear which cramps the front of the foot, faulty attitudes in standing and walking, and whatever weakens the muscles of the legs and feet are the chief exciting causes.

The most common of traumatic causes is Pott's fracture, in which a deformity is the result of inefficient treatment or of a severe and intractable fracture. The deformity is also seen after tuberculous diseases and chronic arthritis of the ankle.

Many of the barefooted races have been considered flat-footed simply because of the strong development of the muscles of the sole, careful examination, however, showing excellent arches.

The most common cause is the weakening of the muscles of the foot by shoes. Shoes as worn by the leisure class or by the class that

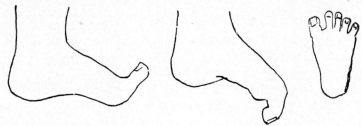

FIG. 343.—Normal Motion of the Front of the Foot.

gain their livelihood (as is the rule in cities) by occupations which require standing rather than strong and vigorous walking, compress the front of the foot. This part of the foot, from compression and from resulting weakness, cannot adapt itself as greater weight is

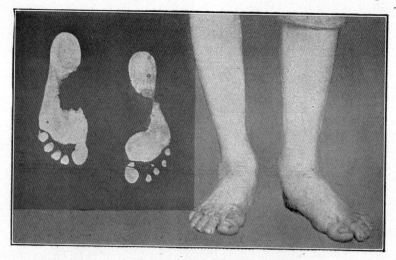

FIG. 344.—Weakened Foot without Breaking Down of Arch.

thrown upon the foot, and the medio-tarsal twisting takes place, which in the strong bare foot is prevented chiefly by the action of the tibial muscles and by the muscles of the first metatarsal and its phalanges. People the front of whose feet have been compressed stand and walk with a greater angle of divergence of the axes of the feet, which increases the danger of the development of the deformity by bringing greater strain upon the inner side of the foot and favoring

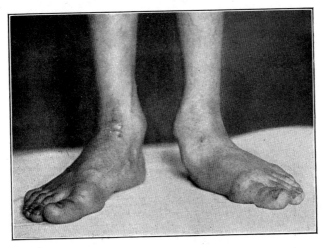

FIG. 345.—Severe Double Flat-foot.

the inward rolling which frequently develops flat-foot. Flat-foot is not developed among moccasined savages who use their feet actively

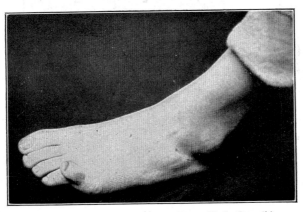

FIG. 346.—Displacement of Little Toe. (H. L. Burrell.)

as hunters, using the muscles of the front of the foot freely, nor among sandal-wearing monks.

Symptoms.—*Flat-foot* is a deformity characterized by a flattened appearance of the sole of the foot.

It can for convenience clinically be divided into two groups:

1. Flexible flat-foot or *weakened foot,* where little or no structural changes have taken place and the foot assumes the flattened position only when weight falls upon it.

2. *Rigid flat-foot* or flat-foot proper, in which the distortion is

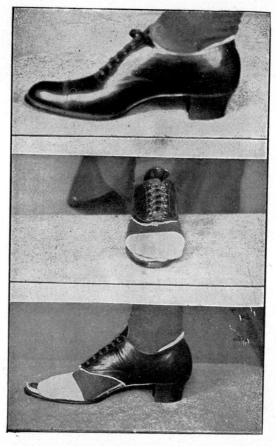

Fig. 347.—Showing Shoe Constriction of Front of Foot, with Normal Foot in Shoe Before and After Removal of Upper.

permanent, some structural change in ligament or bone having taken place.

DEFORMITY.—In the severer cases, instead of the normal arching upward of the inner border of the foot, this border is either less arched than normal or is in contact with the ground.

PAIN.—The first symptom complained of is a sense of discomfort in the feet after standing or walking. This may increase until pain of greater or less extent is present during and following use of the feet. In the milder cases pain ceases when the weight is removed, but as the condition becomes more advanced the pain not only becomes more severe, but continues after the use of the feet is stopped, and in the severer cases persists during part of the night. The severity of the pain may be greater than is to be expected from the amount of distortion; and, again, there may be little disability, although the deformity is marked. The pain is most frequent in the neighborhood of

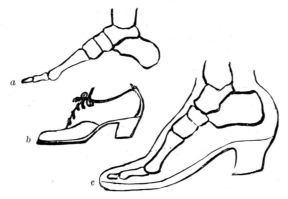

FIG. 348.—*a*, Drawing of Normal Position of Bones of Foot. *b*, Fashionable Shoe. *c*, Tracing of Skiagram of Foot in Shoe, Indicating Cramping and Downward Pressure on the First Metatarsal.

the scaphoid; it occurs also in front of the foot, in the centre of the heel, behind the inner malleolus, and on the outer border of the foot. Pain is also complained of in connection with flat-foot in certain cases in the leg, knee, back, or hip.

TENDERNESS.—Tenderness may be present over points of ligamentous strain.

MUSCULAR SPASM.—In very acute cases there may be irritability and contraction of the peroneal muscles holding the foot in the position of abduction; in this case there is apt to be tenderness over the origin of the peroneal muscles.

STIFFNESS.—Congestion of the foot and swelling of the foot and leg are frequent symptoms. Stiffness or loss of flexibility is a symptom which is gradually developed, and it involves at first and most prominently the mediotarsal joint. The stiffness is such that the front of the foot cannot be adducted actively or passively as much as it normally should be. This is an important matter to recognize, as it prevents an assumption of a correct position by voluntary muscular effort until the proper flexibility is restored. There is also, especially in the later history of the case, some limitation in the plantar and dorsal flexion of the foot at the ankle-joint.

GAIT.—The gait becomes modified as the affection progresses and becomes in a measure characteristic. The feet are generally more everted than normal, and in painful cases it will be noted that in standing the patient deliberately throws the foot over, so that the weight is borne more upon the inner border than is normal. The front of the foot is turned out while the knee is turned in. There is a lack of elasticity to the gait, and this is a symptom often complained of by the more intelligent patients, who find their feet stiff and clumsy. After the patient has been sitting for some time and on rising in the morning the feet are likely to be stiff and clumsy.

Diagnosis.—For examination of the feet, the shoes and stockings should be removed and the patient should stand facing the surgeon upon the floor. The patient's gait should be carefully watched.

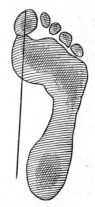

The relation of the foot to the leg should be noted, whether the internal malleolus is unduly prominent and the foot rolled over on to its inner border. The height of the arch of the foot is of importance, and any lowering of the inner border is significant. The rolling of the foot further on to its inner side or the lowering of the arch after the patient has stood for a minute indicates muscular insufficiency under weight-bearing.

FIG. 349.—Meyer's Line in Average Foot.

The imprint of the weight-bearing foot is of interest. This is taken by having the patient step on a piece of cardboard blackened with camphor smoke; the non-weight-bearing position of the foot is recorded first and then the weight-bearing position, the two being superimposed.

The degree of flexibility should be examined by attempting to adduct the forefoot gently with the hands and to flex the foot dorsally with the patient's knee extended. Loss of the first of these movements is of diagnostic importance.

The presence of tender points in the sole of the foot, either under the heel or under the scaphoid, generally indicates static disturbance of the foot. The occasional assumption of the plano-valgus position

does not constitute flat-foot. The deformity is a constant faulty attitude and the inability to bear the body weight without discomfort.

An x-ray examination is of assistance in determining any displacement in the relation of the bones to each other occurring in the
severer grades of the affection and not present in the lighter grades.
It is also of value in giving information as to the presence of arthritis
deformans and the existence of irregular bone growth.

Prognosis.—After a time the foot may become accustomed to its
altered position and painful symptoms cease. In other cases, how-

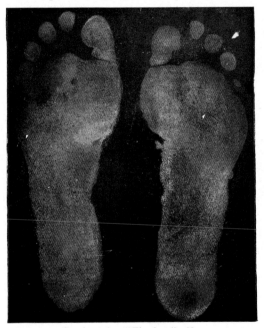

FIG. 350.—Tracing of a " Flat-foot." No symptoms.

ever, the painful symptoms continue and become worse rather than
better.

The condition may persist almost indefinitely, a constant source of
pain and disability.

Treatment.—Treatment of the conditions described should be directed to the replacement of displaced tarsal bones, overcoming midtarsal stiffness and restoration of the muscular strength needed in
sustaining the body weight.

The latter, in lighter cases, can be secured by the exercise of the
feet untrammelled by foot-cramping shoes—moccasin walking on turf,
snowshoeing, or flexible shoe activity on uneven surfaces.

The goose-step gymnastics and marching in army shoes give foot strength to recruits, and the same can be done in civil life; but careful directions as to daily foot exercises, the proper use of shoes, and correct attitudes in standing and walking are usually needed.

Various exercises can be employed. The following simple ones

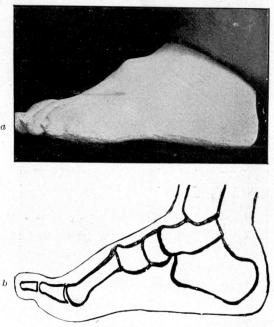

FIG. 351.—*a*, Photograph of Humped Foot. *b*, Tracing of Skiagram of Humped Foot with Irritation Exostosis of the Metatarso-cuneiform Articulation.

will be found of service to increase midtarsal flexibility and foot muscular strength.

1. The patient, sitting forward on a chair, with the feet crossed, and resting on the outer edge, alternately partially rises and sits.

2. The patient, standing, with one foot in front of the other, the front foot turned in, and the rear foot resting behind the front leg on its outer edge, lowers himself a number of times by bending his knee, without changing the position of his feet.

3. The patient walks with the front of the feet strongly adducted.

4. The patient, standing with the feet closely touching, bends the knees as far as possible without raising the heels from the floor, and then spreads the knees, keeping the soles of the feet flat.

5. The patient places his foot with the leg of a light chair between the first and second toe, throws his weight on the ball of the foot, bends the knee and turns the limb outward, keeping the sole and heel flat.

6. The patient sits with the affected ankle resting on the knee of the other limb, the inner edge of the foot directed upward; a weight

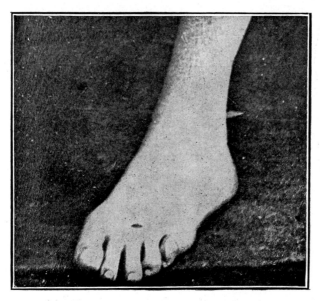

FIG. 352.—Deformity Caused by the Constriction and Confinement of the Foot.

connected to a strap is hung over the front of the foot, which is raised without raising the leg.

7. The patient, pressing hard with the hand upon the front of the foot, endeavors to press the hand up with the foot.

8. The patient, curling the toes over the round of a chair, drags the chair, which can be made heavy if loaded with weights.

In addition to this, rolling heavy dumb-bells with the feet, exercises in picking up small rubber balls, weight and pulley exercises with straps attached to the front of the foot can serve to strengthen the feet and whole limb.

In resistant cases it is necessary to correct midtarsal stiffness by mechanical means. This can be done by a simple appliance. The front of the foot is strapped on to a board, a peg is placed between the first and second toes, and a small block against the outer side of the heel. A rod used as a lever placed against the inner side of the foot and under the head of the astragalus, is made to press this portion of the foot outward.

Patients should be trained in standing and walking so that faulty position should not be habitual, i.e., those in which the weight falls

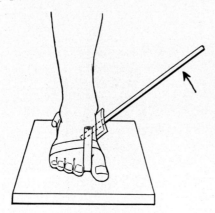
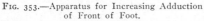
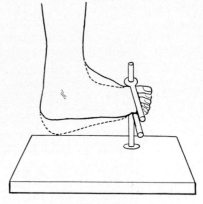

FIG. 353.—Apparatus for Increasing Adduction of Front of Foot.

FIG. 354.—Exercising Apparatus for Use in Cases of Flat-foot.

more upon the weaker or inner than on the outer, stronger foot arch. They should not stand with the feet turned out and the limb turned in, or walk with the front of the foot abducted and not adducted. This latter, common in the weak-limbed, is easily recognized if the gait is watched, and by determining the axis of the patella.

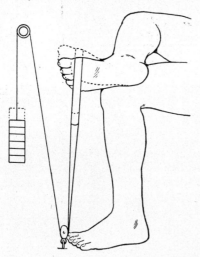

FIG. 355.—Apparatus for Exercising Foot in Flat-foot.

Supports.—When the foot is overweighted and too much strain put on the inner arch, relief is furnished if a firm support is placed underneath the part of the foot. This can be furnished by means of a thin steel plate of a suitable shape placed in the shoe and made from a plaster cast of the foot. The latter should be carefully made. The patient's foot should first be encased in several layers of cheesecloth heavily loaded with plaster-of-Paris cream. While this is hardening, the foot is placed upon the floor with the arch in the best possible position. When this has hardened it is cut off the foot and serves as a mould for the cast.

Another method of preparing casts for plates is to model them from moulds of the foot made in dental wax. If a sheet of quickly hardening dental wax is softened in hot water and placed upon the bottom of the foot, a mould can be taken. When it is hardened it can

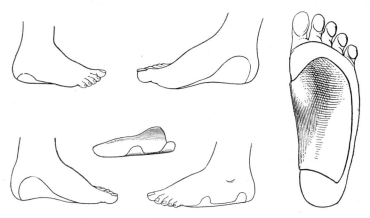

FIG. 356.—Flat-foot Plates.

FIG. 357.—Flat-foot Plate Raised in Front to Support Anterior Arch.

be removed from the foot, and can be cut and moulded to any desired shape by immersion again in hot water. In this way a wax flat-foot plate is made fitted to the boot. A plaster-of-Paris cast can be taken of this, and reproduces exactly the shape and size of the plate desired.

Manufacture and Material.—The best all-round material for the manufacture of plates is a spring tempered steel of a gauge varying from eighteen to twenty, according to the weight of the patient. For the manufacture of plates from this material, the services of an instrument-maker or of a skilful blacksmith are necessary. The cast should be furnished to him and the plate forged to fit the cast exactly. It should then be tried on the patient, before or after which it should be tempered. For final use the plate should be copper-plated and nickel-plated.

By another method the surgeon is able to manufacture the support himself. A celluloid paste is made by dissolving celluloid chips in acetone; this is then painted on to several layers of gauze laid on the cast, between which strips pieces of steel wire are incorporated. The wires are laid on in different directions, giving strength as desired. When the celluloid has hardened, the edges of the plate should be trimmed.

Shape of Plates.—Judgment is necessary in determining the proper shape of the plate in each case, as the deformity varies both in degree and in kind. The shape should be determined by the part of the foot which needs corrective support. As a rule, the scaphoid and proximal end of the first metatarsal and the sustentaculum tali need to be raised. In some cases the tendency of the os calcis to rotate to the inner side of the foot is to be checked, and in other cases side pressure is needed on the head of the astragalus, scaphoid, and cuneiform, with counter-pressure on the outer side of the foot. The most practical way of determining what shape of plate is desirable is to have the patient stand, and by pressure with the hand to see in what place the force accomplishes the best result. In general, a plate should be higher along the inner part of its surface than on the outer, but it should not be made so sloping that the foot continually slides off. If this is the case a counter-point of pressure may be furnished by turning up the outer flange at the outer edge of the plate. Ordinarily it is advisable to have the plate support nearly the whole width of the sole, ending in front behind the sesamoid bones of the great toe and at the back end just anterior to the weight-bearing surface of the heel, or, if desired, running to the back of the weight-bearing surface of the heel.

If the anterior part of the foot is broken down, support to it should be furnished by raising the front of the plate in a dome-shaped rise, supporting the part of the foot behind the heads of the metatarsals. In flexible feet a shorter plate can be used than in rigid feet. The need of an inner flange and its height will be determined by the requirements of the case; the same is true of the outer flange. The plate at its outer border should not project beyond the outer edge of the shank of the boot, or it will push out the leather and destroy the shape of the boot.

Fitting and Use.—The plate should be shaped in such a way as to act as a prop to the portions of the feet which drop to an abnormal position when weight is thrown upon them. In the practical fitting of the plate, if the plate is rightly shaped, the foot when not bearing weight should lie smoothly against the bottom of the plate, not springing off at the front or back. If it springs off, it will exert more pressure than is generally comfortable. When the plate is placed in the boot and the patient stands upon it, there should be a sense of even, well-distributed pressure, and not a feeling as if the patient were standing on a ridge or lump, which will be the case if the plate is too high. If an inner flange is used it should not press too much upon the foot when weight is borne upon it. If sensitive points in the foot are present and cause pain when weight is borne upon the plate, it will be necessary to lower the plate opposite these points. When the plate is first applied it should be worn only for so long a period as is consistent with the comfort of the patient, and should then be taken out to rest the foot if necessary. If the plate is persistently a source of pain it will not give the desired relief, but will cause irritation and must be lowered until it is comfortable. No point is more commonly neglected than this, and the very common use by patients of ill-fitting supports bought at shoe-stores brings much discredit upon the use of plates. The plate should set firmly in the shoe and should not rock, and the front and back ends should be in contact with the sole of the boot.

Misuse of Plates.—The danger of injury to the feet by the too constant use of plates is to be borne in mind. The plate is to be regarded in the same light as is a crutch or cane in the case of any joint unable to bear the strain of use, and is to be discarded when the normal strength has returned and the irritability has disappeared. To continue the plate after the indications for its use have disappeared is to hamper the muscles of the feet and to prolong the unnatural condition.

Pads.—The use of felt or leather pads supporting the arch of the foot is sometimes of use temporarily or under exceptional conditions. Such pads may be cut of the desired shape and worn outside the stocking by being fastened to an inner sole of leather. If they are worn for any length of time the weight of the foot stretches the leather of the boot and breaks down the shank and they cease to be of value.

The Oblique Sole.—Palliative treatment is often attempted in cases of flat-foot by making the inner side of the sole and heel of the boot one-eighth or one-fourth of an inch thicker than the outside. The weight is in this way thrown more to the outer side of the foot and the strain on the inner side is somewhat relieved. The thickness of the wedge which is necessary may be determined experimentally by building up the inner side of the boot till the desired position is obtained, as determined by the diminution in the projection of the internal malleolus.

It is to be remembered that in the correction of flat-foot not only should the body weight fall well on the outer edge of the foot, but the great toe and head of the first metatarsal should perform their normal functions in locomotion.

MASSAGE, GYMNASTICS, ETC.—The supportive treatment of flat-foot should be reinforced by measures to stimulate the local circulation and to strengthen the muscles of the foot. Massage is of the first importance, but should not be pushed to the point of irritation. The use of alternating hot and cold douches or of a local hot bath followed by a cold douche is of much value. Vibratory massage, electricity, and the use of hot air may be of use in especial cases.

It was supposed that by the use of a plate of gradually increasing height tarsal displacement could be corrected, but for this purpose the daily use of a prepared exercising shoe will be found of advantage. A loose broad-toe shoe, with a strong inner edge, heel-less, and with a flexible sole and loose upper opened to the toes, can be furnished with a thick triangular wedge of leather and rubber secured to the sole.

The thick inner edge should reach from behind the head of the first metatarsal to the inner border weight-bearing surface of the heel. The highest point should be below the scapho-astragaloid articulation. This should be from 1 to 3 inches high; the inner border should project beyond the sole, the outer surface should be tapered to a point and shaped so as not to raise the outer arch.

If this is properly attached, the patient walking with this not only has pressure under the lowered scaphoid, but is obliged to attempt to walk with adduction of the front of the foot.

This shoe can be worn with benefit, daily increasing length of time, without interfering with the patient's daily occupation.

As barefooted and sandal-wearing people are free from pes plano-valgus, the footwear should constrict the front of the foot and limit free action of the muscles of the foot as little as possible.

Moccasins and sandals should be worn when practicable, but it is, however, evident that feet weakened by constant confinement in stiff boots must be gradually strengthened before continued free action is possible without some discomfort.

The shape of the shoe has become conventionalized to such an extent that the general use, among the leisure class, of shoes of the shape of the normal foot is not practicable. The people of the city streets will not be shod as hunters. It is, however, practicable to limit the use of fashionable shoes for leisure hours and to furnish working boots for working hours. The boots should be adapted to the gait and use. People who use the front of the feet in locomotion, " front-foot " walkers, and those walking on uneven ground need more room in the front of their boots than heel walkers or those who walk on an even surface.

THE TREATMENT OF PAINFUL CASES.—In certain cases the symptoms of local irritability reach so high a grade that especial treat-

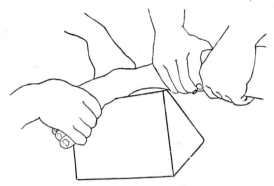

FIG. 358.—Forcible Correction of Valgus on Wooden Block. (Berger and Banzet.)

ment is needed. Spasm of the peroneal muscles may be present, holding the foot in an abducted position and resisting movements of rectification. In this case temporary fixation of the foot in a plaster

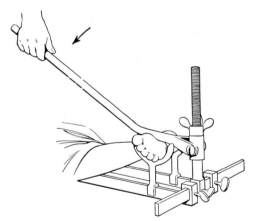

FIG. 359.—Apparatus for Forcible Correction of Rigid Flat-foot.

bandage is the most efficient measure, or the use of adhesive plaster strapping, as in sprained ankle.

Forcible Correction.—In cases in which it is not possible to place the foot in an approximately correct position on account of stiffness and muscular contraction, it is generally unsatisfactory to attempt the use of a support until the position of the foot has been corrected. Such patients should be anæsthetized and the foot forcibly twisted into shape. It must be remembered that there are two elements of deformity to be corrected: first, eversion of the foot; and, second, abduction of the forefoot. This can be done manually in many cases, but in severe cases such an appliance as the Thomas club-foot wrench will be of use in giving better leverage, or the foot can be manipulated over a padded wooden wedge.

The foot should be overcorrected if possible, or in any event placed in the best obtainable position and held by a plaster bandage. It then follows the course of an ordinary sprained ankle, generally of slight degree. As soon as the patient can walk without pain, supports should be applied.

In less severe cases, correction can be gradually accomplished by the repeated application of plaster-of-Paris bandages.

In extreme cases osteotomy of the neck of the os calcis and astragalus may be needed, or the removal of a wedge-shaped piece of bone from the inner side of the neck of the astragalus undertaken; but in a majority of cases, even the severe ones, forcible correction will be found more efficient than wedge-shaped exsection, as the distortion will be found to be distributed in various parts of the foot, and extensive removal of bone will be followed by weakening of the foot. The correction of the complicating deformity of hallux valgus is often necessary for the cure of flat-foot.

CHAPTER XX.

METATARSALGIA AND OTHER DEFORMITIES OF THE FOOT.

METATARSALGIA.

THE name metatarsalgia or anterior metatarsalgia is used to describe a pain more or less spasmodic, situated at the distal end of either of the outer three metatarsal bones.

Causation.—The pain is due to a disturbance in the normal relation of the anterior ends of the metatarsal bones, causing a pinching of the external plantar nerve between the ends of the bones, to pressure of the metatarsals on other digital nerves, to abnormal strain upon the ligaments connecting the metatarsal heads, or to a bruise of the tissues by these bones.

The affection is thus due to the disturbed relation in the position of the metatarsals caused by faulty footwear. Normally the head of the first metatarsal bears a large part of the weight which comes upon the front of the foot. If footwear is worn which gives insufficient room for the toes and at the same time exerts a crowding pressure upon the metatarsals, the heads of the first and fifth metatarsals are unable to drop to the normal plane below the level of the other metatarsals, owing to the narrowness of the shoe. The weight therefore falls unduly on the heads of the other metatarsals, which are crowded downward as the foot slips forward in the boot.

Symptoms.—The condition is characterized by a more or less severe pain, which radiates down into the toes and often up into the leg. It occurs generally between the third and fourth or fourth and fifth toes. It may be preceded by a sensation of slipping between the ends of the metatarsals, or the slipping may occur without the pain. It ordinarily comes on when the boots are on, but may sometimes be occasioned by rising on the toes in the stocking feet. The patient seeks relief instinctively by removing the boot and manipulating the foot, which relieves the acute pain. Some soreness may remain afterward and a tender spot is often found at the seat of the pain.

The attacks of pain may become gradually more frequent and

more severe until a condition of disability is established, the patient dreading walking.

The foot may be normal, so far as can be ascertained on inspection, but on palpation the heads of the second, third, or fourth metatarsals will be found habitually on a lower plane than normal, and callosities may be found under the heads of the metatarsals.

Diagnosis.—This affection is frequently diagnosticated as neuralgia, for which only general treatment is prescribed, yet the diagnostic symptoms are perfectly well marked and definite and not like those of any other affection.

The **prognosis** without treatment is not good; the attacks as a rule become more frequent and painful, though spontaneous recovery does rarely occur. With proper mechanical treatment most patients recover, but occasionally very obstinate cases are seen which resist all the ordinary methods of treatment.

Treatment.—Measures should be adopted to relieve the front ends of the metatarsals from pressing down on to the sole of the foot in finishing the step in walking.

Proper boots with a sole broad at the toes and under the tread of the foot, but holding the foot firmly around the midtarsus, should be worn. High-heeled shoes and shoes with a cross welt pressing the metatarsals down to the sole should be avoided. The normal flexibility of the toes should be developed by proper exercises. In some cases, compression of the shafts of the metatarsals for a time affords relief. In these cases it can be afforded by adhesive plaster, by bandaging, or by a soft leather strap. Removal of the distal end of the fourth metatarsal has been advocated as a measure of treatment, but it is not often necessary.

HALLUX VALGUS.

This name is applied to the outward displacement of the great toe. In the normal foot, as seen in children and people who do not wear boots, the long axis of the great toe when prolonged backward passes through the centre of the heel (Meyer's line).

Causation.—This deformity of the great toe, however, is not necessarily the result of tight shoes, for the deformity may come in people who have worn only comparatively loose ones. The upper leather of shoes, being more yielding than the sole, stretches under the pressure of use, or is stretched to avoid pressure upon the metatarso-phalangeal articulation. The boot is not stretched at its extreme end and it inevitably becomes, in a degree, conical in shape on this account, being broader across the ball of the foot than at the tip end. In the act of walking the foot necessarily slips inside of the boot to a certain extent, and if the shoe slips backward and the foot forward, a certain amount of pressure will come upon the inner side of the end of the great toe, tending to displace it outward.

This deformity may also be occasioned by short boots, and the ordinary pointed-toe boots, or any boot which does not give more room for lateral spreading at the toes than at the metatarso-phalangeal articulation, would necessarily give rise to the trouble. Stockings may be also a factor in its production. The de-

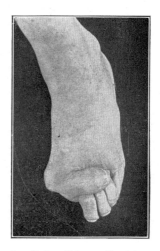

FIG. 360.—Hallux Valgus. Great toe under.   FIG. 361.—Hallux Valgus. Great toe over.

formity is also favored by walking with too great abduction of the front of the foot.

Symptoms.—When the deformity continues for any length of time, alteration in the relation of the bones of the metatarso-phalangeal joint takes place. An exaggerated adduction of the first metatarsal with an abduction of the phalanx, and the head of the metatarsal may become enlarged from growth of the bone due to periosteal irritation. The skin over this prominent joint may grow thick and a bursa form over it. This may become inflamed, giving rise to an extensive cellulitis, which may include the whole dorsum of the foot, which may suppurate and cause necrosis of the bone. This latter termination is, however, rare and occurs only in neglected cases. The inflammation of this bursa is known as a *bunion*. Associated with a hallux valgus deformity, an exaggerated inward divergence of the first metatarsal is sometimes seen. On examination, sensitiveness of the metatarsophalangeal joint is detected on pressure. In its more marked degree it is almost exclusively an affection of adult life.

Treatment.—The treatment of hallux valgus in early cases may be carried out by wearing a splint of steel or hard rubber along the inner

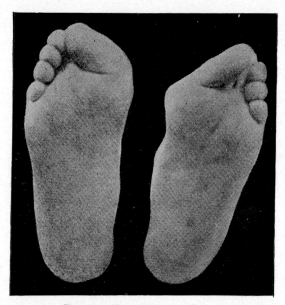

FIG. 362.—Hallux Valgus or Out-toe.

border of the foot fastened behind to the metatarsus. To the front end of this splint the toe is bandaged or strapped and thus pulled inward. This can be worn at night and a " toe post " in the daytime. This consists of a stiff partition (of leather or stiff felt) connected to an inner sole of the shoe and arranged so as to press the great toe to the inside. A stocking divided so as to allow separation of the great toe from the others is also advisable. Broad-toed shoes are essential.

Operation.—In old cases attempts to correct the deformity by such means as those mentioned are generally unsuccessful and operative measures may be adopted. The usual operation for this deformity is the removal of a wedge-shaped piece of bone from the inner side of the head of the first metatarsal, close to the joint, without opening the joint, followed by forcible straightening of the phalanx.

For the best ultimate result it is desirable to avoid removing much of the head of the first metatarsal, which is important in the weight-bearing function of the foot, and in some cases a linear osteotomy on the outer side of the head of the first metatarsal, followed by forcing the toe inwards, furnishes a more serviceable foot, especially if the attachment of the extensor proprius pollicis be shifted so as to pull the toe to the inside.

The use of properly made shoes is essential for after-treatment, and also for the prevention of the increase or recurrence of the deformity.

HALLUX VARUS.

This deformity is not a common one, and is known also as in-toe or pigeon-toe. It is occasionally seen in barefooted people, and has been observed in the Filipinos. This distortion does not generally require treatment, and the use of ordinary shoes is sufficient to correct the deformity.

HALLUX RIGIDUS.

This deformity, a stiffness of the metatarso-phalangeal joint of the great toe, is sometimes seen in adolescents and adults.

The **symptoms** vary with the stage of the disease. Early there may be slight pain over the joint and painful motion, but the cases rarely come to the surgeon's notice at this time. Later there is swelling over the joint, with tenderness, and perhaps an enlargement of the bone itself.

The **treatment** in the early stages will consist in removing the exciting cause. If there is pain, with signs of inflammation, rest with local applications is indicated. A boot with a stiff rocker sole or with an elevation raising the ball of the foot and clearing the toe from striking the ground in walking may be temporarily needed. Operative measures to give motion to the joint, forcible bending, or cutting down on the joint freeing adhesions, and the insertion of flaps of fat tissue or Cargile membrane might be considered, but will be rarely needed.

HAMMER TOE.

This deformity consists of a claw-like contraction of one of the toes, usually the second or third. The condition is one of flexion of the second phalanx, with extension of the third, so that the pressure on the ground is sustained by the *distal* phalanx. Over the upward projecting joint there is usually a callosity, which may cause considerable annoyance.

In the slight degrees and early stages of the deformity the patient experiences but little discomfort, and such cases are not, therefore, commonly seen by the surgeon in this stage. Later, however, locomotion becomes difficult and painful.

In children and adolescents the deformity can generally in all but the severest cases be corrected by simple mechanical treatment. The toe should be bandaged or strapped to a rigid splint, cut from sheet tin or celluloid, placed under the toe and ball of the foot. In children it can be corrected if necessary by subcutaneous section of the contracted fasciæ, forcible straightening, and fixation in a straight position by means of splints and adhesive plaster.

After correction by mechanical means the toe shows a tendency to recontract and must be carefully watched.

In severe cases it is possible to excise the prominent phalangeal joint of the toe which projects upward, and, by taking out sufficient

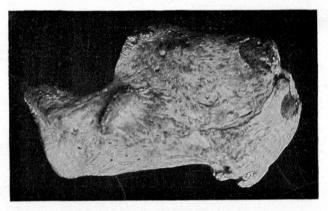

Fig. 363.—Irritation Exostoses of Os Calcis.

bone from the phalanges, to bring two bony surfaces together, which will unite and keep the toe straight and flat. Subcutaneous section of the shortened fasciæ and tendons will be needed in the severe cases.

It also occurs at times in connection with what is spoken of as contracted foot. The tendons and fasciæ will be found shortened.

PAINFUL HEEL.

A tender and painful area under the middle of the heel exists at times, and is spoken of sometimes as " policeman's heel." It seems to be associated with any one of three conditions:

1. The radiograph may show a bony spur projecting forward from the front lower edge of the tuberosity of the os calcis. This may or may not be associated with exostoses elsewhere in the tarsal bones.

2. It may be associated with inflammation of the bursa under the os calcis.

3. It may be the expression of a static disturbance (some degree

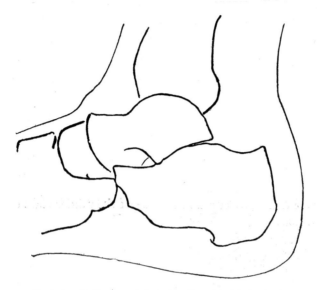

Fig. 364.—Radiogram of Irritation Exostoses of Os Calcis.

of flat-foot), in which the chief strain falls on the posterior insertion of the plantar fascia.

The treatment consists in the relieving the os calcis from pressure by furnishing a thick rubber ring pad under the heel, or by supporting the sole of the foot so that less pressure comes upon the heel.

Local hyperæmia treatment is also beneficial.

POST-CALCANEAL BURSITIS.

(Achillodynia, Achillobursitis, Anterior Achillobursitis.)

A tender swelling at the junction of the tendo Achillis and os calcis is not infrequently met. Plantar flexion of the foot is painful, and the patient walks with the foot everted and avoids rising on the toes. The affection may be unilateral or bilateral, is rather resistant to treatment, and liable to recur when nearly well.

It is caused by the pressure of the leather at the back of the boot pressing on the end of the os calcis.

For treatment it is necessary to remove pressure over the painful area by splitting the back of the boot in the middle line behind and setting in a loose piece of leather between the spread edges.

In resistant and very acute cases the application of a plaster-of-Paris bandage to the leg and foot will be necessary.

An inflammation of a superficial bursa between the tendon and the skin occasionally occurs from pressure of the boot heel. Its treatment consists in the removal of the pressure, and in severe cases dissecting out the bursa if inflamed; in some instances an exostosis of the os calcis is found and needs to be removed.

SYNOVITIS OF THE TENDO ACHILLIS.

Symptoms somewhat like those described occur at times in connection with a tenosynovitis of the tendo Achillis, which is shown by the usual signs of swelling of the sheath of the tendon above the os calcis, tenderness along its course, and silky crepitus. The affection is readily controlled by rest and the use of the milder class of measures mentioned above.

INDEX.